WILLIAM GLASSER

WILLIAM GLASSER

CHAMPION OF CHOICE

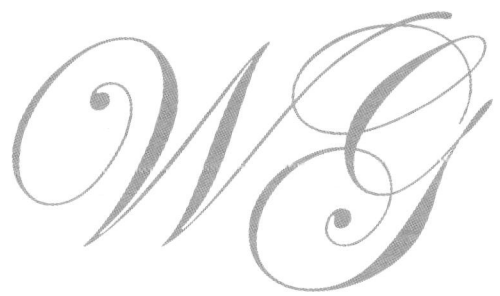

JIM ROY, Ed.D.

ZEIG, TUCKER & THEISEN
Phoenix, Arizona

Copyright 2014
Jim Roy

All rights reserved under International and Pan-American Copyright Conventions. No part of this book may be reproduced, stored in a retrieval system or transmitted in any form by an electronic, mechanical, photocopying, recording means or otherwise, without prior written permission of the author.

Excerpts that appear in Chapter 8 from William Powers, *Behavior the Control of Perception*, published by permission of Benchmark Publications, Inc. (1st ed. 1973/2nd rev. ed. 2005).

Library of Congress Cataloging-in-Publication Data

William glasser: Champion of choice

/ Roy, Jim. — 1st edition
with a foreword by Robert E. Wubbolding

p.   cm.

Includes bibliographic references and index.
ISBN 978-1-934442-47-0 (pbk : alk paper)

1. Biography—William Glasser
I. Roy, Jim   II. Title.

Published by

ZEIG, TUCKER & THEISEN, INC.
2632 East Thomas Rd., Suite 201
Phoenix, Arizona 85016

Manufactured in the United States of America

Dedicated to the memory and work
of William Glasser

CONTENTS

Foreword by Robert E. Wubbolding, EdD .... *ix*
Introduction .... *xiii*
1   Taking Off and Soaring 1
2   Cleveland 17
3   Welcome to the Club 39
4   The Unlikely School Without Failure 73
5   Out of Nowhere 95
6   A Whole New World 125
7   Inside Job 149
8   Trip to Chicago 183
     Photos *207*
9   Making It His Own 215
10 Back to School 239
11 Pain and Joy 267
12 Decision in Australia 293
13 Warning 333
14 Still Looking Ahead 367
Epilogue 409
Acknowledgements 413
Index 415
About the Author 421

Foreword

As someone associated with Dr. Glasser since 1972, I can testify that Jim Roy has captured the essence of William Glasser, his life, his work, and his passion for changing the landscape of counseling, psychotherapy, and mental health. From the very beginning of Glasser's career he had sought ways to move beyond what he believed to be a stalled, unnecessarily limited view of mental health. Rather than treating clients and labeling them as disturbed, disordered, mentally ill, or as victims of their past or of their circumstances he chose to see them as being in possession of at least some ability to choose mentally healthy behaviors. With the help of his supervisor, whom he always referred to as "my teacher Dr. Harrington," he treated patients *as if* they were responsible for their decisions, their behavior, and especially their actions. Glasser's genius was evident in his skill of accomplishing this without the toxic "ABC" behaviors, i.e., without arguing, blaming, or criticizing. And though Glasser continually developed and extended the applications of reality therapy he has always retained and even cherished his central theme: human beings choose their behavior, especially their actions and they are mentally healthy when they experience connecting and caring human relationships.

As a result of his success in treating patients in a mental hospital and with residents of a correctional institution he was sought out to present public lectures on his innovative methods. He called his treatment "reality psychiatry." And yet, the acceptance of his system by the psychiatric profession was less than enthusiastic. In contrast, psychologists, counselors, social workers and educators responded quite favorably. Consequently, he quickly changed the name to "reality therapy" and published his watershed book *Reality Therapy* (1965). Because of the interest demonstrated from educators Dr. Glasser subsequently applied reality therapy to schools and formed the Schools Without Failure program followed by more systemic applications known as the Quality School program. He then adapted control system theory, as developed by William Powers, and extended it by introducing his signature addition—the system of human needs as sources of motivation. He then named it choice theory. This resulted in what is perhaps his most influential book *Choice Theory* (1998). Within the last 15 years he emphasized choice theory/reality therapy as a mental health system and a community issue rather than an individual problem.

Jim Roy has traced the intricacies of this development by conducting hundreds of personal interviews with Bill Glasser himself, his family, and his many associates who have known him intimately. Additionally, he has researched Glasser's teachings through books as well as audio and video recorded lectures. The outcome of this monumental effort is a treasure trove not only of Glasser's progress and process but also the documentation of anecdotes that reflected his appreciation for life in its many aspects and especially his story telling ability and his disarming and endearing sense of humor.

This biography is not merely an authorized commendation or panegyric. Nor is it simply an impersonal or inert narration. Jim Roy writes a lively, engaging story and paints a picture of Glasser that will enlighten readers intellectually and move them emotionally. He appeals to the "total behavior" of the reader who is led to take action, i.e., to learn more, to see the rational and sensible ideas of William Glasser. At the same time the reader will be impacted on the emotional level by realizing that Dr. Glasser was a real human being who himself acted, thought, and indeed felt strongly about choice theory/reality therapy, the organizational issues of The William Glasser Institute, and his own interpersonal relationships, most especially with his wife Carleen.

Moreover, this highly qualified biographer does not shun, but rather faces head on several painful issues that Dr. Glasser attempted to handle as best he could. Roy followed the famous injunction of Oliver Cromwell to his portraitist—to paint him as he is without embellishments, warts and all. For instance, he alludes to the tension between Dr. Glasser and his eldest son. He also summarizes the controversy that involved some instructors' teachings that he saw as external control. This issue was very painful for Dr. Glasser and Jim Roy describes the angst experienced by the founder of reality therapy and the members of his institute.

Such issues illustrate that choice theory is an *explanation* of human behavior. It describes human motivation as well as helpful and hurtful behaviors. Learning it does not automatically bring about behavioral change. It does, however, help the learner to better understand the totality of human nature. The book also shows that even individuals subscribing to the principles of choice theory and reality therapy can disagree about whether specific behaviors constitute internal control or external control.

In this brief foreword I have not attempted to present a thorough explanation of Dr. Glasser's process nor a detailed treatment of specific issues. Jim Roy's superb book *William Glasser: Champion of Choice* has met that daunting challenge. Read on!

—Robert E. Wubbolding, EdD

INTRODUCTION

The story of William Glasser is more than a biography. His was a distinctive voice, one of the most important mental health voices of the 20th century. His message challenged accepted beliefs and practices at every turn and sought to bring people back to what worked—to the life-changing principles of choice, free will, and self-determination. He took on topics like our search for meaning and fulfillment, especially in our relationships with others; the problems of addiction and self-medication; the marriage dilemma and high divorce rates; disconnected families; underachieving students and struggling schools; crime and overcrowded prisons; political oppression and violence around the world; the definition, diagnosis, and treatment of mental illness; and the explosion of brain drugs as the answer to psychological symptoms. Like Toto, Dorothy's little dog in the *Wizard of Oz,* pulling back the curtain to reveal the wizard's fraud, William Glasser sought to reveal the fraud and ineffective practices that society has allowed and perpetuated. Throughout his story we are gently confronted about our own beliefs and assumptions regarding mental health and, put more simply, about how to be happy. Biographies are often inspirational, but some are also transformational. Glasser's story is in this latter category. It will change lives.

I first met William Glasser in August of 2000. We became friends. A few years later when I was deciding on a dissertation topic for my doctorate, I approached him about helping me with a biographical study on the development of his ideas. He said that he would be happy to participate in a study of his ideas, but indicated he preferred the project stay focused on his ideas, rather than on his personal life. "I don't really want to talk to anyone about the details of my personal life," he explained, "but of my professional life I'm more than happy." I agreed to this request and we began a series of interviews together that would span five years, include over 60 hours of recorded conversations between us, and produce over 1,200 pages of interview notes and manuscripts. By the third interview, he began sharing personal stories and referred to our time together as working on his biography and to me as his biographer. From September 2003 to November 2008, I interviewed him 46 times. Often we would meet in his home office, a modest room with two desks and a couch overlooking the Pacific Ocean, but we also conducted interviews in many other locations too. If I attended conferences at which he was presenting, we would meet in the afternoon or evening so that I could keep plying him with more questions. We met in locations like Anaheim and Cincinnati and New York and Nashville and Dublin, Ireland. One of our interviews took place in my home in northern California.

To prepare for the interviews, I read all of Glasser's books—23 by my count, totaling almost 4,400 pages of manuscript—and a host of booklets and published articles in magazines and journals. I reviewed interviews that others did with him over the years and read articles that others wrote about him and the effects his ideas were having on the fields of education and psychology. There is a huge amount of material produced both by him and about him.

To gain an even better understanding of the origin and development of his concepts of reality therapy, control theory, choice theory, and mental health as a public health issue, rather than a medical issue, I also interviewed family members, friends, and colleagues of Glasser.

These additional interviews contributed a great deal to a fuller understanding of his story, and counterbalanced Glasser's own tendency to live in the present and not keep track of details from the past. Those familiar with the principles of reality therapy will know that it is present-focused, and Glasser lives that way every day.

Writing the biography of a person who thinks the past is really not that important can be a challenge. When asked about items or artifacts from the past he would say things like, "I'm not good at keeping things," or "I don't prize possessions that much." He would explain, "I don't have a lot of nostalgia for the good old days or any of that stuff. I did it and I enjoyed it, but I'm much more interested in what I'm doing now than what I did then. I'm not really interested in the history thing."

In one of our interviews I asked him if the changes he has made throughout his life, the adjustments in his choice theory thinking, might be similar to the changes each of us will make as we come to understand the ideas. He agreed, "I think you got a point there." Earlier in the interview, when we talked about how to approach the biography, he admitted that as far as he was concerned, "Where I am now is much more important than how I got there, but to other people how I got there could be very important." When a university student doing a research paper on William Glasser queried Brian Lennon, an important choice theory instructor in Ireland, for information on Glasser's life, Brian responded, "Maybe someday Glasser will do us a favor and write about his early life. Maybe the story of his past would be therapy for us!" The idea that others may benefit from understanding the details of Glasser's journey has been one of the chief motivators for me to write his biography.

As you read you will be seeing Glasser's story through two sets of eyes. The first set is Glasser's own eyes. My hope is that the view through his eyes will dominate this book. During our time together I attempted to be a catalyst for his journey into the past, to jar his memories, to coax experiences and feelings out of his mental storage closets, some of them shut long ago. Our first interview took place when he was 78 years old. He had experienced and accomplished so much by then. So many air miles traveled, so many talks given, so many classrooms visited, so many patients counseled, and so many books and articles written. At times, Glasser himself doubted how well he could remember the past. "I don't hang on to ideas well," he offered. "I write these books and I say a lot of good stuff, but then I move on. I can't always remember everything I say, but it's good stuff." And yet, as I brought up the passages from books written over 30 and even 40 years ago, he seemed to go to the moment the passage was written. He remembered the circumstances surrounding the moment and the reasons he wanted to write what he had written. To be sure, his remembrances are just that, his pictures of how he recalls a particular time period or event. (I have wondered how I would do if someone asked me about events from 40 years ago.) According to choice theory we create our perceptions of the world and like all of us Glasser has created his perception of reality and his place in the world. At times I have discovered inaccuracies or inconsistencies in an event remembered or a detail recalled, but this book isn't about minutia. This story is about how one man came to articulate some of the most important and powerful ideas on earth.

The other eyes through which you will be seeing Glasser's story are mine. As much as I want his perceptions and memories to dominate his biography, my perceptions and views and values also lurk on every page. Yes, the biography is primarily based on his writings and on the interviews we did together, but I will decide what gets in and how it is described, what nuances are emphasized and what subtleties are ignored. I want so much to simply be a conduit from him to you, so that you can see his life and journey accurately. But as much as I may want you to receive his information unfiltered, I am a filter. My life, my experiences, my training, and of course, my choices, have all contributed to who I am. What I interpret and share with you passes through this filter.

I am, what I would call, a friendly reviewer. This is based, I think, on my goals for the biography, my belief in the principles of choice theory, and on the warm and supportive relationship that I have with Bill and Carleen Glasser. As far as my goals for the book, I wanted to conduct a careful study of Glasser's ideas, their origin and development, within the context of his personal life. I wanted to assist him in reviewing his life and the ideas that came out of his experiences. To accomplish this there needed to be a high level of trust between us. None of this would have taken place had Bill Glasser seen me as an adversary. I am an advocate of choice theory and have completed several phases of the Glasser training, which led to my becoming a faculty member of The Glasser Institute (now William Glasser International, Inc.). Prior to meeting Glasser I worked as a school principal and district superintendent, and in those roles I sought to implement choice theory principles with my students and staff. My experience with his ideas through reading, training, and practice contributed a great deal to my being able to ask intelligent questions and further probe his thinking if his answer was less than complete.

The positive relationship between Bill and Carleen Glasser and me has been an important part of our ability to collaborate together on the biography. During the years of the interviewing process I ate with them, slept in their guest room, watched televised Laker games and Super Bowls with Bill, looked through family picture albums, and read through scrapbooks of old newspaper clippings. I attended many of

Bill's presentations at conferences and workshops and breakout sessions, and listened as he visited with people afterward. Occasionally, Carleen would participate in the interviews. Throughout the project I felt welcome to call their home at any time during the day or evening, to visit their home, or to join them on their travel to presentations.

There were two sides to this closeness, though. On the one hand we developed high levels of trust and provided a wonderful environment for communication. On the other hand such closeness created the possibility of accentuating the positive at the expense of reality and balance. As much as I appreciate William Glasser, I didn't want the biography to simply be a rah-rah Glasser review. It was important to me that the biography be credible. Glasser strongly agreed with the need for credibility. "I understand you're not here to write a critical biography," he pointed out, "but you don't want to write a sycophantic biography either." To put it in a familiar phrase, he puts his pants on the same way the rest of us do—one leg at a time. He has been involved in the complex world of the human mind and human behavior for his entire career. He has written books that have called widely accepted beliefs and practices into question, and in the process probably influenced millions of practitioners. He founded and directed a worldwide organization of talented and insightful people. Along the way he changed his mind, set the organization on new paths, and in a few cases made very controversial decisions that led to schisms and pain. There is no getting around the fact that Glasser made decisions with which people in his life, in some cases important people, disagreed. And so while there was much to celebrate as we probed the past, there were also difficult moments in which I simply attempt to lay out what happened. I do not attempt to judge Glasser, or anyone else for that matter. I try to reveal what happened or what was said. The important thing is that these experiences, both the successful and the difficult, the victories and the setbacks, lead us to a deeper understanding of choice theory and the personal responsibility we each possess. Glasser's journey may, in fact, be important to each of our own journeys.

The Glasser Institute* has been a significant part of Glasser's efforts to educate the world about mental health, but this book is not a history of the Institute. The Institute is more present in some chapters of Glasser's life than in others. During some periods it is central to the story, whereas at other times it provides a less noticeable backdrop. It is true that ever since *Reality Therapy* was published in 1965, and *Schools Without Failure* in 1969, people have gravitated to William Glasser. Some of these people actually helped to form the first version of the Institute in 1967—the Institute for Reality Therapy. Through interviews with several of them, I came to admire and respect their quest for truth. One of them actually moved from New York City to southern California just to be closer to Glasser and the organizational center of reality therapy. To the extent they help us to gain insights into Glasser's thinking and into the development of his ideas, I will share stories about people who came into his life. Most of them, once they became a part of the Institute, stayed. But some left, and their story too forms an important piece in the choice theory puzzle.

As I delved into Glasser's history and began to retrace the steps in his development, the richness of his past began to come into focus. One by one the different characters stepped into my view, sat with me, and talked into my recorder. From the earliest stages of this project I recognized the depth of these characters' relationships with Glasser and the length of time they have known him and worked with him. It is important to me that the important people in Glasser's past, the few I interviewed and the many I have not yet met, know that I understand my place as a relative newcomer into Glasser's sphere.

---

*The Institute has undergone several name changes since its beginnings and thus will be referred to accordingly depending on the timeframe of the discussion.

During one of my interviews with Bob Wubbolding, a longtime associate of Glasser and the Director of Training for the Institute, this issue actually emerged.

"I haven't told you this," Wubbolding began, "but I was going to write his biography someday. I'm glad you're doing it, though."

My response reveals that I had been thinking about this already. "I recognize," I began, "that other people go so far back with Bill and have been a part of the battle, so to speak, and I wonder if I should be the one to do this project. Bill was open to the idea. I don't know how others in the Institute feel about my doing it. I'm sensitive to this."

"Well," Wubbolding answered in his upbeat way, "no one else has done it and you stepped up to the plate and are doing it. I think you'll get great support." He was right. Friends and colleagues have been willing and even anxious to share their memories and their insights from being with and working with Glasser over the years. Out of the many people I contacted only one declined to be interviewed.

One of the challenges in the writing of his biography has been how to answer the question: On what exactly should the book focus? As I got into the project it seemed to me that there could very naturally be a three-fold focus, the book being a stool built on three legs. The first leg would be the development of Glasser's ideas. Where did the ideas come from? When did they come? And how did they change over the years? The second leg would center on Glasser's life, the details of his history, and the anecdotes from his past. Initially, he was not interested in talking about his life. "Whatever my secret past is," he said, "is gonna remain secret." I reminded him, though, that he has shared from his personal life when it could help another person better understand choice theory. As it turned out, it just became impossible for him not to talk about his life and the events surrounding the birth, the growth, and sometimes even the death of his ideas. The third leg at first seemed vital to the book, but as time went on it began to bog down under its own weight. The third leg encompassed the fields of psychology and psychiatry and the history of the care of the mentally ill. As I read Glasser's books and interviewed him about the ideas expressed, I became very interested in the idea of mental illness versus mental health, the history of mental illness treatment in the United States, the various forms of talk therapy, the way brain drugs had taken over psychiatry, the way brain drugs have taken over in general, and the way the pharmaceutical companies have become the most profitable companies in the world. It struck me that Glasser could be the poster boy for the new direction in which the field of mental health needed to head. His life surrounds the last half of the 20th century—the era in which psychiatry and perceptions of mental illness so radically changed. In fact, he confronted erroneous ideas about mental illness, and in the process he took on the companies that claimed they could sell happiness in a pill. It seemed natural to include this focus in the biography. Yet the shear amount of the data in this sphere began to loom large and seemed to threaten to take over the project. I could see the biography becoming a very large tome. A tome would not be Glasserian at all, since he likes books to be short and simple. In the end, I decided to focus on the development of his ideas, supported by the details of his life, with just enough of the history and present practice of psychiatry to make the biography come to life, and ultimately to be relevant to any reader interested in a good story, an important story.

I have attempted to be thorough and accurate in the details, but not necessarily painstakingly so. When Glasser says he graduated from medical school in 1953, I go with that. I have not contacted Western Reserve University to confirm it. This is not a *60 Minutes* gotch-ya, although at times I ask him the hard questions. This is not a tell-all, although in the process Glasser tells us a lot. What this is, is the story of his life, from his start in a prison school for girls, to the book that was a psychiatric shot heard around the world, and the way he challenged established thinking. And, of course, especially the way he has urged us to experience freedom through the power we have to make choices.

The novelist Thomas Berger once said that writers write because it isn't there. This biography represents something that wasn't there. Although still very active when I began the biography process with him, Glasser was still traveling throughout the United States and around the world giving presentations—he was still writing, he was still playing tennis—the time was right for him to embark on a purposeful review of his professional journey. This biography invites you to retrace Glasser's journey and put the puzzle together for yourself, and in the process, ultimately, to become more aware of what it means to be loving, powerful, and free.

1
TAKING OFF AND SOARING

"My career just went, well, it was like the Energizer Bunny."
—*William Glasser, describing life after he completed his psychiatric residency.*

"Bill Glasser's work has been a lighthouse in the field."
—*Dr. David Johnson*

Two events in 1954 deserve our notice. The first of these two events occurred in May of that year when the pharmaceutical company Smith, Kline & French introduced chlorpromazine into the U.S. market and began selling it as Thorazine.[1] The second of these two events occurred two months later in July, when a young medical student by the name of William Glasser began his psychiatric residency at the Veterans Administration Center in west Los Angeles, California. Given the national and world news at the time,[2] these events received little attention. Yet for the next 50 years the drug and the doctor would exert an impact on society affecting millions of people.

The development of Thorazine, and its being embraced by the psychiatric establishment, represents the beginning of purposeful choices by psychiatry to affirm drugs as a cure for symptoms it labels as mental illness.[3] More important, this development led to physicians, and in fact, the public in general accepting the idea that people were victims of their own mental states, that they were ill or diseased in some way, and that only a remedy outside of them could help or cure them. In the 1950s this profile of helplessness or "victimness" was further supported by the popularity of psychoanalysis, the therapeutic approach developed by Sigmund Freud, which emphasized the importance of events that occurred in our past, and how these events affect us at an unconscious (and thus, unavailable) level. Thus, psychoanalysis was also an outside remedy. Only someone from the outside could help a person work back into the past and delve into the unconscious to produce a cure.

The young Dr. Glasser, fresh from medical school and just beginning his psychiatric residency, would soon come to represent a belief system in which people, rather than being victims of mental illness, are the architects of their own lives. People, according to this belief system, can begin to take responsibility for their thinking and their actions, and ultimately learn how to improve their own mental health. In the same way that people can know enough about physical health to get and stay in shape, this young doctor would soon be explaining how people can know enough about their own mental health to maintain or improve it.

William Glasser did not set out to take on Freudian psychotherapy, or to take on the psychiatric profession, or to take on the brain drug industry; and neither did he set out to take on the educational behemoth known as the public school system, but that is what he did. His ideas demanded responses. His views, compared to a "kick in the shins" by one writer, formed questions, essential questions, regarding human psychology. Are we, for instance, the victims of mental diseases outside of our control to manage or cure, or do we possess the ability to be self-aware, to be conscious of our thinking, and to make choices, however small, about how we will behave. The mental illness industry would have us accept the disease model, which is the model that current healthcare providers and insurance plans support. The mental health alternative, Glasser's view, would have us recognize the potential in each person to become a self-manager. The stakes being so high and the issues being so important, it was a huge undertaking for a fledgling doctor to take on.

This is the story of that young doctor. This is the story of the development of his groundbreaking ideas, of his mission to teach people how to be mentally healthy, and of the millions of lives that he has touched. It is a story of what it means to be responsible for ourselves and to possess the power to make choices. Along with this amazing choice power, it is a story of love and personal freedom. Ultimately, it is a story of hope.

The plane sits at the end of the runway and waits, its two General Electric jet engines idling a low whine. It is fifth in a line of planes waiting to take off from Los Angeles International Airport. This particular plane, a Boeing 737, is over a 100 feet long and more than a 100 feet wide. In fact, it is wider than it is long. At its highest point the tail is over four stories high. When loaded with crew, passengers, and luggage it will weigh close to 150,000 pounds. It doesn't seem possible that this lumbering conglomeration of metal, steel, plastic, fabric, fuel, rubber, wires, peanuts, and soda is able to fly, but in just a few moments it will. In just a few moments it will make its slow, final turn onto the runway, a long, clear path of cement some two miles long. When the tower clears the plane for takeoff, its engines will come to life and people inside will feel themselves pushed back into their seats. Slowly at first, but then faster and faster, the plane will roar down the runway, until that moment when the airspeed over the wings begins to lift the plane gently into the air. Immediately after leaving the ground, though, its ascent will become steeper as the jets push aggressively toward the sky. Soon the plane will be more than six miles above the ground and traveling at close to 500 miles per hour.

This plane is heading for Kansas City, and one of its passengers, William Glasser, sits in row 12. He is sitting by the window, and as the plane left the ground he could see the Pacific Ocean extending out beyond the horizon. As the plane banks, beginning its gentle turn back toward the east, the city center of Los Angeles comes into full view; its skyscrapers crowded together. The San Gorgonio Mountains to the north provide a beautiful picture frame for the sprawling metropolis below. It is a gorgeous southern California spring day, one of those days that could almost make you want to live there. Glasser himself has lived in Los Angeles for 50 years.

Fifty years. As he soared into the sky that spring morning in late March 2004, it was, in fact, almost exactly 50 years since Glasser had started his psychiatric residency in southern California. As he looked out the window of the plane, he could have spotted the buildings in which he first worked as a resident in west L.A. He could have also spotted the downtown area of Brentwood where his office on San Vincente Blvd was for so long. As the plane got a little higher he could see where his home was in the hills above Santa Monica. And beyond those hills, he could see where his current office was in the San Fernando Valley.

This trip had everything to do with what Glasser had contributed and achieved during those 50 years. In what would be one of many affirmations of his career contributions, the American Counseling Association invited Glasser to their annual convention being held in Kansas City to receive their "Legend in Counseling" award. The year before, in 2003, the ACA awarded him their Professional Development Award in celebration and acknowledgment of his contributions to the field of counseling. In January of 2005, he received the highest honor that can be bestowed on a member of the American Psychotherapy Association—the designation of Master Therapist. Also in 2005, the International Center for the Study of Psychiatry and Psychology conferred on him their Life Achievement Award. Of comparable importance, The Milton H. Erickson Foundation's Evolution of Psychotherapy Conference, held every five years in Anaheim, and which brings together the top 25 therapists in the world for lectures and demonstrations, invited Glasser to be a part of the conference since 1990.

As the plane reached altitude and headed in earnest toward the Midwest, who could have faulted Glasser for recognizing this moment as the 50-year anniversary of an illustrious career, and savoring the success of his efforts. A respected member in his field, he also was the founder of a worldwide organization[4]—The William Glasser Institute. As he looked out the window of the plane and considered the vast landscape, it would have made sense to consider the details of his life, the small and large victories that marked his past. But such thinking is not the way of William Glasser. As someone who has spent a great deal of time with him, in one-on-one interviews, and in observing and listening to him in professional and social settings, I can tell you that at that moment in the plane the upcoming award and his illustrious past were the last things on his mind. Instead, Glasser would be thinking about what he was going to say during the talk he would be giving, and the challenge of convincing counselors across America that talk therapy, not drug therapy, was where they should focus their treatment efforts. Instead of basking in the glow of accomplishments he would be thinking about how he could present the ideas and principles of choice theory in a way that would inspire counselors to join him on his crusade. For Glasser, the invitation to speak was more important than receiving the award.

In the world of psychology and education, William Glasser is a rock star. I have been with him at many of his presentations and I have observed how people approach him and communicate with him. There are the looks that say, *There he is* or *That's him*. There are the deep expressions of appreciation for what he has meant to them. People seek his autograph. Many ask if they can have their picture taken with him, and before he can even answer the person has an arm around him while a friend snaps the shot. So many people, especially in the helping professions, acknowledge Glasser and his ideas in their own thinking. His presence as a speaker or a presenter adds credibility to a conference or convention. His name on the program adds a sense of interest, a buzz of expectancy.

The huge following was not always so. Prior to 1965, Glasser's status was more modest. He had written a very respected book that was published in 1960,[5] *Mental Health or Mental Illness*, and was even invited to the Second Corning Conference in 1961, in which 100 of the best minds in the world discussed topics on the conference theme, The Individual and Society.[6] More locally, he was being invited to speak at California Youth Authority events throughout the state. His therapeutic approach was having a positive impact at the Ventura School for Girls, where he worked as a psychiatrist, and others in the CYA system were interested in what he had to offer. After 1965, though, his modest status changed to something much, much larger. With the publication of his second book, *Reality Therapy*, in 1965,[7] Glasser became famous. Shortly thereafter, the interviews began. *Harper's Magazine*, aware of the growing interest in Glasser, ran an article in 1967 entitled California's Gift to Psychotherapy. "[Glasser] has become an influential young voice in west coast psychiatry," it read, and "among indigenous school administrators, narcotics-rehabilitation agents, and prison matrons, his popularity runs particularly high."[8] The article, maybe the first to comment on Glasser on a national scale, captured the loyalty and commitment that was beginning to grow among those on the frontlines of education, youth centers, drug rehabilitation programs, social work, counseling, and the prison system. The teacher who actually worked with the child in the classroom or on the playground, the caseworker who actually made the visits in inner city neighborhoods, or the staff member of a gang taskforce who was forging relationships with kids on the streets—these were the people using his ideas and seeing the ideas actually make a difference. "Unquestionably," the *Harper's* author emphasizes, "he [Glasser] is attracting serious attention in many parts of the country."[9]

The attention was serious enough after the publication of *Reality Therapy* that Glasser was not able to respond to all the questions and requests for presentations. So in 1967, the Institute for Reality Therapy was formed and a team of support staff and trainers became the nucleus that would help Glasser spread the good news about helping people effectively take responsibility for their own lives. So much was beginning to happen during this time that it is difficult to write about the events in a linear progression. Explosions aren't linear.

In the same year that *Reality Therapy* was published, 1965, Glasser began working in four public schools in the Watts area of Los Angeles. He had begun his career in a school setting and there was something about the potential within classrooms and schools that called to him. Educators were particularly interested in the implications that the principles of reality therapy would have on teaching and learning. And so, even as his speaking engagements were exponentially increasing, even as his own institute was forming, Glasser was writing another book. This book, his third, focused on schools and how they could be places where learning was increased and in which students and teachers thrived. Using the language of baseball, the success of *Reality Therapy*, with almost a million copies sold could be compared to a young, unknown player hitting a grand slam home run. What are the chances of a baseball player hitting two consecutive grand slam home runs? In the world of books, that is what Glasser did when he wrote *Schools Without Failure*, published in 1969.[10] For Glasser and the growing Institute the effect of two grand slam books, published within four years of each other, was fast and powerful.

"*Reality Therapy*," one article began, "challenged some of conventional psychiatry's most hallowed precepts, and *Schools Without Failure*," it continued, "will shake up educators. It should be read by every educator and a copy smuggled onto the desk of every district superintendent." As educators across the country did, in fact, read *Schools Without Failure*, the message of the book resonated at a deep level. Here, teachers thought, was a writer who understood the classroom challenges they faced every day. In an interview in *Scholastic Teacher Magazine*, Glasser is described as a "psychiatrist turned educator whose ideas about education have been sending shock waves through the schoolhouse." Only three years after *Schools Without Failure* was published, *Learning Magazine* credited him with helping to restructure schools serving nearly a million students. *U.S. News & World Report* reflected the countrywide level of interest in Glasser and his ideas when they described him as a top psychiatrist and a nationally noted school consultant. Thirty-three years after *Schools Without Failure* was first published, a respected educational author described it as "one of the most important education books of the Twentieth Century."[11]

In these two books, *Reality Therapy* and *Schools Without Failure*, Glasser took on two huge and powerful establishments, the first being the psychiatric profession, which was even then in tight connection with the pharmaceutical companies, and the second being the education system with its entrenched bureaucracy. An interview in the *Los Angeles Times* captures the phenomena of Glasser's popularity, as well as the tide he was beginning to swim against. Introducing him as a major figure on the U.S. lecture circuit with teachers and mental health workers across the nation flocking to his presentations, the interview acknowledged that Glasser "sounds off passionately against the psychiatric and educational establishments." Anticipating that some might write him off because of his controversial ideas, the author states: "Glasser is not a crank, but a clear-headed maverick who takes an unorthodox approach to nagging problems that have been around a long time—teaching and learning, behavior and discipline." It came out in the interview that Glasser was squeezing up to 20 lectures a month into an already full agenda, further testimony to his growing influence.

Glasser was a popular speaker and a prolific writer. His 24 books, multiple booklets, including his most recent booklet, *Defining Mental Health as a Public Health Issue: A New Leadership Role for the Helping and Teaching Professions*, and the many, many journal and magazine articles indicate that he has gotten the public's attention throughout his career. Of the 14 journal and magazine interviews with Glasser that I was able to locate, 10 included the words "An Interview with William Glasser" in the title. Often this was placed as a title on the cover of the journal as well. Clearly, his name alone could increase interest in reading a journal or buying a magazine.

He came to be known and introduced as a world-renowned psychiatrist and educator. And it wasn't just the frontline, in the trenches, mental health professionals and educators who responded. Sonya Friedman, who at the time had a program on CNN,[12] described Glasser as "one of the most practical and insightful psychiatrists I have ever met." And Robert Schuller, then pastor of the Crystal Cathedral and a television personality in his own right, in an obvious, yet telling moment of over-affirmation, proclaimed that "William Glasser is the world's greatest psychiatrist." I include these testimonies not to make a case for Glasser being the world's greatest psychiatrist, but to reveal the popularity and support that Glasser garnered during the 50 years of his very active career.

WG

Glasser shared a story from his high school years that proved to be a portent of things to come. He described how he enjoyed playing 1st cornet in the school marching band. The band was really high quality in those years, with everyone from the director, to the musicians, to the equipment managers taking their performances seriously. At one of their practices the director was perched on the high school roof, three stories up, directing the band on the lawn below. From such a vantage point the director could really see how the band was working together. Glasser remembers that as this practice was taking place, over some kind of megaphone or speaker system, from the rooftops, literally, the director bellowed, "Glasser, you're out of step!" As a high school student with a trumpet in his hand he actually wanted to be in lockstep with others. That desire, though, did not mark his career. He came to be known, as far as traditional psychiatry was concerned, for being out of step.

Yet, rather than out of step being a problem, many see his views as an invaluable gift. Dr. David Johnson, a prolific author himself, along with his brother, Roger, an acclaimed leader in the area of cooperative learning, feels strongly about Glasser's importance. "He has been a particular type of bridge between theory and practice, from a personality therapy point of view. He's probably been the major person over the last 50 years. I think in the long run he'll be more important than Carl Rogers, certainly more important than Albert Ellis. Especially for people who wanted to work with children and teenagers, Bill's work has been a lighthouse in the field."

It is this ability to alert us to that which is important, and to define and explain the important, that makes Glasser's journey so worthy of our examination. Bob Hoglund, a longtime trainer for the Glasser Institute, points out, "Bill, more than anything, has taken very complex ideas and simplified them. Because he simplifies them so much, you miss the true complexity of what he has to offer. I think that's what Glasser, and choice theory, and the Institute are all about —the complexity. In one sense, he's almost like a comedian. He can take a piece of life and make it totally understandable for people."

Dr. Tom Parish, professor of psychology at Upper Iowa University and a prolific researcher, places Glasser on an even higher plane than that of insightful comedian. "Bill is the intellectual's intellectual. He is the Plato, Socrates, and Aristotle of our time. He has incredibly good ideas and is a wonderful practitioner."

From the beginning, Glasser's approach to mental illness and mental health got people's attention. One author put it in perspective when he stated that the ideas set forth in the book *Reality Therapy* "delivered a kick in the shins to traditional psychiatry."[3] Glasser has been a board-certified psychiatrist since 1961, so he is not an outsider simply making outlandish comments when he suggests that there is no such thing as mental illness, as it has come to be defined, and that psychiatric drugs are a fraud. From the very beginning he saw no sense in a Freudian approach to counseling, and instead believed that people needed to better understand their responsibility for their own mental health. He came to believe that people basically choose their misery and states of depression, and that the mental illnesses listed in the

DSM-IV are the result of a brain's creative response to long-term unhappiness.[14] This is a radically different perspective on mental illness.

The traditional or common perspective on mental health reflects overwhelming agreement, both within the psychiatric profession, as well as throughout the general public, that mental symptoms are the result of an illness or a disease, which is beyond the control of those afflicted and which can only be helped by drugs. The problem is viewed as something coming from outside of you, like a person catching a cold, so the solution is seen as also coming from outside of you, like so many drugs we take for so many conditions. As one writer puts it, "The major psychiatric illnesses are diseases. They should be considered medical illnesses just as diabetes, heart disease, and cancer are."[15] This statement captures the medical model view of mental illness. It is this view to which the medical profession, and especially the psychiatrists, subscribes. Less than altruistic motivation may also be at play here since some see the very survival of psychiatry as a profession tied to the belief that extremes of irrationality and mental disease are connected.[16]

By the end of the 20th century, Glasser's beliefs on human behavior and mental health, as expressed through reality therapy, control theory, and later choice theory, had become a permanent and well-known part of the behavioral science landscape. The principles of reality therapy and choice theory had seeped into the awareness of the psychological and psychiatric professions, as well as the field of education. Not all agree with him, but that is why this biography, this story, is so important. To a great degree, William Glasser's life represents the conflict that has been brewing for decades—the conflict over people's ability or inability to affect their own thinking and make effective behavioral choices.

A 2010 article in *The New Yorker* entitled Head Case[17] focused on the themes Glasser has been trumpeting for over four decades. The article asked more questions than provided answers, but even the questions that were asked would seem to confirm Glasser's concerns. Questions like, Is psychiatry a science? Should depression be categorized as a mental illness or is it a sane response to a crazy world? Are brain drugs a form of valid treatment or are they no more effective than a placebo? Is the *Diagnostic and Statistical Manual of Mental Disorders (DSM)* a medically and scientifically accurate resource or is it simply a product of politics and culture? The stakes are remarkably high in the mega-drama that is playing out right in front of our eyes, right in front of our lives. Financially, the implications are staggering. Whichever direction healthcare heads with regard to mental health treatment, some people and companies, particularly the pharmaceuticals, will stand to make or lose a lot of money. A huge amount of money. More important, though, people will continue to wonder if their mental states and emotions are beyond their control, or if, in fact, they can affect their mental states by their thinking and their choices; they will continue to wonder if negative symptoms occur because of a biological breakdown of some sort in their brain, or if instead symptoms are brought on by their thinking and by their unhappiness; and they will keep on wondering if they are victims of a disease, held hostage to problems and solutions outside of themselves, or if they actually hold the keys to the chains in which they have wrapped themselves. We each have faced, and will continue to face, these conflicting questions. Some of us more than others. Ultimately, we each will decide for ourselves which paradigm we will believe in and invest in. The stakes are remarkably high.

WG

As the plane descends into Kansas City, objects begin to come into clearer view. By now, Glasser is fidgety, ready to land. Over the course of the flight, he has reviewed his talk and is ready to go. Slowly, ever so slowly it seems, the ground gets closer. Individual houses can be seen and individual cars can be picked out on the many connecting roads. The landscape details begin to stand out in sharp contrast. Glasser's professional journey could be characterized in much the same way. Because of his uniqueness, he saw a "big picture" that was different from the picture others were seeing. He then went about connecting the dots, identifying the landmarks, and helping us to understand what makes us tick. Certainly his views on mental health provide a sharp contrast to the perspective the mental illness profession continues to sell us. As the door of the plane's cabin opened to the spring-like air of Kansas City, Glasser is optimistic, expectant, and anxious to share his message.

NOTES

1. Whitaker, R. (2002). *Mad in America: Bad science, bad medicine, and the enduring mistreatment of the mentally ill*. Cambridge, MA: Perseus Publishing.
2. Joe Dimaggio and Marilyn Monroe got married. Hank Aaron hit his first home run in that year, and Willie Mays made his famous over-the-shoulder basket catch during the World Series at the Polo Grounds in New York. The magazine *Sports Illustrated* was born in August. J.R.R. Tolkien published a fantasy series called *The Lord of the Rings*. The big event, though, is the court case known as Brown vs. Board of Education of Topeka, in which the high court ruled that segregation in public schools violated the Fourteenth Amendment, and "that all deliberate speed be used in admitting Negro children to public schools."
3. Whitaker, R. (2002). *Mad in America: Bad science, bad medicine, and the enduring mistreatment of the mentally ill*. Cambridge, MA: Perseus Publishing.
4. By 2000, the Glasser Institute was established in the United States, Canada, Australia, Japan, and Ireland, and was developing strong roots in Croatia, Slovenia, South Korea, Norway, Israel, England, Germany, Spain, Columbia, Russia, Kuwait, New Zealand, Hong Kong, Singapore, and Italy. Since 1967, when the Glasser Institute first began, more than 75,000 people in 28 countries have taken Glasser's Basic Intensive Training. Over 2,000 Irish people alone have taken the training, which is an impressive number for a small country so soon after getting started with Glasser's ideas.
5. Glasser, W. (1960). Mental health or mental illness: Psychiatry for practical action. New York: Harper & Row Publishers.
6. Phillips, M. (1961, May 21). 100 select minds cope 2 days with individual's role in society. *The New York Times*.
7. Glasser, W. (1965). Reality therapy: A new approach to psychiatry. New York: Harper & Row Publishers.
8. Langguth, J. (1967). California's gift to psychotherapy. *Harper's Magazine*, 234, 52.
9. Ibid.

10 Glasser, W. (1969). *Schools without failure.* New York: Harper & Row Publishers.
11 Charles, C. (2002). *Building classroom discipline.* (7th ed.). Boston: Allyn and Bacon.
12 *Sonja Live* ran from 1987-1994.
13 Berges, M. (1974, March 3). William Glasser: A maverick/educator psychiatrist takes a realistic approach to untangling mixed-up kids. *Los Angeles Times Home Magazine,* 40-43.
14 Glasser, W. (2003). *Warning: Psychiatry can be hazardous to your mental health.* New York: Harper Collins.
15 Andreasen, N. (1984). *The broken brain: The biological revolution in psychiatry.* New York: Harper Row Publishers.
16 Breggin, P. (1991). *Toxic psychiatry.* New York: St. Martin's Press.
17 Menand, L. (2010, March 1). Head Case. *The New Yorker.*

2
CLEVELAND

"As far as I could tell with me, my father never used any external control ever in our whole existence together, and I was in my 60s when my father passed away."
—*William Glasser*

Ben Glasser came to Cleveland in 1915 because of opportunity. Soon to be married, Ben had been looking for a business venture that he could call his own, and just such a venture opened up in Cleveland, a city that was emerging as a key business center. By 1920, Cleveland would be the fifth largest city in the U.S., and when the Cleveland Indians won the World Series that same year, things looked bright for this growing metropolis on Lake Erie. The metropolitan growth led to suburban growth, as well, and small surrounding communities quickly grew into small cities of their own, like Cleveland Heights, where Ben Glasser and his wife would settle.

Ben Glasser left Russia and came to America in 1905.[1] He was 13 years old. The eldest of eight children, Ben felt a sense of responsibility to succeed and take care of himself. Although "he never really went to school, he learned English, got a job, and headed to New York City." In search of something better he followed a lead to Minnesota and worked there in 1912, but he returned to New York after that year.

Upon his return, he made two connections that would prove to be permanent. The first was his getting a job at the Hammel & Riglander jewelry supply company; the second was his meeting a young woman named Rebecca Silverberg. Ben ended up working in the jewelry supply and watch business until he retired in 1949, and he and Rebecca formed a marriage partnership that lasted a lifetime.

Only her sisters called Rebecca by that name, and they referred to her as Bec, for short. To everyone else, Rebecca was Betty. Something about Betty would appeal to young Ben, although later in life he would seriously question what he had been thinking when he fell for her. Betty had many qualities, many of them good, but for some reason not all of her qualities endeared her to people. What contributes to the unique qualities that make up the personality of a person? The questions of nature versus nurture play out in each of us. Betty's parents passed on certain dispositions, to be sure, and the way they raised her would also have significance. Betty definitely had a toughness about her that could be interpreted as an ability to attack life. Unfortunately, this toughness was more often interpreted as an ability to attack others. Maybe the toughness was the result of being born on a boat while her parents were leaving Austria to come to America for a better life. The boat was in the harbor at Liverpool, England, when she came into the world, a place that has put the stamp of toughness on more than a few. Whatever it was, when young Ben Glasser saw her, he saw someone whom he wanted to take with him to Cleveland.

He had moved east, to Duluth, once before, only to return to the big city, but this was different. Now, opportunity awaited with a capital O. The jewelry and watch business had been good for Ben Glasser and he, in turn, had been good to it, a fact which was not lost on the Hamel & Riglander people or on the customers whom Ben served. Before electronics and computerization, watches were mechanical. They had moving parts inside that kept them going—tiny springs, screws, and gears. The accuracy of the timepiece depended on the health of the parts inside. Some professions, like the railroad industry, were very dependent on watches that kept accurate time. Ben's New York-based company provided the parts that did just that. New York City wasn't the only place that needed watch parts, though. Lots of people were moving to Cleveland and most of them were wearing watches. So Hamel & Riglander began thinking of westward expansion. Whether owners quietly conferred in the back room about who should head up the new Cleveland location, or Ben heard about the opportunity and said, "I'm your guy," he was soon heading to Ohio.

It must have been exciting for Ben, because the Cleveland business would be totally his. Well, not totally his. The Merit Company (as he and his fellow owner, his younger brother Dave, would name it), would distribute the products of Hamel & Riglander. In other words, Ben Glasser would be independent from the New York company, and while the profits would be his, so too would all of the start-up risks. Starting a business in a new city can be expensive and Ben, as a young man just beginning, did not have anywhere near the necessary capital. But this is where his soon-to-be father-in-law came into the picture to provide Ben with a $300 loan.

Ben and Betty took on a lot of challenge and change within a short period of time. They took on marriage, a new city, and a new business all at once. If that wasn't enough, in less than two years, in 1917, they brought their first child, Henry Earl, into the world. A few years later, in 1921, they would have a daughter, Ruth Janet. And in 1925, they celebrated the birth of their third child, a boy, and named him William. Like most young couples they were made up of one part confidence and one part naiveté. At some point they would look back and wonder what they were thinking, but for now they were young and ready to tackle the world. The Glasser family would have its faults, but they would do many things right, too. One of the best things this family would do is to somehow bring the elements together that would launch one of the children into national prominence. They wouldn't do it on purpose. It wasn't like some of these "tennis parents" today who send their kids off to expensive tennis academies so the kid can become an elite tennis prodigy. No, it wasn't like that at all. In this family the father would go to work and try to provide Cleveland with the watch parts it needed, the mother would stay home and focus on raising the children, and the children would play with their friends, go to school, and slowly take on the world.

How much should be made of the birth order of siblings? Psychologists have studied the impact of birth order and numerous studies have looked for later tendencies in motivation and behavior. Of the first 23 astronauts sent into space, 21 of them were first-borns. Many of our U.S. presidents were first-borns, as well. First-borns, say those who believe in these statistical tendencies, are usually high-achievers and very responsible. They tend to respect authority and keep the rules. Part of their success lies in their spirit of determination and their attention to detail. Middle children learn to negotiate and compromise. They tend to be peacemakers and are generous to a fault. Maybe because siblings surround them, they are known for being social. Last but not least, the babies of the family carve out their own niche. Their brothers and sisters have already established themselves by the time the last-born comes along. Last-borns are often known as idea people with a creative streak. They have a sense of humor (a must for having to cope with older brothers and sisters) and most significant, they tend to question authority.[2] Lists that describe our personalities fascinate us even as we remain skeptical about their accuracy. There is always just enough truth to keep us wondering if our unique, individual mystery has been demystified.³

Miss Hale looked up from the stack of books she was about to re-shelve and saw Billy Glasser looking up at her. As the children's librarian in the Cleveland Heights Public Library she knew a lot of the children who frequented the library. The elementary school across the street, Coventry Elementary School, didn't have its own library, so students made the easy trek to access (remember, this was pre-television and pre-video games) the special world of books. She smiled as Billy placed two books on the counter to check out and then dug into his pants pocket to find his library card. He was only in the fourth grade, but was already asking about how he could get an adult library card, too. The children's section was separate from the grown-up section and each required its own checkout card. She thought to herself that Billy might just check out more books than any of the kids she knew. Actually, she didn't know the half of it. Even when he was just starting in the first grade, Billy often got up at 5:30 a.m. and read two or three of the children's books before breakfast.

"You're going to ruin your eyes," his mother would tell him. Years later he would admit: "I probably did ruin my eyes. I should have never read that much. Your eyes aren't really up to reading then." He didn't come from a home that taught him to read, but his sister, brother, and mother were all voracious readers, unlike his father who "settled for the newspaper, pretty much." As far as reading goes, though, he was more like his mother than his father, because as he remembers, "I was dying to read!" His mother encouraged reading, but she left it to Miss Ferar, Billy's first-grade teacher, to teach him how. Miss Ferar, using phonics as the instructional tool, did just that, and within six weeks Billy was entering a world—the world of reading and writing—that would captivate him for the rest of his life.[4]

Seeing Billy place the card on top of the books, a slight smile on his face, peering up at her through his fairly thick glasses, she wondered what made him tick, what motivated him. But then she quickly realized that he and she were quite alike as far as books went—they both loved to read and just being around books felt good somehow. Billy was in the library literally every day, and especially on Wednesday afternoons when she would tell a story to all the kids who wanted to listen. By the time he was 6 years old, he could walk by himself to the library or elementary school, a distance of less than half a mile. Except for the five-corner intersection, fortunately patrolled by Scottie and Ralph, two big policemen, the route through the neighborhoods was safe. His mother had access to the family car, but unless it was raining, Billy planned on walking wherever he needed to go. The library happened to be a place that he needed to go often.

Billy Glasser loved to learn about all kinds of things, and would even read the encyclopedia, but as far as he was concerned the best kind of learning occurred when the learning was wrapped up in a good story. For him, the epitome of a good read could be found in the books of Joseph Altsheler. His brother and sister introduced him to the books, probably by leaving one lying around their bedroom, but once opened, he read every book he could get his hands on. Titles like *The Border Watch, The Riflemen of the Ohio,* and *The Forest Runners,* were all quickly devoured. *The Young Trailers,* a series of eight books capturing the exploits of five young men, were his favorites, so much so that he read them over and over again. "They fought Indians, and sometimes the British, and traveled down the Mississippi. You learned a lot about geography. They talked about their weapons, flintlocks and muzzle-loaders, and how you could build a fire in impossible conditions."[5] For a boy in Cleveland in the early 30s it was reading you could look forward to. Joseph Altsheler is a popular author to this day. Testimonials on Altsheler's titles in the Amazon.com used book section reveal a deep appreciation for his writing. More recent editions easily go for $25 each, with original hardbound editions going for as much as $200. Billy Glasser was beginning to have an eye for quality.

Later he would get into classics such as *The Three Musketeers,* even though he was still young and didn't understand them entirely. Much later, as an adult, his own daughter would introduce him to the English author, Anthony Trollope,[6] "whom I absolutely loved," he said. "I read most of Thomas Hardy, too. A very great author." He would later come to the conclusion that "to understand human nature you really have to read the great authors of the world. Of course," he continued, "all human nature is basically about love, sex, and the problems with external control."[7] His all-time favorite book, *Raintree County*[8], although written by a comparatively unknown author, had all the elements of a great story. Books and libraries would always be important to Glasser, even when they should have been less important. In college, when he was pursuing a degree, the library proved an unhelpful distraction. "One of the reasons I didn't do well in engineering school is they have a real good library there," he chuckled. "I could sit in the library and read fiction books instead of studying."

Standing at the check-out counter of the Cleveland Heights Children's Library, for Billy, that college library was still years away, though. For now, third-grader Billy Glasser received his library card back from Miss Hale, one of his favorite people, and picked up his new books off the counter. He smiled as he turned and moved toward the front door, and turned and smiled again as pushed the front door open and headed out into the sunshine. Chances are he would start reading after he crossed the first intersection. He knew the way home well enough that he could keep one eye on the book and one eye on the sidewalk in front of him. Books are good partners on walks.

By the time he could walk to school on his own, and definitely by the time he sat in Miss Sheehan's sixth-grade class, Billy Glasser knew that his family had some faults. And to understand Bill Glasser is to catch a glimpse of this family dynamic, especially that of his mother's behavior. As an adult, Glasser would explain, "my mother was different from any other human being that I've ever met." Being different is not necessarily a problem in itself. Most would say that Mother Teresa was different from anyone they had met, too. As a child, though, Billy soon recognized that his mother was different from anything resembling the softhearted, gracious, unselfish Calcutta nun. And Billy wasn't the only one in the family who recognized this difference. Even before Billy came into the family, his father, Ben, realized that the qualities that he had seen in Betty years before in New York City, and that had drawn him to her, had been replaced by something very different. Her drive to control others and ultimately rule the marriage would set the tone, not only for this young household, but also for almost the entire 65 years of their marriage.[9]

As adults it is sometimes difficult to remember the dawn of our awareness and memory. Some claim to have memories from 2 or 3 years of age, while others have no clear recollections until close to 5 years old. Billy Glasser knew by the time he was 4 years old that his parents were not good for each other. He saw his father break things and even hit his mother, events that frightened him, but by the time he was six years old, the violence stopped.[10]

Billy, unlike his brother and especially his sister, learned "that to get along with her you had to go along with her." He saw that his mother got along with no one, and in the process she actually became his anti-role model. Yet in spite of her lashing out at one moment and becoming depressed the next, he had an ability to recognize that she was still his mother. "And while she didn't get along with people, I could see that there was no sense hassling her or things like that. Just go along," he later would explain, "and mostly everything would be okay, which actually my father did with her, too." That a young kid would be able to analyze a painful situation so dispassionately and evenly is amazing. As he described it later, "My mother lashed out all the time, but I loved her and she loved me and it didn't bother me that much. In fact, I thought it was funny some of the time. I understood her when I was a little kid and I just said, well, she's a very unusual person and I may as well make the most of her, because she's the only mother I'm ever going to have."

As a child, when Billy asked his mother why he didn't have a middle name, like his brother and his sister, he was told: "You were an unwanted child and so you only got two names." He was given a similar reply when he asked who he was named after in the family, since both his brother and his sister had that distinction. "You were named after nobody," his mother said firmly. "I liked William and so that's what you were named." It was one more example of Betty Glasser's inability to say or do the loving thing, and maybe even to appropriately connect with another person on an intimate level. Billy somehow felt that it was her way of actually meaning the opposite—that he was indeed wanted. He had learned to go along and to stay out of her way, but her "lashing out" could target even those trying to steer clear of her.

Billy could see that his mother's world had two special people in it—herself and his brother Henry, or Hank as he was called at home. Billy seemed to accept this in much the same way that he accepted other characteristics of his mother. His sister, on the other hand, did not have a good relationship with her mother, or even a neutral relationship with her. As siblings go, Billy was close to his sister, but not so close to his older brother. This was due, to some extent, to the eight years that separated them, but the lack of closeness probably had deeper causes. Billy may not have known or understood the term when he was young, but later he described the "aloofness" of his brother. It wasn't a "big brother looking over the little brother" relationship between the two of them. It wouldn't be exactly accurate to say that Hank and his mother were close, since Betty's form of love always included control, but compared to her relationships with the rest of the family it is easy to see how others would view them as close. To Billy's way of looking at it, Hank got along with people about as well as his mother did, which wasn't very well at all. As a little brother, Billy wasn't being taken under Hank's wing, but one has a sense that he knew early on it really wasn't a wing he wanted to be under.

Hank's aloofness and ability to be critical was not based, though, on his being overly competent. At times, Hank's lack of competence affected his younger sister and brother in very real ways. For instance, by the time Bill graduated from his Cleveland high school, he had also attended school in Miami and in Palo Alto, California. You may recall that Stanford University is located in Palo Alto and while Bill was too young at the time to attend Stanford, it had everything to do with Bill having to be in Palo Alto. Hank attended Stanford, but as his time to graduate got closer, it became apparent that he might not be ready to march as scheduled. Betty's concern, and probably frustration, were great enough that she packed up her two kids still at home and moved to Palo Alto to oversee Hank's success. There was no way, as far as she was concerned, that Hank was going to stumble, regardless of whether he wanted to stumble or not.

The theme of control was always present around Betty Glasser, and while somehow it struck a chord with Hank, it did just the opposite with the rest of the family. She had bravely staked out this territory, the need to rule, and maintained it with determined vigilance. By the time Billy was born this family dynamic had been practiced and refined for nine years. Ben hadn't given in yet or realized the depth of his wife's commitment to controlling him, and so Billy saw brief moments of his dad being pushed to the brink, fighting back at times, and standing up to his wife's relentless domination, although Billy could see that his dad's "heart was not in it."[11] Much later, reviewing his childhood and his parents' uneasy truce, he explained: "My mother had won by the simple tactic of giving my father the message that he would have to kill her if he didn't want to let her rule the marriage."[12] Wherever it came from, whichever was to blame—nature or nurture—Betty Silverberg needed to feel in control and would do whatever it took to get it.

When Billy was 6 years old the fighting and the struggle between his parents stopped. His mother continued in her attempts to control, but his father just stopped making a fight over things. It was a giving in, on the surface at least, but other things may have been at play here. Glasser recalled later: "My father used to hit my mother. It was more than he could stand. She would bait him and bait him and bait him. I saw him do moderate—didn't do violence—like he would break something, when I was a little boy, and he would hit it so hard that it broke on the floor. But, uh, and I think once in awhile my father may have hit her. But, my father—I believe my father had another woman in his life, and I think, I think my mother knew it, too. But I think she knew it would be better for her if she didn't make a fuss about it. My father and the other woman didn't make a fuss about it. And I knew the other woman for years. She worked for my father." Glasser describes his father as a gentle man who fought back at first, but who in the end had no stomach for the battles. For the rest of his marriage, which continued on for another 60 years, Ben never tried to control his wife again.

Bill found the rags and sponges for washing the car next to the cabinet in the garage where his dad kept them and plunged the sponge into the soapy bucket of water sitting next to the car on the driveway. At 14 years of age, he had grown into a young man, and like other young men his age, he was in the midst of negotiating the minefield called high school. He had become independent and confident in his ability, even to the extent that when his father was out of town, Bill would take the car out, sometimes by himself for the practice, and sometimes with his friends. He would not legally be able to drive for another two years, so he concentrated on not getting into trouble and especially not getting into an accident. To the casual observer walking by the Glasser car parked on the driveway in front of their house, the car looked clean enough. But cars were special to Bill and being seen in a dirty car just wouldn't be acceptable. As he pulled the wet, soapy sponge out of the bucket and sloshed it on the hood of the car, his mind recalled a brief talk his father had with him only a few weeks before. Bill was almost finished washing the car, when his dad came out and observed some areas where the dirt still remained, especially the wheels. He could still hear his father's voice gently telling him, "Look, Bull,[13] if you want to wash the car, wash it thoroughly. If you don't want to wash the car, that's okay with me. I'm not going to stop you from driving the car or anything like that, but I just want you to understand that if you do something, do it thoroughly." For Bill, this brief moment on the driveway represented more than a lesson on doing things thoroughly. In microcosm, it symbolized the difference between how his father, on one side, and mother, on the other, approached life. In some small way Bill realized that his father's approach led to much better results. As he washed the car a few weeks later and recalled his dad's encouragement, Bill didn't feel resentment or any anger whatsoever. He could see his dad was right, and as he washed the car again, this time he would attempt to get every spot clean, including the wheels.

No one can know what goes through the mind of a person experiencing an unhappy relationship. The Glasser children certainly saw the uneasy truce at times between their parents, but they also experienced a family that was making it. Life was difficult, they probably thought to themselves, and we don't always agree or get what we want, but we're making it. Mom and dad are as different as night and day, they realized, but we're making it. With regard to understanding human motivation, even our own, it has been said that: "There's the reason we tell others; there's the reason we tell our spouse; there's the reason we tell ourselves; and then there's the real reason."[14] So even Ben Glasser himself may not have totally understood why he stayed in the marriage. In the 1930s and 1940s, divorce was not a part of the culture like it became a few decades later, especially in the Glasser and Silverberg families, even though sometimes an unhappy home can represent a comfortable sameness, a stability. Like other parents in less-than-perfect marriages, Ben Glasser may have given in and stayed in the relationship because of his children, especially because he wanted to be there for his last-born son.

In a way similar to his wife and oldest son having a special bond based on a desire to control and an inability to get along with others, Ben and his youngest son had a special relationship based on their desire to stay away from control and, in the process, get along with others. Ben and Bill were the counterpoint to Betty and Hank. Bill recognized something special in his father, and through some observation and some conversation he slowly learned about life. These lessons had no small effect. Years later, Bill would share, "As far as I could tell with me, my father never used any external control ever in our whole existence together, and I was in my 60s when my father passed away." When asked to describe on whose shoulders he had stood to discover and refine his ideas, Glasser placed his father at the top of the list. "I can say that my father had a strong effect on me my whole life and certainly is the precursor to my psychiatric work and my understanding people."

Ben Glasser had not really gone to school. He had worked since he was barely a teenager, like many other immigrant children, and there was no time for school. He had attended a few classes at Cooper Union College, which in the early days was a kind of community college that charged little or no tuition, but that was the extent of his education. In spite of this, he was a very intelligent man, and while young Bill never saw his father read a book, his father read the newspaper every day and listened to the radio on a regular basis. He also saw how active his father was in politics and came to appreciate his liberal views, especially when it came to steering clear of policies that attempted to control other people. He quietly observed his father work with people and he became convinced that his father was thinking and doing a lot of things right. Young Bill saw the power in invitation, rather than declaration, and the power of leading by example, instead of trying to make someone do something against his or her will.

As a boy, Glasser wondered aloud to his dad why they didn't go to Sunday school like other kids and their families. His father, who was a devout atheist and who thought all religion was harmful, said that if

Glasser wanted to go to Sunday school he could, but to do it for the right reasons. "Don't do it," he warned, "just because other kids are doing it." Glasser felt that if he had wanted to become a rabbi his father would have supported him, because his father loved him. He remembers his father, though, traveling all the way to Chicago on a train to hear his hero, Clarence Darrow, speak. Darrow was a renowned atheist at the time. "I was raised by my father, who I literally worshiped, and he was an atheist. But my father was also a very fair man. He would not push his atheism on other people, including his children. In fact, we were given the opportunity to go to Sunday school and get a religious education and be bar mitzvahed, or whatever it is, but I didn't want any part of it." Given how important his father's influence was on him, it is significant Glasser did not go on to become an atheist himself. Later, as an adult, he would take a neutral position on issues relating to spirituality and religion, since he felt the ideas couldn't be proved one way or another.

When the car pulled up next to the grassy lot where the boys were playing touch football, a few of the football players stopped playing and watched the car pull to the curb. "Come on, ya gonna play or daydream?" one the other players yelled. "Pay attention, let's play."

It was Sunday and the usual guys from the surrounding neighborhoods had come together to play football, just like they did every Sunday during football season. It was just a neighborhood game, yet some of the players acted as if it was for the championship in front of a hundred thousand people, with their reputations hanging in the balance on every play. When Walter showed up in his father's '41 Buick, most of the players acted unaffected, maybe rolled their eyes, or gave each other knowing looks, and kept focused on the game at hand. A few of them thought he might have yelled something out of the open passenger-side window, but when no one acknowledged whatever it was he had said, Walter got out of the car, walked around the back of it and took a few steps onto the field.

"Hey guys," he shouted, but none of the players looked at him. "Guys," he tried again, but still only a couple of heads turned. "Hey!" he continued anyway, "the war's started."

"Get outta here, Walter," one of the serious players shouted back. "We're trying to play."

"You're crazy," another kid yelled.

"No, I'm not. It really has started."

"What are you talking about?" one of them asked.

"Listen to this. I'll show you," and with that he moved around to the driver's door, got in the car, and turned the radio on. He turned the volume up so that all of the guys could hear President Roosevelt's voice describe what had happened in a place called Pearl Harbor. Even the serious players forgot the game as the implications began to sink in. Moments before, when these young men had been lined up for the next play, the most important thing on their mind was whether they could score. Now, as the group stood around the car, it was plain there would be other things on their mind for a while.

The Cleveland years for Bill Glasser encompassed both The Great Depression of 1929 and World War II, each with its national and international impact of indescribable magnitude. During the Depression, which stretched through the 1930s, the Glassers lived in the poorer section of Cleveland Heights, even though they owned their home and had a car. There were some in the neighborhood who were affected by the economic crisis,[15] but to an extent, the neighborhood was buffered from the devastating effects seen in other parts of the country. There were food drives at school, and Betty Glasser made significant contributions to those, as well as to other efforts to relieve suffering.

In 1941, Ben and Betty purchased a new home in University Heights, which was a nicer community right next door to Cleveland Heights. Bill's aunt, who had lived with them for as long as he could remember, had her own room. Hank was on his own by this time and would, in fact, head off to fight in the war, even sustaining a wound during his time there.

World War II helped yank the country out of the Depression, but this solution to our economic woes came at a very high price in other ways. Over 400,000 Americans lost their lives in World War II, and it was a rare neighborhood that did not feel the sting of loss. The Glasser's new University Heights neighborhood was no exception, although to this neighborhood, the war's meaning took on special significance. Like the Glassers themselves, their University Heights neighborhood was predominantly Jewish. Beginning in the mid-1930s there was a growing concern over events in Europe, especially in Germany. This concern was even greater in Jewish neighborhoods. Newspapers, the radio, and letters from relatives in Europe increasingly confirmed the need for concern. On a March evening in 1938, shortly after Germany took over Austria, you could walk down the street and hear Hitler's speech on the radio through the open front doors of every house in the Glasser's neighborhood. The concern was becoming fear. Loved ones were in the midst of a situation that was growing worse by the day. Rumors of Hitler's plan regarding the Jewish people were becoming more than just rumors. But the fear of the '30s led to something worse in the '40s, something that would strike the neighborhood with agonizing frequency.

A few of the young men standing around the car on that Sunday morning in 1941 would eventually head off to the war themselves. The neighborhood sent quite a few to the fighting. Many did not return. Sanford Goodman, one of Bill Glasser's closest friends, was one of those who didn't come home. The Goodman's had the whole upstairs of the double house they shared with the Glassers, so this was a loss that was close to Bill. Tragically, the Goodman's lost another son in the war, as well.

Before America entered the war, though, while events in Europe were getting worse, American families were helping to get relatives out of Europe to safer areas, including the U.S. Betty Glasser knew of relatives who needed such help and threw her energy into getting them out of the danger. It is a wonderful story that reveals the good that Betty often did for people in need. Unfortunately, even this story of Betty has a downside: In part due to her efforts, an entire family was able to escape the cruelty of Hitler's Germany, only to find themselves under her control upon their arrival. Like so many others, even this family that Betty had saved became estranged from her and left to begin again in California. To this day, Bill Glasser is pretty sure he has cousins in California he has not seen since that time in Cleveland.

Bill can remember going to the store as a kid to pick up some groceries for his mother. "The grocer's brain wasn't working too well," he recalls, "and I'd bring back more money than I took in the first place." As he handed the groceries and the change to his mother he said, somewhat triumphantly, "Look at all the money Mr. Purer gave to me." Betty Glasser's response was immediate and firm. "Take the money back," she ordered. "Go to someone in the store and tell them they made a mistake." Betty Glasser had principles that she lived by, in spite of her difficulty in getting along with others. When asked if his mother was religious at all, or if maybe religion played a part in her principles, Bill quickly replied, "No. My mother, as far as anyone could tell, wasn't anything. What she lived by nobody knows, but certain basic things she was very strict about, like you know, cheating people and things like that." People weren't sure where her convictions came from, but they were sure she had convictions. Betty Glasser was intense about these convictions, but unfortunately couldn't leave it at that. This intensity alienated almost everyone who came in contact with her.

On a practical side, little Billy Glasser came to understand the effective strategies for "fighting." He remembers: "Early in life I felt the idea of controlling people is something that I never liked to do, nor did I ever like to be controlled, but I would never fight control to my detriment like some people do. You know, they'll fight to their detriment. So my mother and I would never fight to my detriment." More important, while lessons were being learned about how to live by getting along with others or how not to live by alienating others, Billy Glasser learned these lessons in a home atmosphere in which he felt loved. This he did not doubt from either of his parents. He would later explain, "You know, my mother fought with others, but not with me. It only bothered me that she fought with others, but I never could say that she fought with me or put me down, or anything like that. She was super supportive of me and if anything—if I didn't make good grades—she figured it was the college's fault, which it wasn't. She just had supreme confidence that I would be a success at whatever I did."

By the time Bill Glasser graduated from Cleveland Heights High School in 1942, although still growing, Cleveland would fall one place back to the sixth largest city in the United States. It was a portent of things to come, as Cleveland had reached its zenith as far as comparative size goes. By the 1990 census, Cleveland would stand at number

23 on the population list of U.S. cities. The demographic pull of the coastlines, especially in the West, would be too much for middle American cities to overcome. Still, though, for a city in northern Ohio along Lake Erie with all the weather the Great Lakes could produce, Cleveland had done well. During the early 1900s Cleveland provided an environment for young families to make a beginning. The Glassers were one of those families. Ben Glasser, a young Russian, Jewish immigrant had done well enough selling watch and jewelry parts that he would soon think about retiring and heading to Florida. Ben and Betty survived their disastrous marriage and raised three children through it all. And as the children became adults, they too would set out toward their own horizons. The youngest of the Glasser children would soon put Cleveland behind him, and like his father before him, would head west on his own, confident his future held promise.

NOTES

1. "My father hated the country he came from, Russia, and never would even speak a word of Russian once he got here and would never talk to me about it. What he emphasized was, forget about it, we're in the U.S. now, we are Americans." As quoted during the Wubbolding interview in *Reality Therapy for the 21st Century*, Brunner-Routledge, p. 61.
2. Lorie Sutter, *Birth Order*, Ohio State University Extension Fact Sheet, ohioline.ag.ohio-state.edu
3. Glasser interview, September 26, 2003 - Glasser himself doesn't put much stock in birth-order psychology. His brother was eight years older than him and his sister was four years older, and while he was "pretty close" to his sister when they were younger, none of them are that close now.
4. In the interview he added, "Even though the language isn't very phonetic, phonics is not a bad way to learn to read."
5. As Glasser talked with me about details in the books and the specific names of the characters, like Henry Weir, Silent Tom Russ, Shiftless Saul, and Long Jim, I responded with "You still remember all those details?" He chuckled and explained, "Well I think I read them like seven times."
6. Anthony Trollope wrote in the mid-1800's and used Victorian life as a backdrop. His ability to capture contemporary detail and comment on human nature and human motivation is legendary. When Glasser asked me if I had heard of Trollope, I had to admit that I hadn't. "Oh, my god," he replied, "a great writer." A pang of ignorance swept through me at that moment and I promised that I would meet Mr. Trollope for myself.
7. "Trollope's books all end kind of happily," Glasser pointed out, but "Hardy's books end miserably. Tess of the d'Urbervilles, I mean, I read that when I went to Palm Springs one weekend. My god," he laughed as he said this, "at the end of the book you're suicidal!" Still laughing, "It gets worse and worse."
8. Lockridge, R. (1948). *Raintree county*. Boston: Houghton Mifflin Company.
9. William Glasser, *Choice Theory: A New Psychology of Personal Freedom* (New York: Harper Collins, 1998), p.89,90
10. Ibid.

11 William Glasser, *Choice Theory: A New Psychology of Personal Freedom* (New York: Harper Collins, 1998), p.90
12 *ibid*, p.89
13 His father began calling him Bull, although Glasser couldn't remember why.
14 Roy, J. (2005). *Soul shapers: A better plan for parents and educators.* Hagerstown, MD: Review & Herald Publishing Association.
15 In 1933, almost a third of the Cleveland's workers were without jobs.

3
WELCOME TO THE CLUB

> "I never thought people were so crazy that
> they didn't know what they were doing."
> —*William Glasser*

John Caughey[1] pondered the list on his desk. The names were on a plain, white sheet of paper, handwritten by his own hand. He had been through this process several times before, but each time when it came to the moment actual choices had to be made, it weighed on him. The decisions he was about to make could really change people's lives.

As Bill Glasser drove into one of the parking lots at the Case School of Applied Science on a beautiful fall day in 1942, he felt the same mix of emotions that others experience on their first day of college. He had his sights set on becoming a scientist or an engineer, due in part to the fact that his brother and sister had really done nothing in college. In his view, they didn't learn much and hadn't done anything with the degrees they had earned. Such is the advantage of being born last. Bill would try to improve on his brother and sister's higher education experience. He had done well in high school. He downplays it now, saying that he was a pretty good student in high school, but the record shows that he graduated 55th out of a class of 515, which basically puts him in the top 10%. He chose to pursue a degree in chemical engineering, but would question that decision later. Like many college students who choose a field of study because they may as well choose something and get on with it, Glasser chose chemical engineering, but his heart was not in it. He would later say he'd never known why he took chemical engineering. It doesn't seem like that much of a mystery, though. He was intelligent and thoughtful and could consider problems logically. Science and math came easily to him and he enjoyed dissecting a problem until he understood it. These were traits that would suit a chemical engineer.

The war may have had an influence on his decision as well. Young men were being drafted and sent all over the world to fight. His brother had been wounded and his neighbors had been killed. As a chemical engineer, his draft was deferred in 1943 until he completed that degree. The army, rather than being frustrated with such a deferment, supported degree programs that could be put to use in the war effort. Winning the war would require brain as much as brawn, and college deferments were a part of filling that need. Many of us know about how the manufacturing sector during the early 1940s switched from a civilian production emphasis to a war effort production emphasis, but few of us realize that colleges and universities went into that same mode. As a result, Glasser completed his bachelor of science degree in only two years and eight months. It was a grueling program, running six days a week, including summers and vacations. Glasser was glad when it was over, partly because of having to go to school throughout the week and on Saturday too, but also because he just didn't do well in college. He graduated in the spring of 1945, probably feeling a lot like a young man named George Stephanopoulos would 37 years later. In 1982, Stephanopoulos, who later became an advisor in the Clinton administration, was in his senior year at Columbia and still wasn't sure what he wanted to do with his life. "Law school," he wrote, "seemed like the natural choice: finishing school for ambitious liberal arts majors who didn't know exactly what they wanted to do. It would also meet the Greek standard for achievement. The only problem with law school was that when it was over I would be in real danger of becoming a lawyer."[2] Glasser was now in real danger of becoming a chemical engineer. But while chemical engineering may have clouded his future, there was someone who was about to bring sunshine into his life.

During that same spring, in effect his senior year, Bill Glasser met Naomi Silver. She was two years his junior, but his equal in so many other ways. He was drawn to her, although there were a few things he had to overcome. He was so shy he could barely speak to her, an effective barrier, he would learn, to getting to know her. For the first three weeks he telephoned her home, but declined to leave his name. It is a credit to his creativity that their friendship grew in spite of this obstacle. Naomi's mother, though, confided to her that, "I'm sure he's a fine young man, but do you think you could persuade him to say 'hello' when he comes to the house?"[3] Confident in many ways, Glasser felt less comfortable talking to one person. In spite of his shyness, their friendship blossomed.

The world changed forever on August 6, 1945. That was the day the Enola Gay, a B-29 bomber, dropped Little Boy, an atomic bomb, on Hiroshima, Japan: it was the first atomic weapon ever used on a populated area. It was Monday morning, a little after 8:00 a.m. when the bomb exploded 2,000 feet off the ground. After being released from the plane, it had fallen for a minute before reaching that height and unleashing its searing heat, as bright as the sun, and its incredible wind, stronger than any hurricane experienced on Earth. The minute during which the bomb fell through the sky was the last minute of peace for those below. The devastation was indescribable. By the end of the year, it is believed 140,000 people were killed from the blast.[4] And as superpowers created and stockpiled nuclear might, the world began to live with the feeling that destruction might be just around the next corner.

Glasser had graduated from college only months before, but had quickly started working as a chemical engineer at Case. The head of the chemical engineering department also had a position at a big factory in town called the Lubrizol Corporation, which made additives to make motor oil better. Bill remembers being affected by the bomb being dropped and what it did to an entire city, but he also remembers being concerned as a scientist. He and some other classmates and fellow workers sought out Dr. Marin, a physical chemistry professor at Case. Glasser and the others had not heard about the testing in New Mexico and wondered if splitting the atom could result in blowing up the entire world. He later recalled his introspection about it: "I mean, if these things are gonna blow the whole world up, then we're all gonna be gone. It didn't even frighten me because it was such an immense concept, that we may as well figure that it's not gonna happen. 'Cuz if it happens, what good is worrying going to do? It was more or less the psychology I've had all my life, being that I really find it difficult to worry a great deal about things that I have absolutely no control over." The way he emotionally and psychologically processed the threat of atomic doom was an early evidence of a matter-of-fact approach to life that has marked his personal relationships and professional work ever since.

During the year following his college graduation, some other introspection must have taken place, too. It was a combination of things that led to his thinking about where he really wanted to go with his life. He had trained to be a chemical engineer and now he was a chemical engineer, but something important was missing. Chemical engineering, he realized, would be a job, but would never be his passion; it would call on his logic, but less so on his creativity. More and more he realized how interested he was in people, and in what made them behave in certain ways. As a result, the field of psychology was gently pulling him toward a life of studying human behavior. The pull grew stronger as the months went by. Part of him felt like he had just devoted an entire college career to chemical engineering and that he couldn't just walk away from it, while another part of him looked longingly at the field of psychology. Was it simply a case of the grass being greener on the other side of the fence? To help discover the answer he decided to take a few psychology classes in the spring of 1946. It seemed like a small thing at the time.

If you've ever put on a pair of shoes that felt like they were custom made for your feet, then you can begin to understand the connection that Glasser felt as he sat in those psychology classrooms for the first time. Like a person starting a new job in a company that's a perfect fit he found himself thinking, "I'm home." It was the first time since the days of Miss Sheehan, his sixth-grade teacher, that he looked forward to class. Throughout almost his entire life school had been something you had to do, so you may as well do it. He had rarely, if ever, associated the words useful or relevant to academic experiences in school. That was now changing. By the end of that spring, William Glasser knew what he wanted to do and chemical bonds and valences weren't going to be a part of it. The pull of psychology had won.

At the same time his friendship with Naomi continued to grow. Give her credit for putting the best interpretation on his first, halting efforts at connecting, and give him credit for recognizing the jewel that was Naomi. Things were becoming clear to him—what he was going to do in life and who he was going to do it with—and with clarity comes commitment and action. "When I was going to get inducted into the army we accelerated our wedding plans. I proposed to her right around her birthday, which was the 13th of September, and we got married a week later, on the 20th of September (1946), and I left for the army on the 30th." Their quick decision to get married may have contributed to the wedding taking place in the Glasser home on Fenwood Road. Glasser remembers it as a nice wedding with quite a few people present, although like most weddings it had an unplanned moment or two. When the rabbi got to the part of the wedding where he asks if anyone has anything to say against this marriage, let him speak now or forever hold his peace, a quietness settled over those in attendance as time was given for a response, a quietness that was shattered by Glasser's dog, Snooks, who let out a loud "woof," obviously in protest over his master heading off with someone new. Other than Snooks, though, everyone was for the marriage and the young couple headed off into life together—him to the army and her to finish her degree in speech pathology at Floristone Mather, formerly the women's college at Western Reserve University.

The decision to go into psychology did not come without a price, and while the decision seemed full of positives, there was one little negative ready to have its way. That little negative happened to revolve around his deferment from serving in the army. In choosing to go into psychology his deferment expired and very quickly he was drafted. In fact, a week after he was married he was inducted into the army and began a service experience that lasted for seven months. His first stop was for basic training at Fort Belvore in Alexandria, Virginia. Naomi actually was able to join him there, although she did not have her driver's license yet and a friend delivered her and their old car to the modest housing of Fort Belvore. Soon, though, they were on their way to the Dugway Proving Ground in Utah. The old car was in too bad of shape to make it to Utah and Bill's father bought them a new one.

Bill was a part of the chemical corps, or the comical corps, as the rest of the army seemed to refer to them. Not that what they were handling was a laughing matter. His unit tested the poison gasses the Allies took from the Germans at Normandy, including lethal ones such as Sarin, the same gas that terrorists released in a Japanese subway in 1995, killing 11 and injuring more that 5,500 people. Glasser was part of a study team that killed goats with it, although to this day he remains unclear about their objective. With seven months of service under his belt, and having enjoyed the winter in the middle of nowhere in Utah, he was discharged from the army in March of 1946. Looking back, he says, "I enjoyed my little time in the army there. It was called, you know, military research. I don't think that anyone that really ran the army knew anything about what was going on. Nobody cared, I don't think. We didn't find anything out by killing the goats that I found out." His experience with gas and goats did nothing to dampen his goal of going into psychology, though, and upon his return to Cleveland he resumed right where he had left off.

Having to abandon his psychology studies right when he was gaining some momentum (and immediately after getting married) was not Glasser's idea of a perfect scenario, but many clouds have silver linings, and sometimes even gold ones. For serving those seven months in Virginia and Utah, he would be able to benefit from the G.I. Bill, which proceeded in his case to provide 19 months of schooling toward his psychology degree. He now had the money to complete the master's degree program.

He reentered the master's program in psychology at Western Reserve University[5] in the fall of 1947. As with his earlier psychology classes, he felt that he was in the right place heading in the right direction, and it showed in his performance. Instead of the mediocre grades that he received in his undergraduate program, he did very well in his graduate studies. He was even speaking up in class. He was enjoying school now, even though the traditional teaching practices he had experienced in high school and college were also used in his graduate program. One thing he couldn't figure out was why there was so much Freudian emphasis when no one graduating with a master's degree would be able to use it. Freudian psychotherapeutic counseling took extensive training and only those with the training could use it in a counseling setting.

The curriculum in his graduate program was traditional, but Glasser took the classes and privately selected those materials and ideas that he felt were helpful and useful. He seemed to apply the same rule that he used when working with his mother, that is, not fighting something or someone to his detriment. He asked questions in class, something classmates remembered about him later, and shared his opinions, but he recognized he had much to learn about the human brain and how it operates. He had opinions, though, including ideas on what constituted mental illness. "I never thought," referring to even these early years, "people were so crazy[6] that they didn't know what they were doing."

Those interested in William Glasser, especially those who have studied his theories of human behavior, want to know where he got his ideas from, or in other words, on whose shoulders did he stand so that he could peer a little farther and see a little more clearly. Was it Freud, Jung, or Adler? Were there teachers in his master's program who influenced him in his early thinking? When asked on whose shoulders he stood to peer a little farther, Glasser replied, "No one." He said this without pride, per se. There just weren't teachers in his master's program whom he looked up to or who provided the shoulders on which he could professionally stand. He had not immersed himself in the thinking of those who came before him. He was aware of them to some extent, but they were not his foundation. He was embarking on his own journey. He would be an original thinker, even if all his ideas were not original. He would develop his ideas from his experience[7] and his ability for analysis.

In the late spring of 1948, less than a year after reentering the graduate degree program in psychology, William Glasser stood on the graduation stage and received his Master's degree in Clinical Psychology. He stood on this stage in spite of having headed in a completely different direction in his undergraduate program, and in spite of being newly married with the responsibilities and distractions that comes with, and in spite of the U.S. Army short-circuiting his academic program. He had been able to focus on the goal, almost like a horse with blinders, an ability that was only beginning to show itself. That ability to focus now turned to his next goal of achieving a doctorate in psychology, and a few weeks after marching across the master's graduation stage he entered the doctoral program at Western Reserve University. He was becoming surer every day of the wisdom of his career change, even though he was starting to feel that a potential problem lurked on the horizon.

The problem had to do with his growing awareness that a degree in psychology had its limits. As a clinical psychologist, Glasser could administer various tests (he remembers the Rorschach and the TAT, for instance), and score the results, but he began to feel that he wanted something different. "In those days," he explained looking back, "psychiatrists were the only ones who could do anything." The ability to focus, which he had turned with laser beam intensity toward getting his doctorate, now faltered just a bit for the first time. Picture a horse with blinders struggling to see something off to the side. Deep down, Glasser knew what he wanted, which for him was the ultimate prize—a medical degree. But at this point, he was having a hard time letting himself admit it. And that was because there was another barrier, a barrier that could quickly douse the pilot light of any such hope —that barrier being his undergraduate grades. Grades earned in college were a significant factor in the medical school application screening process. Poor grades, or even mediocre grades, all but eliminated the applicant. Glasser could see the prize he wanted, but now it looked as if this barrier might be too much. He walked past the very building in which most of the medical classes were taught, and saw medical students going in and out of the building, students who looked very similar to him, but theirs was a reality that seemed just out of his reach.

If there was one thing that kept the hope alive, it was his performance in his post-graduate programs. He had gone from earning mostly Cs to earning all As. He had applied at some other medical schools earlier and had not been accepted, but had delayed applying to Western Reserve because he thought he "might actually have a meager chance of getting in and wanted to have the good grades first." With these good grades firmly listed in his transcript he filled out the application to the Western Reserve University Medical School, with a glimmer of hope and a lot of trepidation, and slipped the envelope into the mail. He would never know if he could become a doctor if he didn't try.

When the letter from the medical school arrived at his home, Glasser picked it up, but delayed opening it. He momentarily pondered the probability of the letter thanking him for his interest in applying to the medical school, and that they were sorry, and that his application was being declined at this time, but then his finger slipped under the sealed envelope flap and tore the envelope open. This letter not only thanked him for his interest, it asked him to contact the dean of the medical school to set up an interview. For a moment, Glasser felt like pinching himself to see if this was just a dream. He looked again at the letterhead and sure enough the letter was from Western Reserve University. His hope for medical school had just received a huge shot in the arm.

The interview with the dean went well, although the dean seemed to focus on some specific areas. He asked Glasser about his chemical engineering background. Glasser replied that he did not want a future in chemical engineering and had found a new field which he was pursuing. The Dean spent a significant amount of time questioning Glasser about this new field and Glasser was able to explain that what he really wanted was to be a psychiatrist. The dean seemed to want to be clear about this, which didn't bother Glasser, but did leave him wondering why this point was so important. It is certain Glasser's desire to be a psychiatrist, along with his determination and focus, were on full display during the interview. And, his performance in his postgraduate classes was exemplary even if his undergraduate performance was not.

Almost all of the students accepted into the Western Reserve medical program were accepted based on many of the more traditional measures, including college grades. Almost all, that is, because Dean Caughcy reserved a few slots for students with special circumstances. Each year he mulled over a handwritten list of names that represented the students being considered for those special slots. William Glasser was now one of the names on that piece of paper. The dean saw Glasser as a young man with a strong desire to be a doctor, the post-graduate grades to back that desire up, and high scores on his medical entrance exam. He had been impressed with Glasser during the interview. Additionally, Glasser had expressed his plan to go into psychiatry.

Twenty-five years later at a medical school reunion, Caughey pulled Glasser aside and shared something with him. Glasser was already in *Who's Who in America* at that time, so Caughey understood the value of his decision to admit Glasser to the program decades before.

"Did you ever figure out how you even got into the medical school?" the dean began with a slight grin on his face.

"Well, no," Glasser answered. "I was surprised, but I figured . . ."

"Well, I was allowed to take four or five students who under no circumstances would ever get into medical school, and you were one of them." Dean Caughey apparently had the gift of getting to the point.

"Well, I appreciate that very much," Glasser returned. By his 25th reunion he had published five books, all of them influential and two of them major sellers. "I hope I haven't disappointed you," he told the dean.

"No, no," Caughey laughed slightly. "I think I made a good decision to allow you in. You might have noticed, though, in your interview that I wanted to make sure you were going into psychiatry. I was a bit worried that if you went into surgery you might kill people. I figured in psychiatry you wouldn't kill anyone."

Glasser entered the doctoral program in psychology upon completing his master's degree, and started writing his dissertation, but then the chance to attend medical school appeared before him. He had completed all of his work in clinical psychology and passed his boards, and had only the doctoral thesis to finish. He turned in what he had completed up to that point, but admitted, "The thesis wasn't that good and they didn't accept it." But after getting into medical school his focus changed entirely. Glasser refers to being accepted into medical school as the most significant moment in his life. Everything was different from that moment on. And even though he was almost finished with his doctoral degree, his heart was in a new place. One journalist, writing in 1974, described how Glasser's doctoral advisors rejected his dissertation, and how they were soured by his decision to go on and become a psychiatrist.[8] It's hard to believe that his advisors would begrudge Glasser for being accepted into medical school, but it could be possible. Maybe some of them felt they had invested a lot of time and support into Glasser's doctoral program.

There was much for Bill and Naomi Glasser to celebrate in 1949. He had gotten into medical school and she was pregnant with their first child. But life is difficult and the young Glasser couple was about to face some difficulties, the first being a mere bump in the road, but the second being a real setback, or using road terminology, more like the bridge being washed out.

The bump in the road occurred when Bill's father, Ben, approached him privately and asked for advice. Ben was at his wit's end and Bill could tell his father was too troubled to handle whatever it was by himself. Bill listened as his father described how Betty had "been pushing him to retire and move the both of them to Florida, where they had spent part of each winter for many years."⁹ She really didn't like the weather that seemed to be a constant in Cleveland and she loved the sun and mild temperatures in Florida. Ben liked the freedom his business afforded him, but with Bill going into medical school it was obvious that his son was not going into the watch parts industry. Ben also realized Bill would soon be able to take care of himself. The thought of living in Florida began to appeal to Ben and he went ahead and sold the business. He was 56 years old, and to be honest, he never really liked working that much. Plans were going well until the day he told Betty the business was sold and he was putting the house up for sale. Instead of celebrating and moving ahead with their plans, she responded angrily. "Why have you done all this? What gave you the idea that I wanted to leave Cleveland and move to Florida? I don't want to leave this house and all my friends."¹⁰ Now that Ben was basically giving in and giving her what she wanted, she was acting like she had never said any such thing. It was more than Ben could take and he wondered what he should do.

To Bill the story sounded typical of his mother, although she had carried it to an extreme, in this case. Bill looked at his father sitting in the chair next to him, a bit slumped, and thought of how his mother had treated him for so many years. His father had worked hard to provide her with the things she wanted and he had given in so many times to keep the peace. Now he had given in once again and was willing to sell the business he had started from scratch, only to have her turn on him in her usual way. Bill looked at his dad and when their eyes met he said, "Pop, you're still young. I think you ought to divorce her." The advice took Ben by surprise. Divorce was not really an option in the Glasser clan, yet he considered it. It was plain that Betty was committed to acting the way she acted and Ben would have to totally give in for the marriage to go on. Soon after this, Betty acted like the incident never happened and she and Ben did move to Florida. She encouraged him to play golf and bridge, two activities Ben liked very much, but otherwise controlled their home as she had always done. To this day, Bill Glasser says that if he had to do it again he would offer his father the same advice.[11] Ben Glasser lived for 30 more years after moving to Florida. Bill's sister, Ruth, and her family also moved there within a few years and Ben actually enjoyed life in Florida much better than anyone expected.

The months leading up to the birth of a baby, especially the first baby in a young family, is filled with expectation and activity. A room must be readied, including a crib, clothes, diapers, little toys, nice things on the walls, and the list goes on and on. Bill and Naomi, along with their duties as medical student and speech pathologist, happily busied themselves with these tasks. Their anticipation grew as the due date neared. And then the date passed. Those who have experienced difficulty during childbirth know some of the feelings Bill and Naomi experienced as it finally became apparent that everything was not as it should be. And those who have lost a child during birth know something of the devastation Bill and Naomi felt when they learned that their first child had died shortly before birth. Everything was ready at home, but now instead of the gurgling coos and heartfelt cries of a newborn infant, the room was eerily and sadly quiet. "We cried together," Glasser remembers, but he admits he processed his grief differently than Naomi did. "She was very, very upset. I mean, we had all the baby clothes and everything all laid out. It was hard on both of us, but I don't grieve very much. I would grieve much more if I felt it were my fault or something like that, but, you know, things happen. I had to put the clothes and everything else away." The matter-of-fact approach to life that had served him up to that point continued to serve him now. It had served him in understanding and coping with his mother's behavior; it had served him in understanding his older brother; it served him when he lost friends in the war; it served him when he wondered about the implications of nuclear might; and it served him when he was called to serve in the army, even though newly married. But this was harder than all of those put together. "It was a needless thing," he explains. "Now it would never happen, being that when the baby is overdue the placenta is going to die. Now they understand it, but they didn't understand it then." Further, he says, "You can't let a placenta get old. They die if they get old. So if it goes past term you take it. The baby was born perfectly normal except the placenta was dead and it died of blood deprivation. It died about six hours before it was born. The doctor came to see me with a long face. Well, I've got bad news. Your baby's dead." They did the best they could with what they knew. Years later, he explained: "I don't have the Catholic attitude that all human life is totally valuable and never under any circumstances should you terminate a pregnancy or something like that."

Naomi didn't work after the baby died, which may have made it harder for her to recover emotionally, but Bill was in medical school and it was requiring his full attention. Not that he resented it at all, because this was the first time in his life that he was enjoying school. He would later become famous for writing *Schools Without Failure*,[12] but his first insights into how such a school could exist, he learned at Western Reserve University Medical School. "The medical school that I attended was a school with no failure. I experienced what it is to go to a school where there were literally almost no tests, no grades at all; we never saw a grade. We were told what part of the class we were in, like middle-third, upper-third, and I was in the middle-third for three years and the upper-third for one. I never could figure out why that was, but I was happy I wasn't at the bottom. I was doing okay." Glasser remembers medical school as "just a wonderful experience," because of "the whole idea of not having grades and not having to worry about it or anything. Not that competence wasn't required. Students had to know and understand the material, and had to be able to show they had the required skills, but their competence was revealed through non-traditional assessments.

There was evidence of the maverick Glasser would become even in medical school. He may not have wanted to emulate his mother's inability to get along with people, but he seemed to possess a significant dose of her ability to have an opinion and stand by it. It wasn't that he couldn't be convinced otherwise. He just wanted the proof. His ability to question the *status quo* now had the added confidence that getting into medical school brought to him. At our first interview Glasser pointed out that while he "didn't take for granted" what his teachers were saying, it "wasn't like I was dissatisfied or making trouble." But later when he recalled his 50-year medical school reunion, he said of his classmates, "[They] saw me much differently than the way I saw myself. They were talking about it and when I showed them the *Warning* book, they said, 'well, you made trouble all through medical school.'"[13] Glasser figures that it was such a nice school he didn't get put down for his questioning or his skepticism. "There were just a lot of things in medicine," he continued, "that I thought weren't correct in those days. For instance, I talked to them about cancer, because it was a very interesting thing to study. I said my take on cancer, which is now somewhat agreed upon, but not completely, is that everybody's got cancer. It's a common thing that one of your cells will go bad, but your immune system picks up that cell and destroys it. It's when people's immune system doesn't seem to work very well that cancer comes out." His medical school training broadened his understanding in many ways, and just as importantly it opened his eyes to how learning can best take place. Case Western was good for Glasser, and in

1953, he once again stood on the graduation platform and received another diploma, this time in fulfillment of the dream to be a medical doctor.

WG

Bill Glasser was born in Cleveland, raised there, married there, schooled there, and stayed there all the way through medical school. His roots were deep there but he had his sights set on the West Coast and was anxious to get started in his medical internship. "By the time I moved to California, Cleveland wasn't that familiar to me. My brother, sister, and parents were no longer living there." Other factors, besides family, may have also contributed to his looking west. Maybe it was because of the trips he took to California with his mother and sister to check up on his older brother. Or maybe it was because of the fact that his best friend, Frank Miller, had finished his degree in engineering and had already settled in southern California. And maybe it was because Frank's wife, Joan, was also a very close friend of Naomi. Whether it was the climate or the friends or the professional opportunities, Bill Glasser saw his future before him in the Los Angeles area.

Bill had been accepted for an internship at the Veterans Administration Center in Los Angeles, and was to begin on July 1, 1953. It was an exciting time for the young family, more so due to the fact that they were no longer just a couple. Two years earlier, midway through the four years of medical school, Bill and Naomi had a baby boy they named Joseph. With medical school successfully behind him and his internship in California ahead of him, Glasser had little time to pause and reflect on his accomplishment. He needed to get their few possessions and the family to southern California within a very short period of time. He remembers all of them beginning the drive across country.

Some will remember what it took to drive across the country in 1953. The words "Route 66" come to mind. Interstates were not built yet and it was mostly two lanes the entire length of the trip. Add that it was late June and you can almost feel the summer heat of the Mississippi River valley and the plains beyond. Part way through the trip, Naomi and little Joe got off and hopped on board a plane to finish the journey. It is easy to picture Bill Glasser—with his wife and son comfortably traveling by plane well above the heat—behind the wheel of his car, the driver's window down and his left arm draped outside, feeling more free ever than before. The feelings of satisfaction from completing medical school in Cleveland, combined with feelings of excitement over starting a new life in California, would have created moments of pure joy. In spite of the fact that he was traveling on Route 66, with its two lanes and sparse gas stations and little towns with no business bypasses like they have today, I think the trip sped by for Bill. In some ways it was the kind of trip you would have wanted to freeze in time, and to be able to return to whenever you wanted a sense of pure freedom. That realization, though, would come later. For now, his wife and son already there, and the heat thickly rising off the pavement that seemed to stretch forever in front of him, Bill tapped on the steering wheel and wondered if there was going to be a turnout for the slow truck in front of him anytime soon.

His medical internship lasted one year and he enjoyed the different rotations, yet his sights were always on what came after the internship. From the time he began the master's degree in psychology in 1946, he had visualized the moment that was almost upon him. When he continued with his doctorate in psychology the visualization became even clearer, and certainly when he entered medical school he knew the visualization was only a matter of time. Everything up to that moment had only prepared him to do what he was about to do.

As described earlier, the year 1954 would be a special year. For instance, it is ironic that in the same year Glasser began his career in psychiatry as a resident, the pharmaceutical company Smith, Kline & French introduced chlorpromazine into the American market, selling it as Thorazine.[14] Glasser would go on to advocate for a psychiatric therapy that empowered people from within and tapped into their ability to make better and better choices, while Thorazine would come to represent the beginning of the field of psychiatry's desire to embrace brain drugs as the therapy of choice. As it turns out, of course, these two therapeutic approaches, one based on the idea that people with mental health problems are best helped through effective questioning and coaching, and the other based on the idea that an outside agent, a brain drug, is the best option, continue to battle against each other into the 21st century.

Thorazine's roots go back to the late 1800s when a class of compounds known as phenothiazines were developed as synthetic dyes, and then to the 1930s when the U.S. Department of Agriculture employed phenothiazine compounds as an insecticide and to kill swine parasites. In the 1940s, phenothiazines were found to greatly limit locomotor activity in mammals, without putting them to sleep. French researchers then began to study whether or not these compounds could be used as a part of anesthesia during surgery, and it was synthesized as chlorpromazine in 1950 by a French pharmaceutical company. "In 1951, French naval surgeon Henri Laborit tested chlorpromazine on surgical patients and found that it worked so well operations could be performed with almost no anesthesia. He also observed that it put patients into an odd 'twilight state.' They would become emotionally detached and disinterested in anything going on around them, yet able to answer questions. One of Laborit's colleagues likened this effect to a 'veritable medicinal lobotomy,' an observation that suggested it might have use in psychiatry."[15] Psychiatry was indeed looking for such solutions. In *A History of Psychiatry* (1997), Edward Shorter would later, referring to this family of drugs, write: "Chlorpromazine initiated a revolution in psychiatry, comparable to the introduction of penicillin in general medicine."[16] It would, he continued, "allow schizophrenia patients to lead relatively normal lives and not be confined to institutions."

Even though eugenics had been shamed as a science by the 1950s, due in part to its association with Nazism, psychiatry did not disassociate itself from its therapeutic practices. For instance, between 1950 and 1951, approximately 10,000 patients were lobotomized. Electroshock was a mainstay of psychiatric therapy with psychiatrists reporting successfully "regressing" patients into states of incontinence and muteness; or disrupting memory in patients to the degree that it "cannot well be described"; or to the degree that they could not conceptualize where they were. In addition, approximately 4,000 patients were sterilized in the 1950s. "This was the therapeutic milieu that was still in place—the value system, as it were—when chlorpromazine made its debut in the state mental hospitals."[17] This was the therapeutic milieu that greeted Glasser when he began his residency.

Glasser began his residency at the Veterans Administration Center as a ward doctor in the Brentwood Veterans Neuropsychiatric Hospital in West Los Angeles,[18] the same hospital in which he had completed his medical internship, and was supervised by the UCLA Department of Psychiatry. His ability to question his teachers, as well as his desire to share his beliefs, began early on to cause some difficulty for him with psychiatrists from UCLA. "It's with them that I hassled a little bit. They didn't bother me much when I was in the mental hospital, but when we started going to what they called grand rounds, where they would present a patient and then present all these pathological things and everything else, and I would stand up and say I don't really believe any of that stuff. They also believed and taught that mentally ill people had something wrong with their brain and I said I didn't believe that's so. If it was so, why are we treating them? We don't do anything for their brain, we just talk to them. I said obviously the brain's okay. It's how they're using it that's not okay."

Glasser remembers getting hassled about how he dressed, too. "I don't get frightened at things. Like when I first got my psychiatric residency the chief of the psychiatric program, and I remember his name but that is not important, and I like him, he was a pretty good guy in many respects. But he was one of those psychiatrists who felt inferior as a psychiatrist because he couldn't really use the medicine he had learned. And so what he did, he told the psychiatry residents they had to wear a white coat, like all the doctors in the hospital wore white coats. And I said the white coat is to prevent infection and things like that. Nobody is coming to me who's infected and I'm not infected. And it looked kind of stupid to wear a white coat, so I didn't wear it. And he was after me for a long time, but I wouldn't wear it. The other doctors said, 'Aren't you scared?' I said, 'I'm not scared. I'm a good psychiatrist.'"

Glasser was actually late to the start of his psychiatric residency. "I remember when I started my psychiatric residency, I finished my internship and I went to Florida to visit my parents and take the kids and everything like that. And, you're supposed to be there, back on the first of July. Well, I didn't want to be back there on the first of July. This was a long, expensive trip, so I just, I just, I guess I wrote them and said I'll be back, but I won't be back on the first of July." When I asked him if he was like a day late or a week late, he continued, "I was four days late, and, and they had given all the residents their assignments, and they had given me an assignment, but I didn't know what the assignment was. And so they said 'Did you get your assignment?' and I said 'No, I wasn't here, I didn't get the assignment.' And I said, 'If you give me the assignment, believe me, I'll do it.' So they gave me the assignment. The guy who was the chief resident was really against me for a long time. I just thought he was silly. Fortunately, everyone else thought he was silly, too. But I'm not one that rocks the boat for the sake of rocking it. I won't get involved with things that I think are ridiculous when I've got an MD degree and everything else, and all my education, and a psychology degree. I'm not a fool. I don't want to go places where they do childish things."

It is probable Glasser did not view himself as a crusader and that he did not fully appreciate the fact he was beginning to stand up to the psychiatric establishment. After describing how his medical school classmates viewed him differently than he viewed himself, he admitted: "I've found out since then that a lot of people are uptight about stuff. I'm just not that way." Instead of worrying about the vulnerability of being a young resident or being intimidated by his supervisors, Glasser was inspired and energized by his residency experiences and his new environment. He sees his career, and the way he has consistently challenged the system of psychiatry, actually beginning when he was that young ward doctor in West Los Angeles. "Cuz boy," he chuckles, "from that psychiatric residency my career just went, well, it was like the Energizer Bunny."

The year 1954 brought other reasons to be excited as well. In July, less than two weeks after starting his psychiatric residency, Bill and Naomi had a baby girl. The couple that started in army housing in Fort Belvore, Virginia, eight years earlier was now across the country in a place called California, and the two of them had now grown to four and included little Joe and an even littler Alice.

WG

Like the Energizer Bunny, Bill Glasser seemed to always be on the go. He enjoyed what he was doing, but it was more than that. Although still in the last year of his residency, Glasser opened an office for private practice in Brentwood, not far from the UCLA campus. Opening an office before completing the residency requirements was not how it was supposed to be done, but it wasn't something that UCLA or anyone else policed closely. A few other students were doing it and Glasser's drive and energy were prompting him to go ahead with the idea, too.

It was customary for young psychiatrists who had received their training through the university to get patient referrals from their UCLA supervisors. Glasser had set up a humble office, hung his shingle outside, and waited for the referrals to come in. He was excited to put his skills to use, but there was also the question of money. He was looking for ways to bring in more income. They had recently built a home and with two children money was tight. He set his new office up well, but no referrals appeared. As it turned out, his refusal to buy into the Freudian party line at the university caught up with him.[19] They would supervise Glasser through his residency, but they certainly wouldn't make patients aware of his availability as a therapist. It was a setback, to be sure, in more ways than one. Financially, things were no better once he set up the office, and if anything they were a little worse due to what he had spent to get it ready. But more than that was the sting of being professionally shunned. It was a potential crossroads. He had made a few waves up to this point, questioned a few teachers, disagreed during some grand rounds, and revealed to classmates that he didn't reverence the status quo. But this was different. He had a wife, a house payment, and a family to support. Were his ideas so important that he should risk not only his professional well-being, but the well-being of his family as well?

Sometimes the most important moments appear to be nothing at all. Bill Glasser was about to have one of those moments. He was ready and willing to work, but his opportunities were being derailed before he could get something going. It was during this time of frustration that he became aware of an opening being advertised by the California Youth Authority. The state was operating a school for troubled teenage girls in a place called Ojai, and they needed a psychiatrist to work with some of the girls, as well as functioning as an on-site consultant. There were not a lot of applicants for the opening, as it was not considered a prestigious position among his fellow residents. Plus, the school was more than 70 miles from Los Angeles, one way. To Glasser it was a position, though, and none of his supervisors seemed to care that he was interested in it. When offered the job Glasser grabbed it. It was a position no one else wanted, yet it would prove to be one of the most important decisions of his life. He would work there for 11 years and gain insights that would influence his thinking throughout his career. The girls at this prison school had literally been rejected by society, only to end up in this faraway town. Glasser had experienced a rejection of his own. He, too, would end up in Ojai. No one could know then, especially his supervisors who decided not to send him any referrals, that his Ventura School experience would lead to his developing some of the key foundations of his ideas.

It was the fall of 1956 when Glasser began at the Ventura School for Girls. To him the job was a good one and within a short time he found it to be an interesting and stimulating environment. He had not foreseen his ever working in a prison, especially with teenage girls, but they needed an on-site psychiatrist and he needed the work. It seemed perfect to him. More than that, he was impressed with the way the staff worked with the girls. He could offer the school his expertise, but he was learning from them as well, especially Mary Perry, and later Bea Dolan, both superintendents of the school. He drove up to Ojai at least two days a week and continued in his residency the rest of the time, with occasional private practice patients.

To make a discovery as important as the Ventura School was for William Glasser a rare thing, a once-in-a-lifetime event for some of us, but the year 1956 was not done with Glasser yet. He was about to make another find, and this one, remarkably, would be as significant as the Ventura School.

Finished with his breakfast, George Harrington slid the chair he had been sitting on back under the table and took his few dishes to the sink to rinse off. He had eaten alone that morning, not because he and his wife weren't getting along, but because he had gotten up earlier than usual. He needed to get to the clinic sooner than normal on this winter morning and he wanted to allow for what snow and packed ice did to the roads. His solitary breakfast, besides getting him on the slippery roads earlier, turned out to be significant for another reason as well. He had been thinking about a job offer for weeks and it was during these quiet moments in his kitchen that his thoughts became crystallized and he knew what he wanted to do. He would accept the offer to work in California. He had enjoyed his training and work at the Menninger Clinic in Topeka, Kansas, but he now understood why he would be heading west. On this particular morning, although not a crucial factor in his decision, it did not escape George's notice that it was 12° in the Kansas state capitol, probably significantly different than the temperature in Los Angeles, California, the city to which he had just decided to move.

After 10 years at the Menninger Clinic, Harrington would arrive at his new position in the Veterans Administration Center in 1956.[20] One of the things that would become clear to him as he pondered his future was the realization he enjoyed the practical levels of psychiatry more than the administration and management levels. Working with patients was more satisfying to Harrington than "pushing papers" in a nice office. Upper level leadership and management was accompanied by more prestige, but it also resulted in less contact with patients, or to put it another way, it resulted in less action on the actual frontlines of psychiatry. Harrington was not only willing to make this trade, he had come to the conclusion that he preferred it. As a result, George Harrington became the clinical ward psychiatrist for Building 206 in the Veterans Administration Neuropsychiatric Hospital in West Los Angeles. Along with his position within the Veterans Administration Center he was also part of the teaching and supervising faculty in the Department of Psychiatry at UCLA. These were responsibilities that suited Harrington very well. The fact that he would be able to fulfill a job description that was so perfect for him while living in southern California and its palm tree friendly climate only added to his satisfaction. As he stood at the sink, though, rinsing his breakfast dishes on that cold Topeka morning he couldn't have had an inkling as to how significant his decision to head west would end up becoming.

As fate would have it, Bill Glasser was assigned to Building 206 and G. L. Harrington was his UCLA supervisor. In effect, Harrington was officially Glasser's residency consultant.[21] Glasser would meet with

Harrington on a regular basis and report on how his efforts on the ward were going. The two of them would then discuss treatment strategies. It would have been easy for Harrington to recognize Glasser was as pleased to be within the environment of Building 206 as he was himself. Glasser later recalled the frustration of being limited as a clinical psychologist compared to the excitement of functioning as a psychiatrist. "When I was a clinical psychologist I was very frustrated because in those days psychiatrists were the only ones who could do anything. Clinical psychologists, they could do tests, like Rorschach's and TAT and things like that. But then, boy, when I got on that ward for the first time, in Ward 206 at the V.A. hospital, then I had 54 people and they were all mine." He laughed as he remembered this time, but quickly emphasized, "It was really exciting!"

It would have been obvious to Harrington the passion Glasser had for psychiatry and the energy with which he pursued fulfilling his assignments. But Harrington also began to see much more than that. As he observed Glasser interact with patients and staff on the ward, and as he met with him each week, Harrington began to sense in his student a kindred spirit. It is interesting that Harrington did not affirm this in more obvious ways than he did. It could be that while Glasser was only beginning to appreciate the power of the psychiatric system, Harrington was fully aware of that power, even to the extent that he guarded his words with those he was supervising. Kindred spirits are hard to keep apart, though, and Harrington and Glasser were drawn together by their similar doubts about traditional therapy.[22] Whatever institutional expectations or pressures Harrington may have sensed, it must have been refreshing to him to see similar beliefs in this young resident assigned to his ward. From Glasser's perspective, though, it seems the situation was less clear. Early on in his experience with Harrington, Glasser was comfortable enough, but he wondered where Harrington stood on some of the most basic issues of mental illness. It may be that Glasser almost feared the answer, not from worry that Harrington would then try to change him, but because Glasser sensed something special in his supervisor and hoped he would be different from others within the UCLA psychiatric community.

It was with this hope, tempered with a fear of the unknown, that Glasser brought a specific case to Harrington's attention. He had a patient who constantly talked about her experiences growing up. Her parents were totally out of the picture when she was young and she ended up being raised by her grandfather. She viewed her grandfather as the source of her problems and would go on and on about him. In Glasser's own words: "I hardly could believe my ears. This woman had been three years at that clinic. It was the fourth year of psychotherapy with four different psychotherapists and she is still talking about her grandfather. I thought I had gotten into some kind of time warp or something. So I said to her, 'You have seen psychiatrists and you have told them about your grandfather?' She replied, 'Oh, yes. My grandfather is a big part of my life.' I wondered aloud, 'Is he still alive?' The woman looked like she was thirty years of age. 'No,' she replied, 'he has been dead for a number of years.' So I said to her, 'Look, I can tell you that if you want to see me, I don't have any interest in your grandfather. There is nothing I can do about what went on with him. He's dead. Rest in peace. But if that's what you want, then you'll have to say you want a new psychiatrist, because I think you have some problems, but you have been avoiding them for a number of years by talking about your grandfather. I want to talk about what's wrong in your life right now. I have no interest in what was wrong yesterday. I deal with what's going on right now.'"[23] That mild confrontation encapsulated one of the foundation points of Glasser's thinking and might represent his first real break with traditional psychiatry. It is one thing to think it, and quite another to actually tell a patient you don't care about the past. Glasser had been considering this approach for the first two years of his residency. Now in his third and last year he had made up his mind to follow his instincts. Still, he felt like he was in uncharted territory. He knew the institutional psychiatrists at UCLA would have choked if they had heard him say what he had said to his patient. But he wondered about Harrington and how he would react. He might be sure about the other UCLA supervisors, but he wasn't sure about Harrington.

What happened next is the stuff of lore and legend. The incident is referred to by no fewer than five other writers,[24] including Glasser himself. He met with Harrington and described what had taken place between him and his patient. He went on to explain his disagreements with conventional therapeutic approaches. It would be interesting to know how much silent time passed after Glasser was done explaining his views before Harrington responded, or to see the subtle expressions on Harrington's face in the moments leading up to his reply. It is revealing that in Glasser's own words he says, "When I hesitatingly expressed my own concern . . ." In that phrase "hesitatingly expressed" you can hear his hope and doubt. What a joy and relief it must have been, when describing that moment a few years later, Glasser could write, "When I hesitatingly expressed my own concern, he [Harrington] reached across the desk, shook my hand, and said, 'Chief, join the club.'"[25]

In that instant, both Glasser and Harrington had put their cards on the table for both to see. For Glasser it might have been the first time someone of psychiatric importance agreed with him. Up until then his teachers had tried to help him see the light, reasoned with him, and Glasser probably felt tolerated at times. And while it is considered a highly significant moment for Glasser, it may have been even more significant for Harrington. At the time, Harrington had much more to lose than the student psychiatrist sitting across from him. He, more than Glasser, knew just how small the club was that he had just mentioned. His professionally coming out in that way, though, was about to contribute to the formation of a synergetic relationship that would have significant effects. In hindsight, we now can see that the moment was really the lighting of a fuse that ultimately fired a direct hit (no more warning shots across the bow) on the psychiatric establishment. But neither Harrington nor Glasser was aware at that moment of any fuse being lit. Such fuses are often invisible.

Bill Glasser completed his residency in 1957. He would begin to work at the orthopedic hospital, too, on top of everything else, but such is the life of an Energizer Bunny. He would continue to work with Harrington, continue to work at the Ventura School for Girls, which would also develop into expanded work for the California Youth Authority, and would continue to counsel in his private practice. Without consciously realizing it he was developing the relationships and the experiences that would empower him to create a unique therapeutic approach that would challenge entrenched psychiatric practices for decades to come. The early years, those years when he was still in training, reveal a sense of who Glasser was to become and the way he was going to get there.

NOTES

1. Pronounced Koy.
2. Stephanopoulos, G. (1999). All too human: A political education. New York: Little, Brown & Company. p.15
3. Berges, M. (1974). William Glasser: Maverick educator and psychiatrist. Los Angeles Times Newspaper.
4. Another bomb was dropped on Nagasaki, Japan, three days later, resulting in 70,000 more deaths.
5. Western Reserve University was located right next door to the Case School of Applied Science. The grounds were adjacent and students from each campus could easily move between the schools. In 1947, the Case School of Applied Science became the Case Institute of Technology. In 1967, the two campuses joined to become Case Western Reserve University.
6. To Glasser and Harrington the term crazy was more humane than describing patients as schizophrenic. That has changed now as mental health agencies view crazy as a demeaning term, Throughout this book I use the term crazy in the spirit in which Glasser intended.
7. Barr, N. (1974). *The responsible world of reality therapy.* Psychology Today.
8. Barr, N. (1974). The responsible world of reality therapy. *Psychology Today, 7(9).*
9. Glasser, W. (1998). *Choice theory: A new psychology of personal freedom.* New York: Harper Collins. p. 90
10. Glasser, W. (1998). *Choice theory: A new psychology of personal freedom.* New York: Harper Collins. p. 90
11. ibid. p. 91
12. Glasser, W. (1969). *Schools without failure.* New York: Harper Collins.
13. Glasser had just finished writing *Warning: Psychiatry Can Be Hazardous to Your Mental Health* (2003).
14. Whitaker, R. (2002). *Mad in America: Bad science, bad medicine, and the enduring mistreatment of the mentally ill.* Cambridge, MA: Perseus Publishing. P.141

15 Ibid, p.142-143
16 Shorter, E. (1997). *A history of psychiatry.* New York: John Wiley and Sons. P.255
17 Ibid, p. 142; Rothschild, D. (1951). *Diseases of the nervous system,* 147-150; Cameron, D. (1960). Production of differential amnesia as a factor in the treatment of schizophrenia. *Comprehensive Psychiatry,* (1), 26-33; Cameron, D. (1962). The depatterning treatment of schizophrenia. *Comprehensive Psychiatry,* (3), 65-76.
18 Glasser, W. (1998). *Choice theory: A new psychology of personal freedom.* New York: Harper Collins. p.147
19 Barr, N. (1974). The responsible world of reality therapy. *Psychology Today,* 7(9).
20 *Current Psychotherapies* (1973), edited by Raymond Corsini, p.286
21 *Current Psychotherapies* (1995), edited by Raymond Corsini, p.298
22 Langguth, J. (1967). California's gift to psychotherapy. *Harper's Magazine,* p.54
23 Wubbolding, R. (2000). *Reality therapy for the 21st century.* Philadelphia, PA: Bruner-Routledge, p.49.
24 Evans, D. (1982). What are you doing?: An interview with William Glasser. *The Personnel and Guidance Journal,* April.; Glasser, W. (1965). *Reality therapy.* New York: Harper Collins, p.xxv; Howatt, W. (2001). The evolution of reality therapy to choice theory. *International Journal of Reality Therapy,* (21)1, 7.; O'Donnell, D. (1987). History of the growth of the Institute for Reality Therapy. *Journal of Reality Therapy,* (7) 1, 2-8; Wubbolding, R. (2000). *Reality therapy for the 21st century.* Philadelphia, PA: Bruner-Routledge, p.43-62.
25 Glasser, W. (1965). *Reality therapy.* New York: Harper Collins.

4
THE UNLIKELY SCHOOL WITHOUT FAILURE

*"The Ventura school was where I really developed
the concepts of reality therapy."
—William Glasser*

It would be difficult to overestimate the impact the Ventura School for Girls had on William Glasser. No book has been written about his experiences at the school, yet those experiences are in every book he has written since. Of the different sources of his ideas, Glasser is clear on this point. "The Ventura School was where I developed the concepts of reality therapy."

Glasser had not been interested in education most of the time he was being educated, yet one of his first jobs was at a school. And not just any school, it was a detention center or prison run by the California Youth Authority for 400 delinquent teenage girls from 14 to 21 years of age. The girls were at the school for reasons ranging from incorrigibility to first-degree murder. They usually had a history of repeated offenses and the school represented their last stop before going into the adult penal system.[1] The program consisted of three main parts—the custody program, the treatment program, and the school program. A girl could leave the school when it was believed she could live satisfactorily in the community.

As fate would have it, the needs of both Glasser and the school coincided. The school needed a psychiatrist because the one they had quit and Glasser needed a job.

Although the position was advertised, no one had responded to the opening.

One of the reasons for Glasser's interest had to do with the growing distance between him and the UCLA School of Psychiatry. This was reflected in his disappointing experience with a supervisor. It was common for residents, toward the end of their residency, to be offered an appointment as a clinical faculty member. Glasser received an appointment and was glad that it was such an open place, a place where new ideas could be considered along with the traditional ones. The appointment was canceled, though, at the last minute. Glasser describes: "The worst thing that ever happened to me was when I got a call from a doctor who I had thought was really supportive of me. He was one of my third-year supervisors. He had asked me if I would like to become a member of the clinical faculty. I said yes. I wanted the position. And then when it was all set he called me at home and said they didn't realize that there'd been a mistake, that two people had been hired for the job and that the other guy had been offered the job first. Well, there was no mistake. The mistake was that I was already marching to a different tune, a tune that didn't go along with traditional psychiatry. I said I understand and let's not talk about it any longer."[2]

Another reason for Glasser's interest in the position was that he saw it as "a real opportunity, working with delinquents and everything." He remembers "jumping at the chance to work at the Ventura School." His motivation was further encouraged by the need to support his wife and children. With his father's help they had built a house[3] in

Los Angeles, but he was on his own now keeping the family afloat. And so, in spite of the fact that the school was a 130-mile round trip, and there was no help with mileage or compensation for driving time, or that he made only $35 a day to start (later raised to a mere $75 a day after he completed his residency), Glasser accepted the invitation.

It was the fall of 1956, probably October or November, when Glasser started working at the Ventura School. As he recalled, he didn't have any idea what he was getting into. The buildings were not in great shape. One author, describing Glasser as a "harried, 41-year-old in grey rimmed glasses, dressed with grab-bag neatness," predicted that when the girls at the Ventura School saw their new psychiatrist, "it won't be love at first sight."[4] As the new guy, though, there were several factors in his favor. His predecessor had been totally ineffective, due in large part to the fact she really didn't like the girls. And the school had an excellent administrator in Mary Perry, the superintendent who hired Glasser. With deep respect and affection Glasser recalled how much she identified with the girls. "She was like a 65-year-old delinquent herself." He said this as the ultimate compliment.

On his very first day, Glasser was a part of a significant incident that revealed the impact the school was going to have on him. He had arrived a little late, but Mrs. Perry encouraged him to go down to one of the cottages and meet the housemother and the girls. Since he had gotten there late, it was the afternoon and the girls were either already in their cottage or were drifting back from classes. One of Miss Perry's assistants took Glasser to one of the cottages and introduced him to Mama G. The housemother titles often started with the word Mama and then the first letter of their last name. The assistant headed back to the office, and shortly thereafter a new girl was brought to the cottage. She had just arrived from Norwalk, California. Glasser remembered it like this:

"She came in and Mama G said hello to her. Mama G sat in the day room with the other girls, except she had a little table, about 24" by 24", which she sat behind so she could write notes on it and things like that. They had certain paperwork they had to do. And, the girl, a big girl, I mean, 5'8", like not an ounce of fat on her, must have weighed about 150 or 160 pounds, I mean she was a tough looking girl, and she was angry.

"I've never seen anyone as angry as her. I'd never seen anyone like any of these girls before. I mean, they were all full of tattoos, which I'd never seen before, self-tattooed with India ink. But anyway, this girl, I don't remember if she had any tattoos on her, but she just started to curse Mama G and threaten her, and I, you know, I knew there was nothing I could do, but I was still nervous. Cuz this woman, I don't think Mama G weighed more than, you know, 80 or 90 pounds, 4'10" maybe, and 75 years old. I mean, she was a frail old lady, and this girl is cursin' her. And as I say, the other girls—cuz by that time I was one of the girls—the other girls were watchin' and I was watchin', too. They seemed interested, but no one seemed nervous or upset, you know, as if this is not such a big deal. And so she must have cursed the woman—Mama G, I mean—she must have let her have it for 30 or 40 seconds, which is an eternity.

"And then Mama G got up from her little table, cuz the girl was kind of leaning on her little table and cursing her right in the face, you know, threatening her, and Mama G got up and walked around the table, around the big girl that was standing there leaning on it, put her arm around the girl's waist, which was pretty tall for her, you know, and gave the girl a hug and in a very sweet voice said, 'Honey, is something bothering you?'

"And, then, the girl, dealt with such kindness and total lack of, you know, being angry or punishment, you know, as we would say now, no external control at all, she just started to cry. She cried and cried, and the tears ran down her face, and Mama G had to take a box of Kleenex and kind of settle her down, and the other girls, including me, wanted to help her, and Mama G dragged her over and said, 'Now here are the girls you're going to be with. It's a nice cottage. These are nice girls. They knew you were coming, and they're looking forward to meeting you, and this is Dr. Glasser, our new psychiatrist.' And, I did talk to her a little bit. She wanted to talk to me, and I talked to all the girls, and then I had to leave."

One of the keys to Glasser's counseling approach is recognizing the need for the therapist to establish a relationship with the client, to become involved in an understanding of the client's life and challenges. On his first day at the Ventura School, Glasser witnessed how powerful it can be when the relationship is focused on first.

Glasser would work at the school from 1956 to 1967. For the first five years he worked one day a week at the school, but that increased to two days a week during the last six years. He would usually arrive at 10 a.m. and stay until 4 p.m. He worked straight through, often eating lunch with the girls. And while one author had predicted that "it wouldn't be love at first sight" between the girls and Glasser, another author emphasized how much "his candor disarmed them."[5] There was something genuine about his approach that engendered trust and that minimized the cat-and-mouse games that clients can sometimes attempt to play with their therapists.

Besides working directly with the girls himself, either individually or by facilitating cottage meetings, Glasser oversaw the work of the other counselors on staff. When he started, the counselors were only seeing four girls a day, a number that really needed to increase. Glasser, as he was doing all the write-ups for the girls' counseling sessions, remembers feeling initially that "the counselors were lazier than shit." But he worked with the counselors, encouraged them, and basically began to teach them the pieces of what would become reality therapy. For instance, he explained to the counselors that talking about home with the girls was fine if the girls had good experiences, but not if they had bad experiences. "Life is hard enough without repeating it." Soon the counselors were able to double the number of girls they saw to eight or nine.

That counseling services would be such an important part of the Ventura School program should not be a surprise. Picture a place with 400 girls, each of them there for dysfunctional and, in most of their cases, very bad behavior. Many of them have only street-smart survival skills that are based less on normal coping mechanisms and more on bullying and violence. In almost every case, for as long as they can remember, they themselves have been mistreated. They have been yelled at, cursed at, hit, ignored, exploited, and pushed out of the way. They have been abused—emotionally, physically, and sexually. They had tried to find their way in a world that rarely looked after them, rarely encouraged or supported them, and where helpful life coaching was unheard of. And when they had stepped out of line or messed up they were punished. Get along in society or we will make you behave was the message they experienced from early on. And if you don't behave we will remove you from our midst. And so these troubled girls came to the Ventura School, angry, detached, sullen, wary, abused, violent, and manipulative. Definitely manipulative. To survive they learned to manipulate—on the street, at home, at school, in juvenile hall, with parole officers, and now at the Ventura School. This was the incredible challenge that faced William Glasser and the other staff members—to create a place where very troubled girls could learn the attitudes and skills necessary to make it in society.

Punishment had been a constant presence in these girls' lives. As a result, the girls often arrived at the school with a huge chip on their shoulder; defensive of their own behavior; and ready to make excuses and blame others. Some staff members at the school had recognized, even before Glasser began to work at the school, that punishment was mostly ineffective with the girls. If anything, punishment actually created new problems rather than solving them. However, after Glasser arrived the no punishment strategy gained momentum. Administrators and staff accepted the idea that people could still be accountable and responsible without being punished, and the girls came to understand this as well. Glasser recalled a story: "The girls came to the Ventura School and were angry because it is a prison. They'd be locked up and so we had a rule. They had their own little room and their own little bed and they had to make their bed. And I think what we did there was unique. Occasionally a girl would say that she's not going to make the bed and she would add a few invectives for emphasis. She would add, 'It's your bed, you can take your bed and shove it.' In most places it would never occur to them not to punish her. And at the Ventura School, if a girl wouldn't make her bed, the house mother would come up and say, 'We really want you to make your bed, you know, but if you won't, then we have girls in this cottage to come here and help you make it. The last thing I want to do is punish you.' The new resident would come in and say, 'If someone wants to make my bed, fine, bring her over.' But the other residents would come in and say, 'Look, it is not pleasant being locked in like this. I came here like you. I was angry and everything else, but I'll tell you this is a pretty good place and they don't believe much in punishment. It is hard to get punished around here. But, I'd like to help you make the bed and when we get it done then let's go and meet some of the other girls. I think you'll find this is a pretty good place.' The girl would say, 'I'm not making the bed. You want the bed made, make it yourself.' And the girl would say, 'It's okay, I'll make it, I'll make it for you and then we'll go down and meet the other people here.' And by the time the girl started making the bed, the other girl would chip in and make it with her. Rarely did we ever have a girl just not make the bed. Yet, there was no punishment. We said, 'We're not going to hurt you. We only want to help; we want to be with you, we want to support you. We realize you are upset, we realize you are away from home, locked up behind two-inch steel doors at night.' And when she would go downstairs, the other girls would welcome her and say, 'Look, it's okay, you are going to have friends here.' And then we would have no more trouble. We would go months without even a discipline problem with these really terribly so-called delinquent girls. When you'd visit the school, you wouldn't think they were delinquent girls. You'd say they were some nice young ladies going to a private school, which it certainly was. So this is how we dealt with the girls."[6]

Staff members at the school, in general, were resistant to Glasser's suggestions for changing discipline and teaching practices, yet as they saw where his ideas were going and saw the results with the girls, they came to see his approach as helpful. When counseling with the girls the focus wasn't on the past, the focus wasn't on the symptoms, instead they talked about what they were doing now, and what they were planning to do the next day, and maybe a little bit of what they were planning to do when they left. The girls were encouraged to keep in touch with their parents, and parents were allowed to visit at any time.

Schools of the day, in general, did not focus on students' dreams or their hopes and desires, and this was especially true of the Ventura School for Girls. It was something Glasser noticed right away and that concerned him. "When I went to the Ventura School," he said, "and got to know the girls there, they didn't have any dreams at all. School was a place they hated. It was a place they failed. It was a place they were asked to do stupid work, in their opinion." The role of failure at school was one of the epiphanies for Glasser that came out of his Ventura School experience. If the girls there were going to learn new attitudes and skills to make it in society, then they would have to have dreams and hopes and plans for the future. And dreams don't come out of failure.[7]

The concept of no punishment at the Ventura School was also applied to the school or classroom program, which meant that grades would not be used to punish poor performance. When students completed the course work and demonstrated competence in a subject they were given credit for that subject. Until then their transcript didn't show anything. Through this approach, the girls would do well in their coursework for the first time in their lives. Glasser would talk to them about this very thing and point out how their prior transcripts were very poor. He would ask, "How come you're doing well in our school and you've done terribly in all the other schools?" To that question the girls consistently replied, "Because we don't fail here." Even though Glasser had not enjoyed school that much, he had not struggled with or experienced failure as the girls at Ventura had experienced it. He remembers, at first, asking them further, "Well, have you really failed in school?" They quickly responded, "Yes, we've failed, we get Fs. We do terrible." At this Glasser would say, "Well, you get Fs because you don't do the work or you don't come to class." The girls would not argue this point and instead would agree, "That's right, we don't do the work and we don't come to class. The reason we don't come to class, though, and don't do the work is cuz we failed and we just know we are going to fail again."

The significance of failing in school began to dawn on Glasser. Further discussions with the girls clarified their sense that the common belief is that failure at home leads to failure at school, and that failure at home leads to kids getting into trouble. They would explain that this is their experience—it was failure in school that got them into trouble far more than failure at home. The girls mostly agreed, "Our homes weren't that good; they weren't that bad either." Glasser recalled: "It struck me that it was the school, because very few parents, when a kid is doing bad at home, start saying you're a failure. I mean it just doesn't work that way. The parent might say to buckle down or sometimes parents will threaten punishment if a chore isn't completed. But in terms of almost cold-bloodedly recording a failure after the kid may have worked a whole semester or a whole year in a course, that's only in school. I don't know any other place in the world that does that." That failing in school was more significant than failure at home, that it might be turned around, that it might be the opposite of what society assumed, represented an epiphany for Glasser. More than failure at home, the girls helped him to see it was failure at school that actually caused them to run afoul of the law and societal expectations. As they lost hope for being successful in school, and when they felt that graduating was no longer even an option, they dropped out of school, which basically put them on the street. Their journey into dysfunction was now well underway.

The Ventura School changed the school set-up completely. Failure was not an option. When the work was finished you received credit. The girls responded to this arrangement and attacked schoolwork that had previously intimidated them. Where before they did not think it was possible, and had no interest in making it happen, girls were now completing the requirements for their high school diploma. (Their diploma and transcript actually read Lamaree High School, so that people wouldn't know the girls graduated from a reform school.) That so many girls were successfully completing high school is impressive, not just because it was a prison school with all of its attendant implications, but also because three to five girls were leaving every week and three to five new girls were arriving. If any school had an excuse for students to fail, the Ventura School would have topped the list, yet instead their students were making it.

The school moved from Ojai to a newly built facility in Camarillo (a distance of about 30 miles) in 1962. Each girl had her own room in the new school and a fence surrounded the entire facility, something the old school didn't have. Glasser pointed out that the fence actually increased the freedom within the school. The school was more vulnerable before and much effort was put into cottages being constantly locked up. Their whereabouts was an issue, as some girls would just walk off. Ojai was isolated and rather remote at the time, so the girls were soon located, but it was a problem. The fence eliminated that and created a sense of safety. With the new school also came a new administrator. Beatrice Dolan arrived at Ojai just prior to the move and worked to continue the momentum Glasser and Mary Perry had started. Bea Dolan was an experienced superintendent (she had just transferred from a similar position and school at Los Guilicos) and she arrived with a desire and a plan to start a new kind of program that treated people as if they were responsible for what they did with no excuses. As it turned out, Mrs. Dolan was up to the task, so much so that the new school's program became the basis for what would later become choice theory. Glasser quickly recognized that her beliefs about people were very similar to his and their working partnership strengthened the school even more. "Mrs. Dolan and I," he described later, "it was love at first sight. I loved that woman from the first moment I saw her. She was the best administrator I ever worked with, although Kaye Mentley approaches her. Rather than depending on rules, she would handle things individually. We truly became a school without failure where punishment was not a part of the program."

Change, like the kind of change with which Glasser was involved, does not come without a price. It is true there were many successes at the Ventura School for Girls, yet a state facility as large as the Ventura School was a complex organization with administrative levels within and over the school. It could be that Glasser displayed the same disregard for the status quo at Ventura that he had with his UCLA supervisors during his residency. Or it could be that the head psychiatrist within the Youth Authority just didn't like him. In any case, he remembers that he "ran into trouble at the California facility. And this is an interesting part of my life, too. When they found out that I was really into helping these girls, that things were starting to change, they tried to get rid of me, which hasn't been an uncommon experience, because I was making trouble. You don't want to rock the boat. We were rocking the hell out of that boat. And so they didn't pay me for two and a half years. By that time, they had raised my salary and when I finished my residency I became a full-fledged psychiatrist. They raised my salary from $35 a day to $75 a day. I still had to drive the 60 miles back and forth. No travel pay, no travel time. But at least I didn't have to punch a clock. I just worked without pay and kept sending my bills. I was a contract consultant and Mrs. Dolan would say, 'You keep working, they'll pay eventually.' And they did. I got a check for several thousand dollars. I never got more than $75 a day, but I thought to myself that I am earning thousands of dollars a day because I am getting vast experience." In his defense, Glasser clarified: "It sounds like I was fighting with people all of the time, but I wasn't." Glasser's experience is a reminder to the rest of us that change, even positive change, comes at a price.

From his earliest days as a professional, Glasser has been a teacher. Shortly after arriving at the Ventura School, Glasser began teaching the on-campus counselors and house mothers about basic principles of psychiatry and effective techniques in counseling. It helped that he had a way of expressing complex ideas in simple terms. Miss Perry, the first superintendent with whom Glasser worked, noticed this ability and recommended him to others within the California Youth Authority. She did this with some reservation, as she did not want him snapped up by someone else. In any case, in 1958, Glasser began giving presentations in Sacramento at statewide Youth Authority functions, as well as to staff at other schools around the state. Additionally, the San Diego Probation Department wrote about Glasser in an international newsletter. The young doctor was starting to get a good reputation. The speaking appointments and traveling should not be underestimated. Glasser, you will recall, had been extremely shy as a young man and, as one author put it, literally forced himself into the role of lecturing in the same way that a puny youngster sets out to become an athlete.[8] There was a confidence about him, though, and an understanding of his subject matter that helped to overcome the shyness.

He spoke extensively around the state, and it was while giving these talks that he started to write, by hand, what would become his first book, *Mental Health or Mental Illness?*[9] The book was actually based on the talks he was giving. Many people are not aware of *Mental Health or Mental Illness?* and think *Reality Therapy* was Glasser's first book, even though, as Glasser points out that *Mental Health or Mental Illness?* was the only one of his books to receive a good review in *The New York Times*. John Dollard, a professor of psychology at Yale, reviewed the book and wrote: "If the reader be one of those who has humbly given up the attempt to understand psychology because he has been told that since the human being has unconscious motives the conscious mind cannot comprehend him—if the reader be such, I repeat, let him hope again and try this new work by one of the bright young spirits of psychiatry now practicing on the West Coast."[10] Glasser stated this as his goal in the Author's Introduction: "This book was written so that any interested person could easily gain a basic understanding of psychology."[11] This statement, at the very beginning of his first book, would become the emphasis for all of the books and articles and lectures that followed.

Mental Health or Mental Illness? (1960) was written at the start of Glasser's professional career, shortly after beginning the job at the Ventura School. As such, the book represents his philosophy of psychology and psychiatry at the outset. Those interested in knowing where Glasser's ideas came from and how they have changed or developed over the years would do well to review this book. Glasser himself once told me that the precursors to choice theory occurred in the book *Reality Therapy* (1965), but even he would be wrong to ignore similar precursors in the book published five years prior.

Key points emerge in *Mental Health or Mental Illness?* for instance. Glasser describes how every person is born with a definite set of basic needs and that these needs do not change with age or because of a change of circumstances. He identified both physiological and psychological needs. In fact, of the eventual five basic needs that Glasser would propose, three of them—survival, love and belonging, and achievement (power)—are listed in the first chapter of his first book. He described how we, not the world, must do the changing. Blaming circumstances or blaming our heredity or our environment doesn't help. He suggested the question of heredity versus environment could never be answered and we should not concern ourselves with heredity, since nothing can be done about it. The needs must be satisfied regardless of their source.

Glasser was driven by the need to improve psychiatry's role in society, so it was probably frustrating to admit: "What psychiatry knows and does about poor ego functioning is a mystery to most people, with the result that society either blindly trusts or mistrusts the field."[12] He stated his own philosophy of psychotherapy, though, when he wrote: "It is wrong to construe the task of psychiatry to be the molding of any patient into a hypothetical 'normal' person. The goal of the psychiatrist is only to help the patient establish more effective ego functioning in those areas where his ego function is defective."[13]

Mental Health or Mental Illness? (1960) explained terms like ego, ego reactions, unconscious ego functions, neurotic ego functioning, and ego weaknesses, which are revealed through neuroses. Ego thickness, though, is described as a component of psychosis. These terms are examples of the common psychiatric terms then in place. When asked what ego functioning was all about and how it related to his thinking now, Glasser answered, "Well, the ego, if you talk about the id, the ego, and the super ego, in the psychoanalytic thing, the ego is the source of your present behavior, the way I understood it, and so I was talking about how we shouldn't get involved in the id or the super ego. We can't do anything with that, but we should deal with the person's present behavior and what he's doing now. I developed little diagrams and everything, but it was a step along the way. I couldn't separate myself from some of these terms. I guess that was it. But at the time it was a pretty exciting thing."

The girls' school greatly influenced Glasser regarding discipline and punishment and that influence begins to show up in *Mental Health and Mental Illness?* We see glimpses of what he would later emphasize, but not consistently. At one point he states, "Punishment is futile because it is effective only if it can reinforce built-in anxiety or remorse,"[14] while a few pages later he writes, "Corporal punishment will work only if the person who is punished has some positive feeling toward the person doing the punishing."[15] The girls' school also revealed the girls would sometimes choose pain over their bleak circumstances. "The concept that something, even pain, is better than nothing," he wrote, "is very important in understanding how empty people, typified by juvenile delinquents, struggle to avoid this empty feeling."[16] Such insight began to form the foundation for his belief that people ultimately choose to be miserable.

Glasser wrote things in 1958 and 1959 that he categorically rejects now (we'll get to those things in a moment), yet there were a number of areas in which what he said then represents exactly what he continues to emphasize now, in which he was ahead of his time. "In this book," he began, "the term schizophrenia will be used sparingly because I do not feel that it is a useful term."[17] He noticed that almost all patients in mental hospitals were labeled as some sort of schizophrenic and he viewed such labeling as meaningless. Such labeling also implied the condition would be hard to treat. The early strands of his later beliefs, such as psychotic behavior that walls off the world and creates a reality that actually meets the person's needs, begin to stand out. He described that "a completely psychotic person is not able to fill any of his needs in the world because of the wall thrown up by his ego. This does not mean, however, that his needs go unfulfilled—it means that they go unfulfilled in the world. Actually they are partially or completely fulfilled within the thick-walled confines of his own ego. We call this method of satisfying needs 'crazy' because, according to reality, or our conception of reality, his needs are not satisfied."[18] People involved in this process of behavior he referred to as literally shrinking into their own ego. Psychosis, he explained, could be organic or functional in nature. By organic he meant the psychosis had a known, observable cause—a pathology, as he would say later. By functional he meant the psychosis had no known origin and thus had to do with psychological factors. Already in *Mental Health or Mental Illness?*, Glasser was beginning to explain how the phenomena of a person hearing voices, seeing hallucinations, or having delusions was based on "his own hostile feelings being reflected within his ego, which is unable to modify them."[19] His views regarding depression were not totally formed, but even at this early time he was linking depression to psychosomatic diseases such as peptic ulcers, asthma, eczema, and migraine headaches.

Toward the end of the book, Glasser commented on brain drugs and their use as therapy. He noted how huge amounts of money were being spent to promote them to physicians: "The reason behind the huge push by the drug companies toward marketing these drugs is far from altruistic."[20] While he was becoming aware of the marketing blitz by the drug companies, his position then was tolerant when it came to considering what drugs might do. Describing his view he wrote: "Although these drugs do have a place, many reliable studies have shown that other factors besides the drugs have been responsible for progress which at first was attributed to them. These drugs can render people more comfortable, they can make a bad reality more tolerable, and they can often quiet an agitated or violent patient so that he can better utilize psychotherapy. Not miraculous in the sense penicillin was and is, nevertheless if used with good judgment they can help certain patients."[21]

Glasser later came to reject brain drugs as a necessary or helpful option, but when he started out as the consulting psychiatrist at the school for delinquent girls, he spoke of their potential. He must not have been too enamored with their potential, nonetheless, since he never applied for a license to prescribe narcotic drugs and he wouldn't allow them to be prescribed to the girls while he was at Ventura. He believed the girls were unhappy, not mentally ill. "Anyone at the school who tried to tell me they were mentally ill," Glasser recalled with a certain firmness in his voice, "I wouldn't accept it." While drugs might anesthetize the ego from uncomfortable feelings, he wrote that there were "no psychiatric drugs which will render a defective ego effective."[22]

While the strands, and even the foundation, for the elements of reality therapy and choice theory can be found in his first book, Glasser expressed other beliefs when he was writing *Mental Health or Mental Illness?* (1960) that he would come to reject. For instance, he viewed homosexuality as a neurosis, and in men he felt it represented one of society's most serious problems.[23] The alcoholic, he believed, suffered from a character neurosis. He saw that people experienced depression in varying degrees, but he wrote: "If it continues for a long period of time, it is then a mental illness also called depression."[24] He further pointed out depression was "one of the few psychiatric conditions for which there is a definite therapy,[25] and wrote about the safety and effectiveness of electric shock therapy as one that "appeared to be the most successful."[26]

Glasser admitted administering shock therapy during his residency, but added "he was kind of mixed up on what was causing these things"—these things being depression. Later, he would come to be very clear on the causes of depression and the way to treat it, but at the start of his career he wasn't prepared to identify unhappiness as its root. Even then he recognized that any apparent positive effects from shock therapy were temporary. Patients seemed to forget their problems as their memories were literally knocked out. The memories seemed to return, though. Enmeshed within the psychiatric milieu of his day, Glasser was finding his way. A day or two a week he spent at the girls' school; another day he spent at an orthopedic hospital; the rest of the week he devoted to his private practice. These diverse venues provided a multitude of experiences from which to build and hone his beliefs.

The Unlikely School Without Failure

WG

He had written the manuscript for *Mental Health or Mental Illness?* by hand, as laptops and word processing had not even been imagined yet. As a first-time author, Glasser probably wondered if what he had written was good or not. Robert Glasser, Bill's cousin, related, "He showed me the manuscript of *Mental Health and Mental Illness?* and asked me to read it. He wanted my opinion. I read it and thought it made a lot of sense, although his style of writing wasn't that great. I told him that. He had a neighbor that was a professor of English at UCLA and I told him he should get one of his grad students to edit the manuscript. And he said, 'Would you do it?' I don't know if I thought a lot about it or not, but I said yes. What made him think I could do a good job on it, I don't know." Robert Glasser would go on to also edit his cousin's next three books, including *Reality Therapy* (1965), *Schools Without Failure* (1969), and *The Identity Society* (1972). It may have been Glasser wanted to work closely with someone whom he already knew. He and Robert were cousins together in Cleveland when they were kids. It may also have been Glasser wanted the opinion of a non-psychiatric reader so that he could find out if his views on psychiatry could be understood by the layperson. Robert Glasser, besides turning out to be a very good editor, also met both of these criteria.

With the critical success of *Mental Health or Mental Illness?* and the success from his presentations within the California Youth Authority, Glasser was garnering attention from around the United States. His message challenged traditional psychiatric practices, but it resonated deeply with many of those in the helping professions who worked with those in society most in need of help. Soon after *Mental*

Health of Mental Illness? came out Glasser increased his time at the Ventura School to two days a week. And he began on the manuscript for another book. Written by hand, mostly on airplanes while traveling to speaking appointments, he had no way of knowing how much this next book would change his life.

As mentioned, Glasser worked at the Ventura School for 11 years. The school was "running beautifully," he remembered, and the speaking invitations from around the country seemed to be increasing exponentially. It seemed to him Ventura could carry on without him. When asked if during the 11 years at the school he ever dreaded going to work there, he quickly replied, "Never. I never dreaded going to work at the Ventura School."

Shortly after beginning at the Ventura School, while he was still in his residency, Glasser remembers being so low on money that one time he had to empty his children's piggy bank to put gas in the car. One hundred and forty pennies, to be exact. He chuckled as he explained when gas was 15 cents a gallon you could get almost ten gallons of gas for 140 pennies. By the time he left the school, his fortune had begun to change. When he drove away from the school in 1967, he departed from an important chapter in his life. He didn't know it at that moment, but it would be his last time at the school.

NOTES

1. Glasser, W. (1965). *Reality therapy: A new approach to psychiatry.* New York: Harper Row.
2. Glasser interview, September 26, 2004; Wubbolding interview *in Reality Therapy for the 21st Century,* p 57.
3. When asked how he decided to buy the lot on which to build their home, Glasser said, "I looked for the cheapest lot I could buy. This one was $5,500. The cost of the lot, building the house, and the furniture was $19,600." The house is located in the hills above Santa Monica and overlooks the Pacific Ocean. Glasser has lived in the same house for close to 60 years.
4. Langguth, J. (1967). California's gift to psychotherapy. *Harper's Magazine,* 234, 52-56.
5. Barr, N. (1974). The responsible world of reality therapy. *Psychology Today,* 7(9), 64-68.
6. Wubbolding, R. (2000). *Reality therapy for the 21st century.* Philadelphia, PA: Brunner-Routledge.
7. I'm not talking about setbacks here. I'm not talking about the inventor who tried something that didn't work, but kept on trying; nor am I talking about the business venture that went bust, but the owner kept trying until he met with success. Instead, I am talking about society, in one way or another, placing an F on your forehead, or a school placing an F on your transcript.
8. Berges, M. (1974, March 3). A maverick educator/psychiatrist takes a realistic approach to untangling mixed-up kids. *Los Angeles Times Home Magazine,* 40-43.
9. Glasser, W. (1960). *Mental health or mental illness: Psychiatry for practical action.* New York: Harper Collins.
10. Dollard, J. (1961, January 22). *New York Times Book Review.*
11. Glasser, W. (1960). *Mental health or mental illness?* New York: Harper Collins. pg. ix
12. Glasser, W. (1960). *Mental health or mental illness?* New York: Harper Collins. pg. 10.
13. ibid. pg. 12.

14 Glasser, W. (1960). *Mental health or mental illness?* New York: Harper Collins. pg. 24.
15 Ibid, pg. 29.
16 Ibid, pg. 25.
17 Ibid, pg. 121.
18 Glasser, W. (1960). *Mental health or mental illness?* New York: Harper Collins. pg. 114
19 Ibid, pg. 126
20 Ibid, pg. 154
21 Glasser, W. (1960). *Mental health or mental illness?* New York: Harper Collins. pg. 154
22 Ibid, pg. 158
23 Ibid, pg. 103.
24 Ibid, pg. 30.
25 Ibid, pg. 134.
26 Glasser, W. (1960). *Mental health or mental illness?* New York: Harper Collins. pg. 153.

5
OUT OF NOWHERE

"All of my writing basically started with *Reality Therapy.*"
—*William Glasser*

In spite of it being vacation it had still been a busy day, a busy week, and for that matter a very busy few months. In one way it had been a terrible month. The conference in Sacramento at the end of October was very good, but the usual busyness and fun of the holidays was shattered by the death of John F. Kennedy, shot in broad daylight during a very public motorcade through Dallas, his wife sitting at his side as the awful event unfolded. A decorated war hero, he represented a can-do energy for the present and hope for the future. Yet, in a moment, all of that hope seemed to disappear. In its place a national numbness, tinged with deep anger, settled in. The Christmas season had helped to distract, but who could know what the new year would bring?

It was the Monday following Christmas and Donald O'Donnell had gone to his office at the Pershing School, an elementary school in Orangevale, California, to get a few things done. He wasn't planning on staying long, but he did want to get a letter written and mailed. The conference he had attended at the end of October turned out to be very significant to him and he wanted to follow up with the presenter. He was alone at the school that morning, the quiet undisturbed even by secretaries and custodians, the usually bustling hallways and breezeways now empty, as he put a piece of paper into his manual typewriter and thought about how to begin. The letter was short and to the point, yet it turned out to be significant in several ways. The exact letter went like this.

>
> Pershing School
> 9010 Pershing Avenue
> Orangevale, California
>
> December 30th, 1963
>
> Dr. William Glasser
> Consulting Psychiatrist
> Ventura School for Girls
> Camarillo, California
>
> Dear Doctor Glasser,
>
> I had the pleasure of attending the workshop presented on October 30th in Sacramento. Since that date my teachers and I have read with interest your speech presented to the Governor's Conference on Youth, Chicago, Illinois, May 9, 1963.
>
> We are trying to understand and apply some of the concepts you have developed in Reality Therapy. I am interested in two items for the further development of Reality Therapy concepts in our school.
>
> 1) When may we expect your book, Reality Therapy, to be published?
>
> 2) Do you have a syllabus available to purchase that you use with your college class at San Fernando State College?
>
> Is it possible for anyone outside the Los Angeles area to enroll in your extension class for the Spring Semester?
>
> My teachers and I are most interested in the concepts you and Dr. Harrington are developing. We are interested in securing more materials in this subject area for our own personal background.
>
> Sincerely,
> Donald J. O'Donnell
> Principal

Every rainfall starts with one drop and this letter was one of the early raindrops preceding the deluge that would soon engulf Glasser. While his own field of psychiatry was less than supportive of his ideas, the other helping professions, and especially the field of education, began to pursue Glasser's ideas with surprising commitment. Glasser remembers, "The psychiatrists dealt with me by ignoring me, rather than trying to discredit me. Hardly anybody tried to actively discredit me. But ignoring me and my work was rather common. And then, interestingly enough, I became more and more known in the schools." Another way in which the letter was significant had to do with Donald O'Donnell himself. He would go on to become a close friend and advisor to Glasser, and in the process would become a vital connection between Glasser and the K-12 educational system. As he signed his name to the bottom of the letter O'Donnell could not have imagined that he would be prominent in one of William Glasser's highest selling books. And lastly, the letter was significant in that it heralded Glasser's next book, which focused on an approach called reality therapy. Almost unknown when O'Donnell wrote his letter of inquiry, reality therapy was about to create a wave of its own.

When George Harrington reached across his desk in early 1957 and invited Glasser to "join the club" of non-conventional therapists, he could not have known that within a few years Glasser would write the club manifesto. Glasser began working with Harrington in the fall of 1956, around the same time that he began at the Ventura School for Girls. The starting dates at these new positions were so close that Glasser couldn't recall which came first. He figures that one began in October and the other began in November. He had a year left on his residency when he began with Harrington. After finishing the residency, he continued working at the Ventura School, but switched from the Veterans Administration Hospital to the orthopedic hospital. In spite of his leaving the Veterans Administration Hospital, Glasser continued seeing Harrington on a weekly basis.

Bill and Naomi's third child, Martin, was born in 1958, the same year that Bill began lecturing in schools within the California Youth Authority, and just prior to *Mental Health or Mental Illness?* being published. On top of this, Glasser became a board-certified psychiatrist in 1961. While the lecturing and the writing and the accomplishments were all good, the fast pace of Glasser's life was starting to be felt at home. Glasser's cousin, and the manuscript editor for his first four books, remembers that Naomi eventually put her foot down. "When he was writing those early books, and he had three small children, Naomi said no work at home. When you're at home you're a family man. And he was an excellent family man. So he had to write these books in his spare time. He was doing a fair amount of traveling then, and while everybody else was on the airplane reading magazines or having drinks, he was just working like mad the whole time. A lot of those books, both the writing and the editing, were done on airplanes. To me it was impressive at the time, and still is." Glasser helped around the house and with the kids. He says of this time, "When the kids were little babies, you know, Naomi didn't like to get up in the middle of the night and I always got up because she liked to get up early in the morning and I like to sleep a little bit in the morning."

He was writing books while traveling in planes and often caring for his kids in the middle of the night, even as he was figuratively holding an increasing number of pans over an expanding fire. Along with his responsibilities at home, maintaining a private practice, serving as psychiatrist at the Ventura School for Girls, working at the orthopedic hospital, lecturing throughout the state, Glasser was also beginning to work with Donald O'Donnell and others within the public school system in the Sacramento area.

WG

Still nervous as a speaker, yet getting more polished with each presentation, Glasser began to realize that his approach would benefit from having a name or title. About this time a fellow psychiatrist in Los Angeles remarked to Glasser, "I was going to send you a patient for your private practice, but I thought you were too reality-oriented for her." And although Glasser thought this was a strange reason not to refer the patient, the word *reality* stuck in his mind as he prepared for an upcoming talk in Seattle.[1] The Seattle talk took place in September of 1962 and was given to the American Correctional Association. The newsletter distributed by the San Diego Probation Department, along with his work within the California correctional system, had created quite an interest in his ideas and there was a big audience in Seattle when Glasser introduced his approach as Reality Psychiatry. The talk went well, but on the way back home Glasser kept thinking about Harrington and his saying "if all the psychiatrists in the world disappeared, no one would notice they were gone." It was true, he thought, that so few people in the world were directly involved with psychiatry, while huge numbers of people are involved in counseling, social work, corrections, and education. A month later, in October of 1962, Glasser had been invited to speak in Vancouver to the British Columbia Correctional Association. Keeping in mind the need for a name change, it was in Vancouver that he first referred to his approach as Reality Therapy. "Reality Therapy," he explained, "is teaching people to deal more effectively with the reality they live in." Reminiscing later, he remarked, "It was a very fortuitous title. Still is a good title."

Glasser has often been asked where his ideas came from. As people experience its effectiveness, they want to know more about reality therapy's roots and history. When asked about the people who influenced him, rather than citing great names in psychotherapy, he credits his father, Ben Glasser; his supervisor and teacher, G. L. Harrington; Mary Perry and Bea Dolan from the Ventura School; and even Donald O'Donnell for helping him form and shape what was to become reality therapy. These people were the most significant mentors in his life. Glasser had heard vaguely of some of the big names—for instance, Alfred Adler and Adolf Meyer—but he had not read any of their works and consequently was not directly influenced by them. There was a similarity, though, between Glasser's ideas and the approaches of other therapists. That William Glasser and others were on similar tracks, even though they had not spent time together or read each other's work, represented a kind of cultural parallelism.[2] More than one person can be in the process of discovering a good idea. Good ideas have a way of attracting creative thinkers.

Reality therapy was based on eight essential pieces, none of them particularly startling, and most of them not even new. Others before Glasser had written or modeled compassionate therapeutic elements. In the early 1900s, Paul DuBois, a Swiss physician, developed an approach called Medical Moralizing. One writer described, "DuBois held conversations with his patients and taught them a philosophy of life whereby they substituted in their minds thoughts of health for their customary preoccupations with disease. He insisted that the physician treat the patient as a friend, not merely as an interesting case. Also, the physician must be sincere in his conviction that the patient would get well."[3] While a date for the invention of psychotherapeutic common sense cannot be identified, an argument can be made that Paul DuBois was an early version of what William Glasser was to become. Others picked up on the strength of DuBois' ideas—Jules Dejerine and Joseph Pratt, most notably—and embraced the concept of the therapist as a friendly counselor. Alfred Adler, Adolf Meyer, and Abraham Low all built on the DuBois tradition. Psychiatry needed to be more rational and less mystic. People needed to be helped toward trusting their own judgment, rather than being led to believe that only another person, a psychiatrist or counselor, could unravel the mystery of their lives.

The approach DuBois believed in and modeled did not become a torch that, over the years, was passed directly from one therapist to another. Instead, there was a method of counseling people that made sense and seemed to work better, and many different therapists tapped into the elements of this method. The history of the treatment strategies for those struggling with mental and emotional dysfunction clearly bears out the fact that some approaches work, while others do not. Robert Whitaker, in his important book, *Mad in America*[4], describes this evolution and how different approaches vied for supremacy. Early efforts to deal with the mentally ill were barbaric enough that they are difficult even to read about. In the early 1800s, though, a humane, compassionate approach developed that came to be known as Moral Treatment. The results indicated Moral Treatment was quite effective, however medical physicians were threatened by the treatment's non-medical success and worked politically to "gain control of the asylums."[5] As Whitaker concluded, "A reform that had begun a century earlier as a backlash against the harsh medical therapeutics of the day had clearly come to an end. A scientific approach to treating the mentally ill was now ready to return to the center of American medicine, and that would lead, in fairly quick fashion, to a truly dark period in American history."[6] *Mad in America* refers to the period between 1900 and 1950 as The Darkest Era. The point in sharing this historic perspective is that therapists have always had choices about how people are best helped to overcome their mental and emotional difficulties, and that personal treatment philosophies are drawn to certain treatment approaches. Some are drawn to what they believe is scientifically and medically valid; while others are drawn to what they believe is humanly effective and morally defensible. One person who was drawn to the latter of the two approaches was Helmuth Kaiser.

Helmuth Kaiser came to the United States from Israel in 1949. Kaiser began his career as a psychologist and psychotherapist in Germany in 1930. He moved to Spain and then to France and then to Israel. By the time he left Israel and moved to Kansas, though, to become the training analyst for the Menninger Clinic, Kaiser's views on traditional psychotherapy had changed dramatically. It was at the Menninger Clinic that Kaiser became G. L. Harrington's supervisor. Kaiser's "ideas were radical by the standards of that day, and his departure from the rigid rules of classical analysis was shown in his supervision of Dr. Harrington."[7] As a result, by the time Harrington left the Menninger Clinic and headed to southern California to work at the veterans' psychiatric hospital he had been drawn to elements of the non-traditional approach. In this case we might even say that a torch had been handed from one therapist to another.

When he arrived at Building 206 in 1962, Harrington inherited a stable mental hospital ward where each day an unspoken contract was fulfilled. The staff would do all they could to provide the patients with what they needed or wanted, and the patients would stay peacefully psychotic. Harrington decided to break this contract.[8] Where before patients were expected to remain at the hospital, much as vegetables being stored on a shelf in a kitchen, Building 206, under Harrington, instituted a program from which patients would actually be released from the hospital to reenter the real world. As part of the new approach, each staff member in the ward needed to be trained in the principles that would ultimately become the basis for reality therapy. Harrington conducted this training with the entire staff and emphasized that staff members needed to forget concepts like schizophrenia and mental illness; that patients with crazy behavior should be viewed as doing the best they could; and staff should not respond to abnormal behavior and thinking. All patients should be treated as if they were capable of not being crazy. Glasser came to see that "if we ask a person about his hallucinations, then we're just as crazy as he is." He also remembers thinking "these people are not mentally ill, but they're terribly lonely, they're terribly frustrated, and they haven't succeeded. They're expressing their unhappiness and they're expressing their frustrations differently, but basically all of them are literally disconnected and in need of a good relationship." Somehow, these patients needed to be nudged and invited and pulled toward success. Glasser was convinced that a positive relationship in their lives must be a part of this nudging and inviting.

One of the psych technicians on the ward, Mr. Bland, seemed to have a special skill at connecting with patients and Glasser described how important he was and how much he learned from him. "I became very close to Mr. Bland, because I realized that he knew an awful lot about people who were diagnosed with schizophrenia, as almost all my people were. I don't particularly believe in that diagnosis, but at the time I did believe in it, at least to some extent. I recognized he had skills, though, so when a patient would come in with that diagnosis on a Friday afternoon, and I knew he was going to be working over the weekend, I would say to him, 'You have these skills and I would like that patient, if you could work with him over the weekend, to be relatively sane by Monday, perhaps not to be hallucinating or delusional, to be more comfortable on the ward, and to be willing to talk with me during the coming week. Tell him Dr. Glasser will be back and that I would like to talk with him.' And by the time I talked with the patient the following week, in terms of their hallucinations and delusions, most of them were relatively sane and seemed to be more under control. Because I was doing it, Mr. Bland was doing it, and the nurses were helping with it. Everyone was cooperating a lot to reach out to patients who were lonely and make a relationship. I learned a lot from Mr. Bland, which I used for the rest of my life. I especially learned when dealing with people who have symptoms, all of them are basically lonely and in need of companionship. These people are not unreachable."

For Glasser, several factors were now coming together, like ingredients marinating in the same pot, to begin to form a picture of a distinct therapeutic approach. Among these factors were his previous beliefs. From his earliest behavioral science classes at Case Western, Glasser had questioned conventional psychiatric views. His views were enough a part of him that Harrington, after being around Glasser for a while, could reach across his desk and invite Glasser to join the non-traditional psychiatric club. Certain things were clear in Glasser's mind before the specifics of reality therapy began to develop. "I realized before I even wrote the book," he points out, "that a good relationship is at the core of all psychiatric or psychoanalytical help."[9] And it is important to remember Aaron.

Early in Glasser's residency he was treating a boy named Aaron, who turned out to be a very significant patient. Putting it in perspective, Glasser wrote: "Dissatisfied with traditional therapy as early as my last year of training, I was groping for a better way to treat people than what was being taught. It was during this period that a small, unhappy boy was assigned to me for treatment. It was to be many years before I was able to understand why this boy changed so drastically, but if there was a time when reality therapy began for me, it was with Aaron."[10] In simple terms, Glasser described Aaron as "the most obnoxious child I ever met." He was at times aggressive, nasty, and destructive, and other times he was critical, complaining, and withdrawing. An important breakthrough occurred with this young patient, though, and Glasser was able to later write, "It was with Aaron that I first discovered the dramatic force of confronting a child with present reality."[11] Getting to this breakthrough was not immediate, though, and Glasser had to confront the psychiatric practices on which he had depended. The following excerpt describes his internal struggle: "I realized dimly that in following the principles of orthodox therapy I was contributing to Aaron's present desperation rather than relieving it, and I made up my mind to change my approach. Against all my training and reading, and without telling anyone what I planned to do, I began a kind of reality therapy. The explaining was over. From now on we were going to emphasize reality and present behavior."[12]

Predictably, there came a moment between Glasser and Aaron, therapist and patient, when Glasser's new approach would be tested. Glasser recalled: "He whined and tried to get away, but I held him and faced him toward me. I told him to shut up and for once in his life to listen to what someone had to say. I informed him that the play was over, and we would sit and talk in an adult fashion, or if we walked we would walk as adults. I explained clearly I would not tolerate any running away or even any impolite behavior while we were walking. He would have to be courteous and try to converse with me when I talked to him. He was to tell me everything he did and I would help him decide whether it was right or wrong. When he immediately attempted to leave, I forcibly restrained him. When he tried to hit me, I told him I would hit him back!"[13] Glasser didn't describe this moment to serve as an example of how treatment sessions might go. In fact, this strategy would be unacceptable now. He was a young resident. The ideas and practices were just forming. The approach did work with Aaron, though, and he experienced a breakthrough in his behavior. Glasser had a breakthrough, too. He admitted as much when he wrote, "Not only had Aaron benefited greatly from the therapy, but I had learned the valuable lesson that breaking with teaching and tradition as I had done could be beneficial."[14]

Of the several factors in Glasser's life that were now marinating together, another was his connection to the Ventura School for Girls. It was at the school that Glasser saw firsthand the value of involvement—of staff having a positive personal connection with the girls; he saw how a management plan, even within a prison environment, could be effective without relying on punishment; he saw the importance of the girls being able to make a plan for their future behavior; and he saw the incredible difference it makes when people experience success, or when people believe they can achieve success.

The third factor in this marinating pot was his involvement at the veterans' hospital and, more specifically, his work with G. L. Harrington. Glasser witnessed Harrington put a program in place that incorporated different levels of patient responsibility and that ultimately enabled them to be released back into society. He saw the importance of not referring to patients with the usual therapeutic labels. Harrington emphasized positive regard for patients and the need to accept them, even as their symptoms were rejected. In other words, within this supportive environment, patients were asked to give up their crazy symptoms.

Much like a chef leaning over a pot on the stove and enjoying the aroma of the simmering ingredients, Glasser was coming to see the potential and the importance of this new psychological arrangement. You can picture him in early 1963 as he decides to put pen to paper, probably on an airplane, with the excitement and commitment of an evangelist. He had made a discovery and people needed to know about it, especially people who worked in the mental illness field.

As the manuscript took shape, Glasser explained that when we are unhappy or are acting crazy, it is because we are unable to fulfill our basic needs. Our basic needs—the need to love and be loved, and the need to feel that we are worthwhile—are fulfilled through involvement with other people. He had come to appreciate we can be successful in involvement with others as we become effective self-evaluators, knowing when to correct a behavior or when to credit ourselves when we do right. Problems sometimes occur because, while humans are born with a set of unchanging needs, we don't arrive with a set of behaviors to fulfill those needs. Such behaviors must be learned.[15] One of the things he was absolutely sure of was neither our past nor our unconscious holds the key to living successfully now. A word he kept coming back to was "responsibility." In fact, he hoped the reader would come to "substitute responsible for mental health and irresponsible for mental illness."[16] Rather than depending on terms such as psychotic and schizophrenic, he suggested these labels be viewed as descriptions of irresponsibility. Responsible[17] behavior was the key and teaching it was the most important of all human tasks.

"Responsibility," Glasser emphasized, "is thrown at the patient in every possible way,"[18] including patients being required to pay for group therapy treatment by taking on some work detail. Positive and negative reinforcement were a constant part of Harrington's program. One writer, referring to how the concept of responsibility was applied to the recreation room, described it this way: "Glasser moved all the pinball games into one corner of the ward, and made a clear line with a sign to mark the entrance to this section. He informed staff, and told all the clients on the ward that 'no crazy behavior' was allowed in the games room. They could act crazy if they chose to, outside the game area. However, within the games area, they had to suppress crazy behaviors or they would be asked to leave."[19]

When I asked Glasser about this anecdote, he quickly replied, "No, no, no, no. I didn't do that. Harrington did that." Later he denied either of them doing it, even when I told him how much I liked the story and how much I wanted the story to be true. He insisted it was apocryphal. Whether this story about the recreation room is accurate or not, though, in general, Building 206 was dependent on such strategies. Harrington himself emphasized, "The place of the learning theory procedures should not be minimized; over and over again behaviors are identified, discussed, and then either rewarded or punished."[20]

In his first descriptions of reality therapy, Glasser emphasized the importance of involvement, or connection between therapist and client; the need to reject unrealistic behavior while accepting the client; and the need to teach the client better ways to fulfill his/her needs. He explained that behavior is more important than attitudes and present behavior is the key, rather than studying past behavior. He wanted people to understand happiness most often is the result of responsible behavior. These are themes he would build on for the rest of his career, themes his readers would become very familiar with over the years.

PRINCIPLES OF REALITY THERAPY
Positive Involvement
Present Behavior
Self-Evaluation
Make a Plan
Commitment
No Excuses
No Punishment
Never Give Up

Glasser clearly delineated the differences between conventional psychiatry and reality therapy. In general, conventional psychiatry proposed a series of related beliefs, including in the existence of mental illness and that people who suffered from it could be meaningfully classified; a focus on the patient's past life was essential in the treatment process; that the patient must transfer to the therapist attitudes that are held toward important people; that the patient must gain insight into his unconscious mind; that morality must be avoided since deviant behavior is the result of a mental illness; and that teaching people better behavior is not an important part of the therapy. In contrast to conventional psychiatry's approach, reality therapy does not accept the concept of mental illness; works in the present and future, and does not become involved in the patient's past; it also does not

The Differences Between Conventional Psychiatry and Reality Therapy

Conventional Psychiatry	Reality Therapy
Mental illness exists and treatment must be based on meaningful classification.	The concept of mental illness is not accepted; therefore the patient cannot act the role of a mentally ill person who is incapable of responsibility for his behavior.
The patient's past life, which contains the psychological roots of the problem, must be understood for change to take place.	Focuses on the present and the future, not the past. The past cannot be changed and, therefore, should not limit present behavior.
Maintains that the patient must transfer attitudes she holds toward important people to the therapist. Through transference, the therapist relives the difficulties with the patient so that the patient can gain insight.	Therapists relate to patients as themselves, not as transference figures.
The patient must gain understanding into his unconscious mind, which is more important than his conscious mind.	Does not focus on unconscious conflicts and does not accept excuses based on unconscious motivation.
Avoids the problem of morality and whether behavior is right or wrong. Deviant behavior is considered a product of mental illness.	Emphasizes the morality of behavior and issues of right and wrong.
Teaching people better behavior is not considered an important part of therapy.	Desires to teach patients better ways to fulfill their needs.

look into unconscious conflicts; emphasizes the morality of behavior; and teaches patients better ways to fulfill their needs.

Glasser was dogged on the point regarding mental illness and wrote, "We believe that this concept, the belief that people can and do suffer from some specific, diagnosable, treatable mental illness, analogous to a specific, diagnosable, treatable physical illness, is inaccurate and that this inaccuracy is a major roadblock to proper psychiatric treatment."[21] He used the term "weakness" rather than "illness," and believed there was a world of difference between being cured of an illness and helping oneself overcome a weakness. The fulcrum was between responsible and irresponsible behavior, and even behaviors like schizophrenia, neurosis, depression, and sociopathy were a part of this spectrum as examples of irresponsibility. From his point of view, it was only necessary to know whether the patient was struggling with irresponsible behavior or suffering from an organic disease.

As described previously, the girls' school in Ventura was significant in helping Glasser discover and refine the ideas of reality therapy. The need for positive relationships, or involvement, was emphasized at the school. When giving talks he would consistently emphasize this point: "Whether you are dealing with truants or mainliners, the vital thing is to be personal. Tell the addict or the delinquent in every way you can, 'It's important to me what happens to you. I care about you.'"[22] Present behavior needed to be the focus, and excuses were not accepted. What the girls did was more important than what they felt.

The case of Jeri, a 16-year-old runaway, who became a shoplifter, illustrates this approach. After her attempts to manipulate the staff at Ventura failed, and she finally realized she needed to truthfully face her behavior, she poured out the story of her deceitful life and the ways she had hurt others. Glasser had fostered a positive relationship with her throughout the difficult early stages of her stay at the school, in spite of the terrible things she said about him and to him. Yet when Jeri revealed the details of her destructive past, he wrote, "Instead of forgiving her, which used to be my natural impulse before I discovered how wrong it is therapeutically, I told her she was right to feel miserable and probably would continue to feel bad for the next few weeks."[23] He continued, "In reality therapy it is important not to minimize guilt when it is deserved."[24]

When I questioned Glasser on that stance, he replied, "Yah, yah, I think guilt is a perfectly good emotion. I have nothing against guilt." He added: "Well, the girls used to ask me this question, 'Dr. Glasser, will you forgive me for the things I've done?' You know they have a little religious background, some of them, and I said, 'That's not up to me to forgive you. I won't hold what you've done against you, but in terms of forgiving that's something you have to work out with your own self. I can't forgive you. You did something wrong. You did it. The best way, if you've done something wrong, is to stop doing it, and maybe even treat the people you wronged, if you treated people wrong, better. That's my advice, but that's again up to you.'"

But if someone, like a person may come into my private office and say, 'I feel so guilty, and I don't know why.' I said, 'What have you done wrong?' And that came as a new concept. Guilt without sin is a very common concept among people. It's like you carry around the sin of the world or something like that. I said, 'Well, if you can tell me something you've done really wrong, then I could certainly appreciate that you feel guilty about it, and I think that's good. The guilt will prevent you from doing it again. But if you're all upset and worked up and you've done nothing wrong, then I have no interest in it. It's up to you.'"

Glasser developed a matter-of-fact toughness that was an important part of his caring and desire to be positively involved with his patients. He was clear though this toughness must never be a part of a contest between two people. "Patients want you to correct their irresponsible behavior, but they want it to be done in the genuine spirit of helping them, not to satisfy yourself by winning a power struggle."²⁵ The environment at the Ventura School fostered this spirit.

WG

One of the goals of this biography is to examine where Glasser's thinking has changed over the years. The way in which his ideas developed may be significant for others who are also developing in their understanding of choice theory. I mentioned earlier how much Building 206, under Harrington, was dependent on positive and negative reinforcement. Glasser, while he cooperated with Harrington in the reward/punishment program, would later move away from this emphasis, clarifying instead the need for appropriate boundaries and how boundaries could be compassionately applied. When asked about Harrington's program where patients paid for treatment through work details and the use of reward and punishment, he replied, "Well, the problem with that whole concept is, I wouldn't, I probably wouldn't support that today. If you're going to assign people a job, and associate the job with their privileges, I think you have to talk it over with them and see if they'll accept it."

There are other areas in his early reality therapy thinking in which Glasser has since made changes. He would come to emphasize the concept of happiness and that its absence is the cause of poor mental health. In *Reality Therapy*, he wrote, "We must never delude ourselves into wrongly concluding that unhappiness led to the patient's behavior, that a delinquent child broke the law because he was miserable, and that therefore our job is to make him happy. He broke the law not because he was angry or bored, but because he was irresponsible. The unhappiness is not a cause, but a companion, to his irresponsible behavior."²⁶ Glasser admits responsibility was the big contribution that Reality Therapy made to the literature, however he later retreated somewhat from this emphasis. Lennon affirmed this when he wrote, "Even the core idea of responsibility is one Glasser uses with care nowadays."²⁷ Glasser explained: "I pulled back from it because people were using responsibility as an external control." When he heard teachers saying that the best part of reality therapy was they could come down hard on kids, Glasser knew he needed to change that perception.

He later clarified *Reality Therapy's* position on morality, as well. When asked about the emphasis on morality and right and wrong, he said, "I do do that, but not, not global morality. I think each person has to make some choices, and to me the moral choice would be the choice of the behavior that would bring him closer to the other important people in his life." For Glasser, morality is a personal matter that should not be imposed on another person.

Homosexuality is another area in which Glasser has since changed his thinking. In 1965, he wrote: "The psychiatrist, however, must not fall into the trap of helping them become better adjusted homosexuals, as many patients initially desire, but work in the opposite direction, helping them accept themselves as men so that they can gain a male identity and thereby find love and self-worth in their proper role."²⁸

When I pointed out that he had referred to homosexuality as an example of irresponsible behavior, he responded, "Right, that was a mistake." When I probed further as to his current thinking on homosexuality, he continued: "With homosexuality I'm at the point where I consider it to be a statistically abnormal behavior, but not in any other way. Any more than Shaquille O'Neal is abnormal. He's statistically abnormal, but he's a normal human being otherwise. I mean by size, you know. So some people are homosexual, you know, completely homosexual. Some people are completely heterosexual, and a considerable number of people go both ways. And I don't think there's any, there's no, as yet, discovery in the difference between a homosexual's brain, and or, or, or a heterosexual's brain, although there's been many things reported, none have held up. It's the same as the mental illness argument. Many things reported, but, but none have held up."

Less than two weeks after Glasser and I discussed the topic of homosexuality, he received an e-mail from a person interested in whether or not choice was involved in a person becoming homosexual. Glasser's reply included the following: "I have counseled homosexual people. In the beginning, I thought that maybe I could help them to become heterosexual. But after treating a number of them, I realized that homosexual was what they were or what they wanted to be. I can't tell the difference between the two. I used to say in my lectures that I could no more help a homosexual person to become heterosexual than I could help a heterosexual person who came to me and said they would rather be homosexual. I can only help with counseling and people who are choosing a behavior or even people who, like psychotic people, offer very creative behaviors like hallucinations and delusions. But still, if these people build a relationship with me, they can begin to understand that these behaviors are the way to deal with the basic unhappiness they have, which all people have. Unhappiness is what brings people for counseling. When someone's unhappiness is physically based, for example if a man comes to counseling with Parkinson's disease (because there is something wrong with his brain) and asks me to counsel him so that I can help to rid himself of the Parkinson's, I can't help him because there is really something going on in his brain. I really can't even say that much for homosexuality, that there is something going on in their brain. That is the mystery. They are different. Is anyone able to explain why some people are born left-handed, as I am, or right-handed, as most other people are? I am not abnormal. I am just different. That is the way I view homosexuality."[29]

Although a bit hesitant at first, Glasser would become a gifted public speaker, able to connect with large groups and seemingly hold them in the palm of his hand for hours. However, he seemed much less able or interested in connecting with people on an individual basis, at least in non-counseling situations. Later in Glasser's career a mutual friend wondered aloud to me if Glasser might be socially autistic. Glasser would come to be viewed as a conference celebrity, with people coming at him from all directions, some of them wanting something from him or wanting to "hitch their car to his fame train," so some of his distant ways are understandable. Plus, it can be just plain tiring to deal with people, even friendly people, for hours at conferences. Still, though, Glasser's lack of interest in connecting with people socially may be the result of a personality trait, a trait that evidenced itself during his time with Harrington.

Looking back, Glasser seemed to recognize this inability to connect as he thought about Harrington. It was because of their association that the ideas of reality therapy emerged; yet they were different in significant ways. Glasser recognized in Harrington the personality to be good friends with the psychoanalysts, to be connected with them and to garner their support and receive referrals from them. "If they couldn't deal with a patient, they sent him to Harrington knowing he could. And he was one of those people—I've never been able to do that—who had enough of a presence and a skill to do a different kind of thing from what most psychiatrists were doing, but still gain their respect."[30] Glasser seemed to lack the personality to make and keep those social connections.

Harrington, while he was able to nurture important connections with others in his field, recognized what Glasser possessed that he himself lacked. After reading *Reality Therapy*, he admitted: "He's much more disciplined than I am. I could never have got it organized and in print. Besides, I'm from an earlier generation that was born and will die with Freud. I thought Glasser's book was beautiful, but I told him, 'You can't say that. It's almost sacrilegious.' Bill felt free enough. He had guts enough."[31]

The relationship between Glasser and Harrington was more complicated than the way in Glasser publicly framed it. Publicly, Glasser consistently and quickly, even affectionately, referred to Harrington as "my mentor" or "my teacher." During later interviews a slightly different picture emerged. Harrington began meeting with Glasser in the last year of Glasser's psychiatric residency in late 1956 and continued meeting and consulting with him until 1964, just before *Reality Therapy* was published. During an interview in 2000, Glasser remembered, "I stayed with him for seven years. Once a week I came to his office and talked over my patients and my struggles. He was like a supervisor. But we never really became personally very friendly. I didn't see him socially. . . . I don't remember why I stopped seeing him. Whether I got too busy or he got too busy or whatever it was. . ."[32] But during an interview in 2004, when pressed on this point, more of this story came out.

It became apparent that Glasser was a young man who had a deep respect for Harrington, even looked up to him, and that as *Reality Therapy* began to take shape, Glasser wanted to include Harrington and have him be a part of it. But as this shaping and development took place their two roles were becoming clearer. "Harrington was more supporting me and encouraging me," Glasser explained, "than he was teaching me something I didn't know. He never really strongly supported. . . Harrington was a very popular guy. He was a big, good-looking guy, very jovial, very friendly, and he was sent a lot of patients by psychiatrists in town, because it was okay for Harrington not to be a psychoanalyst. He could still do good work. But Harrington was kind of cautious of supporting me for fear he would lose some of his psychiatric support. And I lived with that. I understood that."

Interestingly, he added, "Harrington's wife kinda thought that he was giving me stuff and I wasn't giving him credit for it. But the truth of the matter is he wasn't giving me much credit for anything. He was giving me credit for saying that he worked with me. But he never came out, that I know of, and even supported the title, *Reality Therapy*. He didn't deny it, but he didn't, he didn't really support it."

As Glasser recalled what really happened, a picture emerged of what must have been his disappointment and frustration, as his mentor, the man who had reached across the desk and said, "Join the club," began to distance himself from Glasser and reality therapy. In his consistently matter-of-fact manner, Glasser emphasized, "I understood Harrington didn't really support reality therapy and that he was still at the VA, and still among the psychoanalysts. I was already becoming *persona non grata* for the way I was thinking and, and so, I thought that rather than put him in an uncomfortable position, I didn't need him anymore and I knew he really didn't want to come out strongly and support the term reality therapy so I just kind of said, you know, 'I think that, that you helped me a great deal and I appreciate it, and, you know, we'll keep in touch,' which kind of we did a little bit."

When mentioned in an interview that it sounded as if Harrington had supported the term, Glasser interrupted and responded, "If he had supported the term reality therapy I would have continued to see him." Glasser wanted to be close to Harrington, wanted to continue to work together, but Harrington didn't feel the same way. "Reality therapy was becoming a big thing, like psychoanalysis, or Jungian therapy, but he didn't want to restrict himself just to be known as my kind of a person. So, I just did it by saying I learned a lot from him, but that, basically, I won't be coming anymore."

Glasser's positive regard for Harrington throughout his career is well documented. When questioned on his referring to Harrington as the one who "introduced the concepts of reality therapy," Glasser replied, "Well, I think he did come up with many of the concepts, and taught them to me. I give him credit for that." Harrington did inspire or confirm in Glasser the idea that mental illness did not exist in the traditional way it had been viewed up to that time, and that labels such as schizophrenia and psychosis are not helpful when working with symptomatic patients; he also emphasized the importance of responsibility, although for him responsibility involved levels of reward and punishment. But it was Glasser who put the reality therapy package together. Harrington was well aware of some of the pieces, yet he never embraced the package. Mrs. Harrington may have felt Glasser didn't give her husband enough credit, but in the end it may have been otherwise.

Glasser had challenged the theories and practices of his own field, which would not have been that big of a deal had the book not sold so many copies and become so well-known. He remembers it as a "boom heard around the world," which in the psychology community may have not been that far from the truth. When I wondered how professionals within his field treated him after the book was published, he explained that fellow psychiatrists ignored him rather than trying to discredit him. Some psychiatrists were amused that a technique called reality therapy would come out of Los Angeles, the illusion capitol of North America. One New York psychoanalyst said there wasn't much in Glasser's approach that would be useful to him, while a Beverly Hills analyst referred to Glasser as a social worker. It was intended as an insult. One fellow psychiatrist proclaimed the ideas and methods in *Reality Therapy* to be "irritatingly prosaic, devoid of brilliance or intellectual excitement."[33] If the book hadn't done so well these comments could have been discouraging. When Glasser was asked why one more form of therapy was needed, he responded, "Because reality therapy seems to work and a lot of the others don't."[34]

While his own field ignored him, though, other fields, especially the field of education was beginning to take real notice of Glasser's ideas. Donald O'Donnell, introduced at the beginning of this chapter, was one such educator. Another was Adrienne Nater, whose story exemplified both the power and the danger in Glasser's methods. Ms. Nater was a vice-principal at Oxnard High School in southern California when she came under administrative attack for her methods in working with the students sent to her for discipline. The story was well-documented in the local paper, the *Oxnard Press-Courier*, and reveals the issues at stake that led to her forced resignation at the of the 1965-1966 school year. An editorial in the paper explained: "Miss Nater's chief task has been to discipline girls sent to her because they were causing some sort of trouble in the classroom. The complaint against her is that she has not followed the traditional methods of discipline, rough talk and suspensions, but has 'counseled' the students." She tells how she came on the book, *Reality Therapy*, by accident and that Glasser's techniques were far more formalized than her own. Yet she was trying to apply the important principles of the theory in her work with the problem girls at Oxnard High School. "If a child is sent to the office," she explained, "I try to find out why. I let her relate what happened and then I try to show her why she can't be disrespectful. I don't mete out punishment without letting the child know why. Control by fear and hatred is bad. I think the only way is through respect and understanding." The principal of the school, a Mr. Powell, said her forced resignation was "just a case of not being suited to her job." The *Oxnard Press-Courier*, in its editorial, felt differently and described Nater as "one of those rare adults who can talk on an adolescent's level and straighten them out, rather than throwing them out." The editorial also suggested: "It may be that what some people resent is that Miss Nater is successful with a different method, one that others have not always been willing to try." Students and parents led a campaign to reinstate her, but in the end she was forced out.

There was a quality to Glasser's ideas that seemed to divide people and force them to show their cards, so to speak. The ideas of *Reality Therapy*, which challenged the concept of mental illness and confronted readers and listeners with involvement and responsibility, would not let them settle into comfortable compromise. Glasser had put everything on the table. He had revealed exactly what he thought and his act of professional honesty called on others to do the same. And because his ideas called into question, even attacked, accepted practices in fields throughout the caring professions, not only he himself, but others who responded to his ideas, who shared his worldview, and who tried to implement his approach came under counterattack. *Reality Therapy* had struck a chord, discordant to some, but in perfect harmony to others.

NOTES

1. O'Donnell, D. (1987). History and growth of the Institute for Reality Therapy. *Journal of Reality Therapy, 7*, 2-8.
2. Zunin, L. and Glasser, W. (1973). *Current psychotherapies*. Itasca, IL: F. E. Peacock Publishers.
3. Wolberg, L. (1954). *The technique of psychotherapy*. New York: Grune and Stratton.
4. Whitaker, R. (2002). *Mad in America: Bad science, bad medicine, and the enduring mistreatment of the mentally ill*. Cambridge, MA: Perseus Publishing.
5. *Ibid*.
6. Ibid. p. 38
7. Zunin, L. and Glasser, W. (1973). Current psychotherapies. Itasca, IL: F. E. Peacock Publishers.
8. Glasser, W. (1965). *Reality therapy*. Harper Row. (Although it should be noted that G. L. Harrington wrote most of chapter four.)
9. Wubbolding, R. (2000). *Reality therapy for the 21st century*. Philadelphia, PA: Brunner-Routledge.
10. Glasser, W. (1965). Reality therapy, p. 165, 166
11. Ibid, p. 170
12. Ibid, p. 170
13. Glasser, W. (1965). *Reality therapy*. New York: Harper & Row, p. 170, 171
14. Ibid, p. 173
15. Glasser, W. (1965). *Reality therapy*. New York: Harper Row, p. 16.
16. *ibid*, p.18.
17. On page 15 in *Reality Therapy*, Glasser defined responsible behavior as the ability to meet one's needs without depriving others of the ability to fulfill their needs.
18. *ibid*, p.158.
19. Howatt, W. (2001). The evolution of reality therapy to choice theory. *International Journal of Reality Therapy, 21(1)*, 7-11.
20. Glasser, W. (1965). *Reality therapy*. New York: Harper Row.
21. Glasser, W. (1965). *Reality therapy*. New York: Harper & Row, p. 55
22. Langguth, J. (1967). California's gift to psychotherapy. *Harper's Magazine, 234*, 52-56.

23 Glasser, W. (1965). *Reality therapy*. New York: Harper & Row, p. 96
24 Ibid, p.96.
25 Glasser, W. (1965). Reality therapy. New York: Harper & Row, p.113.
26 Glasser, W. (1965). *Reality therapy*. New York: Harper & Row, p. 36, 37.
27 Lennon, B. (2000). From reality therapy to reality therapy in action. *International Journal of Reality Therapy, 20(1)*, 41-46.
28 Glasser, W. (1965). *Reality therapy*. New York: Harper & Row, p. 186.
29 Glasser email, May, 2004.
30 Wubbolding, R. (2000). *Reality therapy for the 21st century*. Philadelphia, PA: Brunner-Routledge.
31 Langguth, J. (1967). California's gift to psychotherapy. *Harper's Magazine, 234*, 52-56.
32 Wubbolding, R. (2000). *Reality therapy for the 21st century*. Philadelphia, PA: Brunner-Routledge.
33 Langguth, J. (1967). California's gift to psychotherapy. *Harper's Magazine, 234*, 52-56.
34 Ibid, p. 52

6
A WHOLE NEW WORLD

"So, at this time, I consider myself a psychiatrist who is desperately trying to become a school teacher in order to help all the school teachers who are trying to become psychiatrists."
—*William Glasser, 1969*

As Fitzgeorge Peters stood on the balcony of his flat overlooking the East River, across to the boroughs of Queens and Brooklyn, he couldn't believe what he was about to do. New York City was his life. His work was there. His friends were there. Yet he was thinking about heading west, to California of all places. Peters was a counselor in the New York City probation system and, along with Sam Buchholz and Alex Bassin, worked with drug and alcohol impaired clients who were trying to be successful in life outside of the penal system. Even before the publication of *Reality Therapy*, Buchholz had brought Glasser to New York to begin working with a group of counselors. Peters remembered, "We were an enthusiastic group of people. We saw the ideas working." The ideas of reality therapy struck Peters at a deep level and he recalled, "I found myself saying, 'Wow, this is almost like a way of life.'" He described how at first he used the reality therapy ideas with his clients, whether in individual or group sessions, but soon he also began to apply the ideas to his own thinking and behavior. He would always be in the front row taking notes whenever Glasser came to town to give presentations. The success of the ideas when they were offered to his clients, as well as the impact the ideas were having on his personal life, led Peters to his balcony and to the real possibility of a coastal change. He remembers the conversation going like this: "What is important to me? And I thought reality therapy is important to me, and Bill Glasser is important to me. And then I thought, where is Bill Glasser? And I answered, well, he's in California. And then I asked myself, where are you? Well, I'm in New York. I said, wow, what the hell is this? Once I discovered that connection, there was no turning back."

Shortly after the balcony epiphany, Peters loaded his car and headed west. "I got into my Volvo and drove all the way to California. I still have the same Volvo, by the way. I drove up to the very house they still live in now. Bill offered me Joe's bed. I think Joe was in college at the time. He just opened his home to me. I didn't know where I was going to go, but he said, 'Come into our house until you can find your own place.' We'd go around together looking at apartments, but he would say, 'Nah, nah, nah, you don't want to be here.' Finally, I found a place. And then I started working in the schools, along with Bill. I was a therapist doing what I loved."

Of Peters it can be said that he was there at the beginning. Along with Sam Buchholz, Alex Bassin, and soon to join them, Al Katz. Fitzgeorge Peters was a part of an early group of professionals who, even before *Reality Therapy* was published, recognized something special, something effective, something needed, in Glasser's ideas. Others may not have gotten in their cars and driven to California, Peters level of passion was unique in that way, but they similarly experienced a heightened awareness of their own beliefs when confronted with the beliefs of reality therapy. In many cases, Glasser's writing affirmed people's ideas or gave them permission to follow the direction in which their beliefs pointed. Al Katz said as much when he shared,

"Many of us who have come to follow Bill were leaning in that direction anyway." Peters and Katz were deeply moved by the principles of reality therapy. Katz was taking a Basic Concepts in Counseling course from Alex Bassin, who had just recently finished reading *Reality Therapy*, and when Bassin challenged his students to apply *Reality Therapy* to their own lives and make a plan, Katz decided to give up smoking.

Fitzgeorge Peters is further unique in that he left the early group of "first responders" in New York City and arrived in California in time to become a part of the first responders on the West Coast. He explained, "When I first moved to California, Glasser used to meet on Wednesday nights on Olympic Boulevard—that place would eventually become our Educator Training Center—and we'd have educators come there and run with the ideas. He would give them drafts of what was coming up. I would joke about how we met in the upper room. Ideas would be tried out and people would come back and have a discussion." Peters had wanted to work closely with William Glasser and moving to Los Angeles put him at the epicenter of reality therapy's growth.

Donald O'Donnell and Doug Naylor had a lot in common. They both were young principals of elementary schools within the California public school system—O'Donnell worked just north of Sacramento in Orangevale, and Naylor worked at an inner city school in south central Los Angeles. They both became very interested in the ideas of William Glasser and they both got in touch with Glasser as a result and began to work with him so not only teachers and students within their own schools would benefit, but others outside of their schools would benefit too. It isn't unusual for listeners, after hearing a great presentation, or readers, after reading an important book or journal article to say, "Man, I'd like to talk with that guy." It is less usual to actually go for it and make the connection happen. Something within the reality therapy ideas was important enough that both O'Donnell and Naylor did just that.

Doug Naylor was the principal of the 75th Street Elementary School near the Watts area of Los Angeles. Naylor first got in touch with Glasser during the spring or summer of 1965, which is significant in that the Watts Riots ignited on August 12th of that year. Although almost all of the students were black, Naylor and many of his teachers were white. Suffice it to say this would not have been an easy time to work at the 75th Street School and the environment there would have been especially challenging. Glasser remembers Naylor getting in touch with him and wanting to consult with him on how the reality therapy ideas could be implemented in an inner city school environment. The visits must have struck an even deeper chord in Naylor, as he introduced Glasser to Robert Purdy, who was then a superintendent of elementary education in Los Angeles. Purdy recognized that it wasn't just the 75th Street school that needed the help and support Glasser could provide and hired him to work in three other area schools—Ascot Avenue School, the 112th Street School, and the Weigand Avenue School. At the time Glasser was still working at the Ventura School for Girls and at the orthopedic hospital, where he began making good money once he figured out how to bill the insurance companies. The needs of the schools, though, were a powerful draw to him and he left the money to work with the teachers and students. "They paid me a $100 a day," Glasser explained, "so at four schools, two days, $200, which was, as far as I am concerned, they were getting a bargain." Compared to the orthopedic hospital he was taking "a $900 pay cut for a job that was a hell of a lot harder."

In a talk that he would give several years later, Glasser recalled: "The first thing I noticed was that the situation in the public schools was a lot rougher than in the school for delinquent girls. It was much, much rougher. There was no way you could keep your finger on some of those kids; they were vibrating all over the building. It was a really difficult situation, and I became very frightened. Like anyone else who is frightened and feels inadequate about the problem he is faced with, I started to hunt for excuses for my ineffectiveness."[1] He would come to understand "the school was making it difficult for kids and the kids were fighting back," but at the outset he was overwhelmed with the challenges. He remembers during this time, after a day of work in the schools, he would arrive home with headaches on a regular basis.

He doesn't remember feeling unsafe in that area of Los Angeles, but he does remember being confronted regarding his work in the schools. "I only had one problem," he began. "They were criticizing me for being a white guy coming to tell them how to teach their kids. They liked what I was saying, but they still criticized me for being there. You know, there's no logic to this, to prejudice with these kinds of things. So, anyway, there were a couple of people talking to me like this and I just rolled up my shirtsleeve and said, 'See this arm, this arm is white and it's never going to be black, and if you don't want a white man in here helping, you tell me and I'll leave. I'm trying to help these kids to learn more and if you think that they're doing as well in school as they could be doing, then I'll go.' Well, then they shut up and I never heard another word."

Glasser was beginning to be more known for his work in the schools and it was a reputation for which he paid his dues. In spite of the challenges and the headaches, he created a routine in which he spent a half-day at each of the four schools "teaching teachers and demonstrating classroom meetings and talking about no failure and let's stop punishing kids."[2] It was not commonplace for schools to hire psychiatrists, and even less commonplace for psychiatrists to accept such invitations, but Glasser was getting in the habit of doing the uncommon. Leaving a job that paid him up to $1,000 a day for a job working in an inner city school near a riot-torn area of L.A. at $100 a day is what his decision boiled down to. While people who heard his views of mental health and human motivation often resonated with the ideas at a deep, personal level, it should be noted Glasser himself resonated with his ideas at a deep, passionate level, as well. He was on a mission to improve mental health, to demystify the psychiatric process, and he was following leads as they arose. It is true educators, more than in any other field, initially approached him for help and support. But Glasser himself began to see the need for prevention rather than cure and was drawn to working with children and teenagers in the school setting, partly because the schools were in such need, and partly because he recognized the earlier people began to understand the principles of reality therapy, the better off they and society would be.

Remarkably, beside his work at the orthopedic hospital, his two days a week at the Ventura School, two days a week at the Los Angeles elementary schools, his private practice, and increasing travel due to the success of *Reality Therapy,* Glasser was also involved with two other important projects. The first project was his work in Palo Alto, where he and Superintendent Harold Santee were beginning to see the need for a demonstration school. People could hear about the school program Glasser envisioned, and even believe in such a program, but they often left his talks wanting to see such a place in action, an idea that he and Santee wanted to oblige. The second project was closer to home. In the evenings, Glasser was teaching classes to people interested in reality therapy. One place he taught was at San Fernando

A Whole New World

Valley State College, a new school that had been built on farmland less than 10 years earlier (and that later would become Cal State-Northridge). Glasser also remembers teaching a class in west Los Angeles, at a small, private school with approximately 30 people in attendance, almost all of them educators from various regions and levels of the Los Angeles school system. Doug Naylor and his vice-principals were a part of this class. This particular class was important because it was out of this group that the Institute for Reality Therapy was formed in 1967. The interest and commitment and passion of the group were an encouragement to Glasser, however for the ideas to really take off a more tangible form of encouragement was needed. As it turned out, tangible encouragement from an unexpected resource was on the way.

Billy Sharpe looked nice enough and sounded nice enough, but Naomi Glasser didn't think they should accept what he was offering. Sharpe had come to the Glasser home as a representative of the Clement Stone Foundation, which wanted to give Glasser money, a lot of money, to help disseminate his ideas on a wider and larger scale. Donald O'Donnell was present at the meeting too, and like Naomi, he didn't really like the sound of it "I don't want anything to do with these people," Naomi emphasized. "Something is wrong." The Stone Foundation, funded through the insurance business, was on the lookout for ways to help public education and due to the success of *Reality Therapy,* Glasser popped up on their radar screen. They sponsored Glasser to come to Chicago and give a talk outlining his vision for improving public schools. Glasser explained to Naomi that he wanted to at least talk with them. And to the Foundation he responded that if they wanted to give him money, they should come to his house.³ Shortly thereafter, Billy Sharpe flew to Los Angeles to discuss a grant that could help Glasser get his ideas into the nation's schools faster and on a wider scale. And the Foundation was not talking small change. They were prepared to give Glasser $300,000 to jumpstart the effort. (To put this into perspective, the median household income in 1967 was $7,200; 20% of households made less than $3,000 a year.) With money comes control, though, and Naomi Glasser and Donald O'Donnell felt that accepting the grant wasn't worth the risk of the strings that likely would be attached.

When asked by the Foundation how much money he wanted and what he would do with the money once it arrived, at first Glasser didn't know the answer to either question and said as much. In spite of this, the Foundation was adamant they would provide backing for this cause. In the midst of his hesitancy and the Foundation's pledge to move ahead, the answer came to him. The fledgling Institute for Reality Therapy would be improved and stabilized so that an entire new branch, the Educator Training Center, could be developed to start working with schools. And so in 1968 the Educator Training Center was created and Doug Naylor, the young principal from the 75th Street Elementary School, became its director, a position he would hold for almost 30 years. The ETC would soon become a very busy place. Interest from school districts around the country would require more and more trainers to meet the growing demand for help. This was especially true after 1969, when *Schools Without Failure* was published.

It is noteworthy Donald O'Donnell was in the Glasser's living room when a representative from the Stone Foundation presented the idea to fund the implementation of Glasser's ideas. O'Donnell was there at Glasser's request. He was a good friend of both Naomi and Bill, and in this particular case he was siding with Naomi. Ultimately, Glasser would decide to accept the money and jumpstart a program that would help schools be places without failure, but the point here is that of all the people within Glasser's growing circle of friends and colleagues it was O'Donnell he asked to be there. The two had worked closely since his letter to Glasser inquiring about *Reality Therapy* material at the end of 1963, so closely that Glasser would come to refer to him as his psychological brother. (As far as I know, Glasser would come to refer to just one other person in similar terms.) O'Donnell was informative and even inspirational to Glasser regarding the needs and possibilities within the public school system, however their friendship, both personal and professional, also revealed Glasser's tendency throughout his career to collaborate with someone else in the development of his ideas. This collaboration seemed less about the joy that can come from working with another person and more about needing the added credibility someone else's voice would bring to the project. Glasser involved George Harrington in the writing of *Reality Therapy*. (Some might say having Herbert Mowrer write the foreword for Reality Therapy is another example of this need for credibility, but Glasser explained later he did not have anything to do with Mowrer getting involved.) And now Donald O'Donnell was collaborating on *Schools Without Failure.* This tendency would reveal itself again during his work with William Powers, David and Roger Johnson, Brad Greene (and even W. Edwards Deming), and later with Jon Carlson. During a day in which I was working with Glasser at his home, he became excited when his fax machine produced a letter from Wayne Dyer. He proceeded to explain they were in communication about something, but I could tell he thought Dyer paying attention to him was a big deal. Dyer was a successful author and his presentations on the power of intentions and inner beliefs could be seen on cable channels. Yet in spite of Dyer's writing and presenting, he was not on the same level as William Glasser. He had not affected as many people or had the same level of impact on society as Glasser, but Glasser didn't see it that way. When questioned about this he admitted that Dyer had given him credit for some of his most significant beliefs. Still, Glasser seemed unable to recognize the significance of his own importance.

Glasser quit working at the Ventura School for Girls in 1967. In his own words, the school was "running beautifully and could carry on without him." The school had been significant in the sculpting of the ideas he was now forming, but with the success of *Reality Therapy* he was consistently bombarded with speaking appointments. He was also very involved in public school projects in Los Angeles, Sacramento, and Palo Alto. In Palo Alto, district superintendent Harold Santee and Glasser wanted to move ahead with the creation of a *Schools Without Failure* demonstration school. Glasser lobbied for Donald O'Donnell to be the principal of the "new" school, another indicator of Glasser's closeness to O'Donnell and of his confidence in O'Donnell's leadership skills, and not only did O'Donnell come to Palo Alto, he also brought with him three of his teachers from the school in Orangevale. Ironically, the demonstration school in Palo Alto was set up in an already existing school known as the Ventura School.

Glasser began writing *Schools Without Failure*[4] immediately after finishing the manuscript for *Reality Therapy*. The girls at the Ventura School for Girls, his work in public schools, and his association with educators like Donald O'Donnell and Doug Naylor, all convinced Glasser of the need to create schools built on a different approach, an approach in which failure was not even an option. The success of the girls at the Ventura School and Glasser's own experience at Western Reserve University Medical School were the most influential toward forming his no failure ideas. Glasser credits the girls at Ventura for emphasizing the idea of schools without failure. "The girls encouraged me to incorporate the idea of getting rid of failure in my next book. It was the girls at the Ventura School, as much as anyone else who said this is an important thing. Because they said that what causes us to be locked up in this juvenile prison really isn't our families, it's failure in school. So what we need is a book called Schools Without Failure." And regarding his medical school training, he described: "On the first day we were there, the dean spoke to us. We didn't believe him, but this is what he said: 'We selected you to become doctors, and everybody in this room is going to be a doctor. We hope you enjoy your four years. You are all going to make it. There's no problem. Don't worry about anything. Just relax and learn a lot and that's it.'"[5] Both of these schools, so disparate on the surface, with one being a prison school and the other being an elite medical school, were very similar at their core. Both of them greatly valued individual students and wanted to create an environment in which students wanted to learn; both wanted their students to look forward to coming to classes; both schools valued relevant, authentic learning, rather than memorized learning that would soon be forgotten; and both wanted to convey the idea that students, if they did not want to fail, would not fail.

Glasser became convinced when students were unsuccessful in school it led to them being unsuccessful afterward. When students came to see themselves as unable to succeed it had the effect of limiting their efforts outside of school. The situation in the schools was so significant Glasser shifted his own direction: "It is with the crucial importance of the school system in mind that I have moved from the traditional but limited psychiatric practice of working in prisons, mental hospitals, and clinics into working with children and teachers in school to see whether the concepts of reality therapy, especially involvement and responsibility, applied to the public schools, can work as well there as in reform schools and mental hospitals."[6] The question for Glasser was: Could children be taught in such a way that it would really lead to their success in life and prevent the emotional and mental problems that attend dysfunction and failure? He felt if schools could become places that focused on student success, rather than places that identified and tracked their failure, it would be a huge help to society. The eventual cost of dysfunction to taxpayers and businesses is beyond staggering. For instance, in 2010 the amount the state of California spent on each minor in its juvenile detention system was $224,712. (The amount spent on each student in the Oakland public school system was $4,945.) Glasser became convinced that the best place to combat societal ills—more and more people taking drugs, both legal and illegal, to handle stress and unhappiness; higher crime rates; increasing prison populations, high divorce rates—was in the schools. For him it was simple and he insisted, "We must develop schools where children succeed."[7]

In *Schools Without Failure* he pointed out "there are factors within the education system itself that not only cause many school problems, but that accentuate the problems a child may bring to school."[8] Rather than helping children, well-meaning educators often made the problems worse. The education system needed to be reviewed, but systems are resistant to such reviews and instead of recognizing student failure as a wake-up call, these students were seen as a problem and separated from others so that they could be treated by a specialist. According to school leaders of the day the school system couldn't be the problem; the low-achieving students were the problem. Glasser saw firsthand the large numbers of students who were being cut off from success, and who were reacting by tuning out and then dropping out. Even those who were ultimately deemed successful by the educational system had simply learned to play the memorizing, testing, non-thinking games that led to a diploma. He felt that 75% of children did not receive a satisfactory elementary education, and that failure in the inner city schools was at epidemic proportions. This failure then led to thousands of young people being unprepared for anything except the most menial of jobs. This failure had contributed to the need for places like the Ventura School for Girls.

When it was published in 1969, along with its *Schools Without Failure* title, Harper & Row emblazoned in large letters across the top of the book cover "The controversial new book by the author of *Reality Therapy.*" Some would see the word "controversial" on the cover as simply the publisher's attempt to sell more books, however a closer examination of the book's contents reveals that Glasser's points were indeed controversial.

He proposed:
- The grading system, as we know it, be abolished.
- Schools focus on being warm and inviting; the kind of place about which a kid would say, "I want to go to school."
- Educators be more interested in the idea of involvement, rather than in the idea of motivation.
- Schools no longer use poor home environments as an excuse for low student achievement.
- Schools eliminate punishment as a way to control student behavior.
- Learning based on memorization does not lead to thoughtfulness or understanding.
- Closed-book, objective tests should be eliminated.
- Student progress reports reflect what the student knows, not what the student doesn't know.

There were five educational mediocrities on which Glasser especially focused: ABCDF grading, grading on the curve, objective tests, closed-book tests, and homework. Objective, closed-book tests did not value thinking skills and instead emphasized the importance of memorizing information. Such tests embraced the principles of certainty and measurement, two ideas with which Glasser took exception. The certainty principle is based on the idea there is only one right answer and either the teacher knows the answer or it can be found at the back of the textbook; the measurement principle is based on the belief that only that which can be measured is valuable, therefore learning must be turned into a number or a letter. While these approaches have obvious flaws, Glasser added that a dependence upon memorizing information offers a very shallow potential for developing a healthy, personal identity. "Little of a success identity can be attained by using one's brain as a memory bank," Glasser explained. "Merely retaining knowledge, without using it to solve problems relevant to oneself and to society, precludes extensive involvement with other people and with the world. The certainty principle emphasizes isolation rather than cooperation and involvement."[9] In other words, people are able to create a success identity as they successfully solve challenges that are relevant to themselves or to others. Glasser felt strongly "the school practice that most produces failure in students is grading."[10] While a sacred part of American education and revered as utilitarian and necessary, he saw ABCDF grading as a very ineffective way to portray a student's learning and very effective way to kill motivation. He pointed out how grades had become moral equivalents, with good grades being correlated with good behavior and bad grades being correlated with bad behavior. In the process, grades had "become a substitute for learning, the symbolic replacement for knowledge. One's transcript," he continued, "is more important than one's education."[11] The result of such a shallow system of accountability was that standards were lowered rather than raised. Grades were actually a part of the problem. Grading on the curve made matters even worse, since the curve showed no interest in what was learned, only in dividing students into arbitrary categories. And sending students home with more schoolwork, usually irrelevant busy work at that, only contributed to the negative educational spiral.

Schools needed to be places where students were taught, really taught, the content and the skills. Schools had become sorting machines, identifying those who could and those who could not, rather than instructional centers where all students learned to be successful. For educators wanting to create such schools the principles of reality therapy were helpful. Reality therapy emphasized that no excuse is acceptable to not following through. Punishments, usually the first response to poor performance, were recognized as ineffective and destructive. Instead, students should be helped to form (or re-form) a plan and commit to it. This process of discipline, which is much different than punishment, builds responsibility and ultimately a success identity.

After *Reality Therapy* was published Glasser was referred to as reality-oriented and non-traditional. After *Schools Without Failure* came out he began to be referred to as get-tough, no-nonsense, and tough-minded. It is true he believed children could be held responsible for their behavior and they should achieve competence before moving on to higher learning levels, but such labels were misleading. Referring to his ideas as a get-tough approach caused people to overlook the importance of involvement and the idea that students need to experience a strong connection with their teachers and with the school program in general. It downplayed the fact that involvement could only be fostered in a psychologically warm and loving environment and within an academically meaningful and relevant curriculum. Glasser's "toughness" was dependent on these elements being in place. Such labels also caused people to misunderstand the "toughness" in

Glasser's approach. The toughness or no-nonsense perspective in reality therapy lies in students being lovingly, yet firmly, confronted when they misbehave, and then helped to understand their misbehavior and develop a plan to channel their energies in a better direction. Through this process students learned to become self-evaluators who were capable of making a reasonable plan for improvement and then making a commitment to the success of that plan. Rather than being manipulated through punishment, students were invited and persuaded to change by teachers who conveyed that we would never give up on them.

Glasser himself may have intentionally contributed to the toughness aura being attached to *Schools Without Failure*. When asked about his statement in *Reality Therapy*—"warmth never supersedes discipline, nor discipline warmth"—he explained that he said it then because he didn't want *Reality Therapy* to be dismissed as a touchy-feely kind of thing. In a talk he gave to school administrators in the same year that *Schools Without Failure* was published he admitted, "Toughness is a part of the procedure." He proclaimed, "You have to be tough in this business. People can be warm and friendly and loving and involved, but that doesn't mean you have to be easy or permissive." He summarized his emphasis by stating, "You have to be tough enough to let children make their own decisions." In *Schools Without Failure* he exhorted educators to keep in mind, "Neither school nor therapist should attempt to manipulate the world so that the child does not suffer the reasonable consequences of his behavior."

Applying the principles of reality therapy to the school environment Glasser described how children, like all human beings, are constantly trying to fulfill their need for love and belonging with others and their need for self-worth, which is based on their ability to be successful in school. When they are unable to meet their needs through traditional school approaches students will shift their need-satisfying behavior strategies to either rebelling against the system that has labeled them or by giving up. These dysfunctional student behaviors could develop to the point that the school system would further label such students as mentally ill. Glasser reminded educators, "These students suffer and withdraw because they can't find the successful pathways to a success identity. We wrongly label variations of this suffering and withdrawal as 'mental illness.' Such people are not ill; nothing has happened to them that they can't remedy themselves. Illness implies that a person has been attacked by a bacteria, toxin, or chemical imbalance over which he has no control. In helping children, we must work to make them understand that they are responsible for fulfilling their needs, for behaving so that they can gain a successful identity."[12]

It is interesting that *Schools Without Failure* can be read 40 years later and still feel relevant and up-to-date. Educators can get a bit discouraged that systemically so little has changed. It is interesting, too, that *Schools Without Failure* continues to be accurate in terms of Glasser's message. Other than in one area, *Schools Without Failure* explained the important themes of *Reality Therapy* in a way that has stood the test of time; that one area had to do with emotions. In *Schools Without Failure* Glasser wrote: "Emotion is the result of behavior." When I pointed that out, he quickly responded, "Well, that's wrong. I hadn't figured out total behavior then. Emotion is one of the four components that make up behavior. It's not the result of behavior. That's wrong. That's a mistake." To carefully read through a book written over 40 years ago, a book covering the complexities of human behavior, and discover only this one change, this one difference, is impressive. Glasser would go on to modify his views on how emotion and behavior relate to one another and in the process develop the concept of total behavior, which he felt was one of his major contributions. Overall, however, *Schools Without Failure* was an accurate portrayal of his ideas as they stand today.

WG

Shortly after arriving at the Ventura School for Girls, Glasser began conducting cottage meetings with the girls. There were usually over 50 girls at a time involved in these meetings. The meetings were designed to convey to the girls that they had a voice and their needs and views mattered. The meetings also helped them to communicate better with each other. Glasser would get the girls into a circle and then throw out a question to get the discussion started. The question was usually open-ended, maybe something like, "What could schools do to do a better job?" or "What makes some teachers better than others?" While he sought to foster a discussion on whatever the subject was, he remained non-judgmental, a key, throughout the meeting. His goal during the meetings was not so much to influence or teach as it was to listen and help the girls become aware of their own thinking. He also wanted them to begin to appreciate the views of others.

When he began working at the four elementary schools in Watts, Glasser brought this practice with him, only now referring to them as class meetings. He saw these meetings as absolutely essential in the process of a school becoming a school without failure. There were three different kinds of meetings—social problem-solving, open-ended, and educational diagnostic—and it was important that teachers knew how to engage students in each of them. These meetings really did form the backbone of the *Schools Without Failure* approach. In other words, if schools were to become schools without failure and to become schools that students wanted to come to each day, then students would need to experience class meetings on a regular basis.

And because of their importance Glasser spent time each day at the four elementary schools modeling to teachers how to conduct class meetings. During his Las Vegas talk to the school administrators, he stated, "I estimate that I've had somewhere between 1,500 and 2,000 class meetings in the last five or six years."[13] It was clear he was quite willing to get in the trenches with teachers.

Glasser learned a lot about what students were thinking during the class meetings and this knowledge fueled his desire to improve schools. Somehow the public had to get a sense of what schools could be, of what they needed to be. And so he sounded the call. "When one asks students," he pointed out, "whether their school work is in any way related to their lives outside of school, most of them reply incredulously, 'Of course not.' By the tenth grade, students are firmly convinced school is a totally different experience from life." More than 40 years later, has this changed? Do students feel differently now than they did then? Or is this wake-up call as applicable to us now as it was when Glasser penned this passage?

The success of *Schools Without Failure* would seem to indicate that educators were listening to this call and wanted to head in the direction Glasser was heading. Yet wanting and doing can be two different things. Teachers, constantly in the midst of complex and demanding challenges, were always on the lookout (this continues to be the case) for quick, helpful ideas. Though not a part of any written code, teachers exude the mantra: Give me something today that I can use tomorrow. Glasser's approach, while tangible, was more about heart change and thinking change than it was about what to do to students when they misbehaved or under performed. The ideas had great appeal for teachers, but their implementation required a change of thinking. Only an internal thinking change, a paradigm shift, would lead to a change in the way the system operated. As most of us are aware, systems don't like to change. When I asked Glasser about the degree to which *Schools Without Failure* affected the system, he acknowledged, "It sold widely, but people didn't really do it. Still don't." Class meetings did not have to take that much time, yet teachers, unable to shake traditional beliefs or pressured by schedules, did not create and maintain time for them.

One of the remarkable things Glasser did throughout his career was to conduct class meetings in front of an audience. When a school district or school arranged for him to come and present the SWF ideas, as a part of his presentation Glasser would request that a group of students be available for him to interview. Such interviews often involved a group of four to eight students, but he sometimes interviewed an entire classroom of students. The interviews usually took place on the stage of a packed gym or auditorium. Other than asking the district or school to select a representative group of students from various academic and social stratas, Glasser had no control over which students he would interview. There was no rehearsing or communicating beforehand. It wasn't unusual for schools to want their "best" students on the stage, but Glasser seemed ready for that possibility too.

At one of these meetings, in front of a gymnasium audience filled with parents, community members, teachers, principals, and district superintendents, Glasser was on the stage with an entire class of sixth-graders. The topic was grading and Glasser introduced the topic by pointing out that some educators thought eliminating grades would lead to better schools. He then asked them if they would be willing to participate in such an experiment. While students at previous schools could see value in this idea, the students on the stage with him at that moment rigidly defended grades, something they were sure their parents preferred as well. Half of the group felt so strongly about it that they said they would transfer to another school if grades were done away with. Glasser tried to pull them in his direction, but they remained firm as they explained that grades were necessary to tell students how they were doing, and that without them students would stop working and no one would learn anything. Almost every one of the 35 students had something to say about the need for grades.

Glasser let them fully air their convictions and then he asked a question that changed the direction of the meeting completely.

"The climax of the evening came when I asked, 'Since you believe grades are so valuable and so important, would you like to have your teacher grade you tonight?' The response from the class was immediate and loud. Every hand went up, even the hands of two girls who had said nothing all evening. There were groans and moans, and as fast as I could call on students they protested. One boy who had been a vociferous defender of grades said if the discussion had been graded, he would not have come. Child after child who had earlier spoken openly and thoughtfully said if the discussion had been graded, they would not have spoken so freely. One child said, to the nodding agreement of the class, that it is impossible to have free discussion when it is graded. Although she had spoken only briefly, one girl said, if her comments were to be graded, she would not have spoken at all. She said, 'I have found out that the safest thing in a discussion is never to say anything.' The two girls who had not spoken had a kind of smug I-told-you-so expression on their faces when she made this statement. There was complete agreement this had been a wonderful, happy, and open experience. There was also complete agreement that discussion of this type would never occur if they were graded. After this dramatic demonstration of the effects of grades, there was little more to say. The point had been so well made that in the short time remaining, the audience's comments centered around how we could get the school board's permission to do away with grades. Not one voice was raised in defense of elementary school grades."[14]

Schools Without Failure had a similar impact on the field of education as *Reality Therapy* had on the field of psychology. Glasser began to be known on a national, and even international stage. He was referred to as a nationally noted psychiatrist and school consultant and affirmed for his original ideas. His ideas, one writer admitted, would shake up educators, which he thought was a good thing since he wanted a copy of *Schools Without Failure* smuggled onto the desk of every district superintendent in the country. He was complimented as controversial and even his critics admitted Glasser was immensely influential in shaping education philosophy.[15] With the immediate interest in *Schools Without Failure,* the Educator Training Center, which was started the year before the book was published, became busier than ever. The Center had been created due to the interest of educators in the ideas of *Reality Therapy,* however now that Glasser had written *Schools Without Failure,* a book that specifically applied the principles of reality therapy to the classroom, the requests for SWF training were arriving in great numbers. As a result the Educator Training Center expanded significantly. Glasser's decision to accept the money from the Stone Foundation and start the Educator Training Center was paying off. The word was indeed getting out on how to create better schools.

Glasser entered the decade of the 1960s as a young psychiatrist working with severely impaired veterans and delinquent teenage girls, venues not associated with the fast track to making a significant impact. He left the decade of the '60s having published three books, each critically acclaimed, and the last two headed toward great success in terms of numbers of books sold. He entered the decade unknown and left it famous.

NOTES

1. NEA publication, 1971 reprint from 1969 talk in Las Vegas.
2. Wubbolding interview with Glasser.
3. Wubbolding interview with Glasser in Wubbolding's book, *Reality Therapy for the 21st Century*.
4. Glasser, W. (1969). *Schools without failure*. New York: Harper & Row.
5. NEA publication, *The Effect of School Failure on the Life of a Child*, 1969.
6. Glasser, W. (1965). *Reality therapy*. New York: Harper and Row. Pg. 7
7. Glasser, W. (1969). *Schools without failure*. New York: Harper and Row. Pg. 6
8. *ibid*, pg. 8
9. Glasser, W. (1969). *Schools without failure*. New York: Harper and Row.
10. *ibid*. p. 68
11. *ibid*. p. 70
12. Glasser, W. (1969). *Schools without failure*. New York: Harper and Row.
13. NEA publication, 1971 reprint from 1969 talk.
14. Glasser, W. (1969). *Schools without failure*. New York: Harper and Row.
15. Sykes, C. (1995). *Dumbing down our kids: Why American children feel good about themselves but can't read, write, or add.* New York: St. Martins Griffin. Pg. 72

7
INSIDE JOB

"A pill can never replace a friend."
—*William Glasser*

The March 1969, edition of *Playboy* magazine was a bit different from the rest in that Penny James, the model on the cover, was fully clothed. In fact, she had on a winter coat and long pants. Inside the magazine she had taken the coat off, along with a few other clothing items, but on the cover, she was laughing and looking over her shoulder toward the camera, one leg thrust up behind her, like she was jumping for joy, a carefree image that invited readers to check out the contents inside. In this March edition, besides pictures of Penny with her coat off, there was also an interview with Marshall McLuhan. By the late '60s, McLuhan, an English professor at the University of Toronto, had "won a worldwide following for his brilliant theories about the impact of the media on man."[1] Hailing McLuhan as the high priest of pop culture and the metaphysician of media, the article probed his views on technology, the alphabet, tribal culture, the printing press, and education, to name a few. It was a long interview, not all of it easy to follow, but something caught the attention of one of Glasser's friends and the friend recommended the article to Glasser.

Glasser was aware of McLuhan's emphasis on "the medium being the message," but it was McLuhan's comments on the growing crisis of identity in society that prompted Glasser to pause and consider the concept of personal identity through the lens of reality therapy. "From Tokyo to Paris to Columbia," McLuhan declared, "youth mindlessly acts out its identity quest in the theater of the streets, searching not for goals but for roles, striving for an identity that eludes them."[2] Glasser's tuning fork resonated with the idea that people were on a search for identity. He had said similar things to people involved in the fields of psychology and education. In fact, in *Mental Health or Mental Illness?*, Glasser had written, "The most important ego function is that of establishing identity."[3] But McLuhan wasn't talking to a specific field, he was talking to and about everyone. Every human being was struggling on a personal quest to really discover and savor his/her own unique beliefs, values, and purpose. Glasser especially noticed the idea that humans are searching for roles instead of goals, identity instead of achievements. Had McLuhan stopped there it would have been enough—his comments about identity and roles and goals had gotten Glasser's attention—but he went on to say more, and that more felt like a direct challenge to Glasser. After McLuhan referred to the crisis of identity the interviewer asked, "Do you relate this identity crisis to the current social unrest and violence in the United States?" McLuhan answered, "Yes, and to the booming business psychiatrists are doing."[4] One can picture Glasser reading that and feeling a bit like them's fightin' words. This fightin' feeling was not aimed toward McLuhan. Glasser would have been thankful someone else was singing the same song he had been singing for the last decade. No, instead the feeling ignited the inspiration to go into action. There was something very important in the concept of identity versus goals and Glasser's full creative forces would now focus with laser-like intensity on what that something was.

By the late 1960s society was indeed trying to find its balance. The euphoria after WWII and the optimistic growth of the '50s had been replaced by the tumult and tension of the '60s. On the home front we were rocked by the assassinations of the Kennedy brothers and of Martin Luther King; the growing debate over our involvement in Viet Nam; and the convulsions that arose out of our attempts to settle the issue of civil rights for every American. Fear seemed never to be in short supply. The Cold War and the nuclear arsenal that Russia and the United States now aimed at one another only added to this fear. And on a much different, but very real level there was the terror that many adults felt about where kids were headed nowadays. For many, Woodstock, the 1969 summer rock music festival in upstate New York, with its pulsating rock music, drugs, and kids swimming naked, epitomized this world of youth gone bad.

Billy Joel, who was 20 years old in 1969 and would go on to become a prolific pop star in his own right, would later write a song, *We Didn't Start the Fire*[5], that captured the angst of the times, much of it well-founded, and also pointed out that it wasn't his generation, the Boomers, that had started this angst. The angst, he reminded us, had been going on ever since the world began turning. Regardless of its source, though, the angst was a problem and Americans (along with pretty much everyone else on the planet) were searching for answers, or at least relief. American adults may have had disdain for the ways in which "kids" found relief—with things like marijuana, LSD, and promiscuous sex—but they had as much of their own drive to find relief in drugs and sex as the kids they criticized. An excellent example of this can be found in Milltown, New Jersey.

Frank Berger, a Czech emigrant working in England in the 1940s, could not have known what he stumbled onto during his search for a penicillin preservative, which was much in demand during the war. Working with a chemical called mephenesin, he noticed it had a tranquilizing effect on mice. After the war he moved to the United States and continued working with mephenesin, ultimately synthesizing it into a drug to relieve anxiety.[6] The tranquilizer was called Miltown, after the New Jersey hamlet where it was manufactured in 1955. Even though there was virtually no advertising (the FDA did not approve direct-to-consumer advertising until 1985), the release of the drug set off a consumer stampede. Within two years, Americans had filled 36 million prescriptions for Miltown, more than 1 billion pills had been manufactured, and these so-called "peace pills" accounted for one third of all prescriptions.[7] Not as cynical about drugs as they would come to be later, people referred to Miltown as "psychiatry's penicillin." In business terms, Miltown was incredibly successful. Even so, it would soon be eclipsed by two new drugs—Librium and Valium.

Valium, an anxiolytic, or anti-anxiety drug, was as one writer put it, "wildly popular," but that might have been putting it mildly. Introduced in 1963, by 1968 it was the most prescribed drug in the Western world. In 1972, the same year Glasser's next book was published, Hoffmann-La Roche stock, the manufacturer of Valium, traded at $73 per share.[8] Valium stayed at the top of the most commonly used drug list until 1982. In 1978, the peak of its popularity, 2.3 billion pills were sold. In the corporate world, Valium was so common that it was referred to as "Executive Excedrin."[9] The numbers would indicate we were desperate for something, desperate for answers. Whether it was the kids seeking escape in marijuana or the adults seeking escape in pills, a lot of people were in search of tranquility and coming to grips with who they were. We couldn't say we hadn't been warned. At the end of 1965 the Rolling Stones produced a song that went to #8 on the 1966 hit chart. The song was titled *Mother's Little Helper* and it captured this seemingly overlooked, yet powerful trend with barbiturate drugs.

Kids are different today, I hear ev'ry mother say
Mother needs something today to calm her down
And though she's not really ill, there's a little yellow pill
She goes running for the shelter of a mother's little helper
And it helps her on her way, gets her through her busy day

Society was indeed in search of answers. Some attempted to fast track the process of personal discovery through anger-filled, rage-prompted demonstrations against societal injustice, while others sought to shield themselves from the personal discovery process through drugs, which included alcohol. In either case, society in the late '60s could use some help.

Glasser, inspired by McLuhan's comments regarding identity and goals, and fueled by McLuhan's accusation that psychiatrists were a part of the problem, became even more convinced that reality therapy held the answer and that a book, written for the general public, which described the reality therapy process was needed. "The concepts of reality therapy," he wrote in 1973, "are not specifically psychiatric concepts. They are a way of life. They are a way of living your life or working with people or large groups of people. If you live this way, whatever you do can become more effective."[10] Glasser was convinced that people, anyone, not just mental health professionals, could apply reality therapy to their lives and in the process become mentally healthier.

Glasser's first book, *Mental Health or Mental Illness?*[11] appealed to those primarily in psychiatry; his second book, *Reality Therapy,* identified his unique therapeutic approach and expanded his audience to all of those in the helping professions, not only those in psychiatry, but also counselors, social workers, law enforcement and corrections professionals, and teachers; *Schools Without Failure,* his third book, applied the concepts of reality therapy specifically to the school setting. Now, though, due in part to the great need McLuhan had articulated,

Glasser felt clear it was time for reality therapy to be shared with everyone. From the beginning of his career, he had wanted to tear away the mask of mystique that covered the psychiatric process. His next book would describe how anyone, from the waiter in San Diego to the fish warehouse employee in Seattle to the executive in New York City to the parent of two toddlers in Miami, could become more responsible for his or her own mental health.

Schools Without Failure hit bookstore shelves about the same time Glasser read McLuhan's article in *Playboy*, which gives us a sense of how quickly things were moving then for him. No sooner had one book been published than Glasser was off and running on the writing of another. The writing he did was no small thing when you consider the backdrop of his life. The Institute for Reality Therapy had just been created in 1967. The Educator Training Center, due to the interest of educators in applying the principles of reality therapy to the school setting and spurred by the support of the Stone Foundation, was created a year later in 1968. Both of these organizations required the development of a supporting infrastructure, with all the challenges that go with creating a national, and even international network. Both organizations needed to respond to a growing number of phone calls and letters asking for information and training. This meant work sites needed to be located and employees needed to be hired. Within months after *Schools Without Failure* was published it became apparent the Educator Training Center needed to be a bigger organization than first envisioned.

Sue Reilly,[12] who did an article on Glasser during this time, provides a lens into the explosive growth of the Educator Training Center. Less than four years after it had really been established, the ETC became a force. "Today," Reilly wrote in the spring of 1973, "the ETC is a growing beehive of offices on the fifth floor of an office building in downtown Los Angeles. It employs 25 people, including 10 who do nothing but fly around the country teaching teachers how to create schools without failure. The other 15 are still answering requests for information and materials which now include feature films, film shorts, cassettes, books, magazines and a mound of other printed materials."[13] At the core of this explosion was Glasser himself, who, she pointed out, was now managing two institutions, providing training called Intensive Weeks for professionals wanting to implement his ideas, giving up to 75 speaking presentations a year, making short movies demonstrating his approach, consulting on several projects, and writing journal articles and books. On top of all this he even wrote and produced a play called *Beehive*, which ran for six months in 1975 in a Santa Monica theater. (The sitcom, *Three's Company*, which first aired the year after *Beehive's* run, and featured Santa Monica as a backdrop, had very similar themes to the play.)

The Intensive Weeks took time and energy, but Glasser saw them as critical to reality therapy's long-term success. Bob Wubbolding, who later would become the Director of Training for the Institute, remembers these early days fondly. "My involvement," he began, "goes back to the early '70s, maybe 1972. After finishing my doctorate I was investigating different counseling theories and I attended a workshop in Youngstown, Ohio. The approach I learned about at this workshop made the most sense to me and I wanted to know where I could go to learn about the approach in greater detail. When I asked Ed Ford, the instructor, he told me I would need to go to Los Angeles, since that is where the Intensive Weeks were conducted. So I started going to Intensive Weeks. One year I went four times. I had a brother who lived out there and I would stay with him and he would let me use one of his cars to go in from Northridge to the Educator Training Center on West Olympic Boulevard. All the programs were conducted in a room about 20' x 20', about the size of a small meeting room in a hotel. Glasser conducted all of them. And they all were done in Los Angeles."

Beginning in 1973, people could become certified in reality therapy, a process Glasser oversaw. Other training was taking place, too. Al Katz remembered going to Los Angeles during the summer of 1968. "We would work in the local schools in the morning and then had a workshop from Fitzgeorge Peters from 1-4 p.m. every afternoon where we reviewed the concepts of reality therapy. The training, which took place at the Educator Training Center, lasted for three weeks." If the figures in Reilly's article are correct, Al Katz was one of 90,000 teachers to receive training from the ETC during its first four years of existence, training in which the insights gained were then passed along to their 3.2 million students.[28] Glasser and those working with him were indeed busy. The *Reality Therapy* and *Schools Without Failure* message was being spread. People were reading his books and articles, they were listening to what he had to say, and they were being trained in his methods. This was good for the individuals and organizations, like schools, which were being helped by the ideas. It was also good for Glasser, since in 1974 royalties from his books were bringing in $5,000 to $6,000 per month and his standard speaking fee was $500.

Like his first three books, *The Identity Society*[14] was written by hand on a yellow pad, much of it while flying to speaking appointments. Like McLuhan, he believed something new was happening, and that while the traditional struggle for a goal—a job, a diploma, a home, a secure family—still existed, it had been replaced by the struggle to find oneself as a human being. "It is my argument," he explained, "that today almost everyone is personally engaged in a search for acceptance as a person."[15] Earlier he described identity as the totality of a person's unique beliefs and values, his distinct sense of I AM I. Glasser felt this change was due to major shifts in society, shifts that occurred over millions of years, and that this change had brought us to a point where we could, as a society, seek personal understanding and fulfillment. In the first part of the book Glasser became the anthropologist, wanting readers to grasp the background. He described how there have been two different kinds of society—either Primitive or Civilized—and each of these societies had experienced a Survival phase and an Identity phase.

Primitive Survival Society—Lasted three-and-a-half million years; man's primary goal was survival in a rigorous and hostile environment; those who cooperated with others survived; slowly the need for intelligent cooperation became a part of the human nervous system.

Primitive Identity Society—Occurred approximately 500,000 years ago; successful cooperation led to increasing moments of rest and freedom from stress; people were helping one another not just to survive, but also to experience pleasure; people lived peacefully in a fairly abundant, non-stressful environment; people had time for rituals, symbols, and religion.

Civilized Survival Society—Lasted approximately 10,000 years up to around 1950; as population increased, land became more valuable and people began to prey upon one another; conflict became the rule, rather than the exception; to survive, individuals became subservient to the group; hierarchies existed in which a few strong people occupied the top while many more people grubbed for existence at the bottom.

Civilized Identity Society—From 1950 to present (for Glasser it would have been from 1950 to 1970, since he was writing *The Identity So-*

ciety in 1970); affluence made it possible for more people to become politically concerned with human pleasure; people became focused on their identities and how they might express them; intelligent cooperation and involvement became essential skills; those who, through involvement, can match their roles and their identities, develop a success identity; those who are unable to achieve a satisfactory role end up developing a failure identity.[16]

Whether or not the anthropological emphasis was helpful, *The Identity Society* went on to explain some of the most important concepts in Glasser's reality therapy approach to life.

Even before the book was published Glasser began floating the ideas to his audiences in talks and articles. In 1970, in an interview with *U. S. News & World Report,* he explained, "When a student begins to depend on memory rather than on thinking, it provides him with a very thin potential for identity, for discovering the world and his place in it."[17] There were problems with rote learning, memorization, and irrelevance that were more serious than people realized. When students withdrew or tried to distance themselves from this kind of teaching format it was wrong, he added, to label them as mentally ill. People withdraw into a world of their own choosing, a process that has everything to do with identity. Glasser gave a talk that summer at a science teachers' workshop, under the direction of Harry Wong, at Stanford University. A year later the talk appeared as an article in *The Science Teacher* journal. He explained that we are constantly evaluating ourselves and we either see ourselves as successful or potentially successful, or we label ourselves as failures. He urged readers to consider that a healthy identity is based on being accepted for one's basic humanity, rather than being judged for what one does or accomplishes. In an environment where failure is so much a part of the system, like a school, for instance, it is to be expected that students will cope by either agitating or withdrawing. Schools had a preoccupation with making these judgments, which prompted Glasser to provide his own definition of failure. "If you are fishing 25 miles off shore," he began, "and you drop your camera overboard—that is failure. The options are all over. In 2,000 feet of water, that camera is gone. There is no way you are going to get it back. That is what failure is like. All paths to success are closed." His point was that schools don't have to be like boats 25 miles off shore. He added, "The outside world doesn't operate on a failure system nearly as much as schools do."[18] The importance of whether one sees oneself as either a success or a failure cannot be overstated. As Henry Ford once said, "Whether you think you can or can't, you're right."

A month before *The Identity Society* was published, *The Saturday Review* ran an article entitled "The Civilized Identity Society: Mankind Enters Phase Four." Glasser used the article to more fully explain the anthropology of the book—from Primitive Survival to Primitive Identity to Civilized Survival to Civilized Identity—which may have put some off, or at least shielded some from examining the real points of the book. He felt it was important, though, to propose a rationale for how we came to that moment in history. If this emphasis did put off some or distracted some from seeing the message of the book, it's a shame because *The Identity Society* described and explained key points regarding the principles of reality therapy.

The book was dedicated to Donald O'Donnell, which confirmed the esteem in which Glasser held O'Donnell both personally and professionally. In 1968, O'Donnell became principal of the Ventura School in Palo Alto, California, bringing along three of his teachers from Orangevale with the plan the school would become a *Schools Without Failure* model. Glasser and O'Donnell had worked together closely for seven years by the time the book was published. Their relationship embodied a concept Glasser emphasized in the first chapter: "The only way you can maintain a successful identity is to accept and be accepted by others whom you respect and who believe you are worthwhile."[19] Positive, caring relationships are vital for every human being to be mentally healthy. Glasser acknowledges that people may not always experience support and acceptance, relationships can break down and even be destructive, but he reminds us when we feel bad we must learn to reduce the pain in a way that does not separate us from others. Whether a wife fretting about her unloving husband or a student bummed about the way his school treats him, both search for ways to cope with the frustration. Often they turn to various forms of self-medication. People want to feel good, whatever it takes.

In *Reality Therapy* Glasser introduced and emphasized the significance of involvement or a positive, caring connection between two persons. For him, involvement between therapist and patient was a key. In *The Identity Society*, though, he was expanding the concept of involvement outside of the therapeutic treatment room to anyone struggling to cope. "In the new Identity Society," he explained, "the most common cause of pain is the failure to get involved, which we experience as loneliness." Our basic needs, the need for worth and the need for love, are met through involvement or connections with other people. There are different reasons to feel bad, he pointed out, but "none is as painful as becoming directly aware that we are alone, rejecting and rejected by others around us." When I asked him during one of our interviews what his definition of involvement was, he said simply, "making a relationship that's satisfying to both parties." Because it sounds so simple, some view the concept of involvement as unimportant, a mistake it turns out, that continues to have a serious impact on individual well-being and ultimately our personal and national healthcare costs.

Of the new Identity Society, Glasser wrote, "fraught with loneliness and failure, is more concerned with relief of pain and suffering than any previous time." As support for this statement he reminded readers that one-fourth of all prescriptions were for tranquilizers or pain relievers, and more than half of the people who see physicians do so for non-specific complaints, rather than for a specific ailment. Newspapers advertised dating services to match one lonely person with another lonely person. Hotlines and help lines were available to the despondent, and help groups like Alcoholics Anonymous, Gamblers Anonymous, and Synanon were thriving as people turned to others dealing with the same pain, frustration, and failure. Glasser made his case for widespread loneliness and failure because he was setting the stage for several key beliefs of reality therapy. In fact, the collection of statements that follow form a cadre of essential readings for those wanting to understand the reality therapy approach to life. One of these keys centered on the belief that when a person is unable to become involved or connected with others, especially the important people in his or her life, the person will start to focus on being self-involved. To help us comprehend this behavioral dynamic Glasser wrote, "To avoid the fact that we are really involved with ourselves, we have learned to focus our attention on a creation outside ourselves. We create and then concentrate on an idea, such as an obsessive fear of germs; a behavior, such as compulsive gambling; a physical symptom, such as migraine headache; or an emotion such as depression. We focus on these self-creations as if they were real and separate from us. Keeping overly clean, gambling, suffering and treating a headache, or being depressed then becomes our problem in place of our true problem—that we need others. We have chosen to act as we do because we desperately hope the symptom or the behavior will provide enough involvement to satisfy what we should get from others."

These small inward steps are coping responses, a defense against the implications of failure. "A little depression from time to time is normal," he continued. "Most people recover and again move toward others. Staying depressed for a long time, however, signifies our inability to gain new involvements to replace the old ones. The depression now becomes a friend, not a good friend, but a faithful, foul-weather friend whom we can always count on, a friend who, if we are incompetent, may consume all of our time to the point of immobilizing us with his friendship." Of course, the implications of statements like these are very significant. Rather than softening the implications, Glasser declared, "I believe every psychologically diagnosable condition is an example of involvement with one's own idea, behavior, symptom, or emotion, or some combination of them." Such statements left no room for doubt as to his beliefs regarding how people cope with loneliness and failure.

Rather than being attacked, so to speak, from some condition or circumstance outside of ourselves, and rather than having to deal with something biologically wrong in their brain, people were constantly in the process of setting up their lives to be as pain-free as possible. Rather than being passive recipients of mental and physical symptoms, people were active participants in the pursuit of that which felt good, while consistently deflecting and dodging that which felt bad. "A person may say, 'My headache is back,' as if it had gone on vacation and then suddenly returned." Glasser may have chuckled while he wrote this, however it was a point he really wanted his readers to get. The responsibility for our mental health lies within us.

He may have declared in *Mental Health or Mental Illness?* that he wanted any interested person to be able to "easily gain a basic understanding of psychology," but comparatively few people read the book, and certainly very few of the general public read the book. Now, though, the situation was changed. He had become a well-known author in the fields of psychology and education. His last two books were significant sellers. Now when he wrote so that any interested person could understand the psychology of the human mind there was a better chance that interested people would read it. *The Identity Society* was written for that reason.

An emerging issue revolved around Glasser's commitment to the idea of personal responsibility and the implication that a person has control over his or her mental health. It was a thorny topic and frequently drew responses from audiences. Glasser's position that there was nothing wrong with a person's brain was in direct opposition to a growing majority who believed that neurotic and psychotic symptoms were the result of a mental illness. While Glasser had to address this, it was his trainers, the reality therapy and schools without failure instructors who probably had to deal with this topic even more. The people who flew into Los Angeles to receive training directly from Glasser himself, and who paid for the plane fare and arranged for the hotel, probably already were in significant agreement with what Glasser was saying. It was the instructors out in the hamlets of the South or the cities of the Northeast or the towns of the Midwest who had to face the cynics and skeptics. Usually the person who challenged this concept had a brother battling schizophrenia or a spouse in deep depression. There is no way, they would often passionately argue, their brother or their spouse was in control of this illness. Forty years later this debate continues.

Glasser, wanting to address this issue and wanting to explain it in a way that any interested person could understand, wrote: "Obsessions, compulsions, psychoses, and most long-term symptomatic illnesses that have no presently known medical cause all serve the same purpose as depression. They act as companions that lonely people choose because they are unable to tolerate the knowledge that they have only themselves with whom to become involved." Glasser went on to acknowledge, "Many reasonable people take exception to the word 'choose.'" It was hard to believe people would choose crazy and outlandish behaviors. Even so, if one was to understand the concepts and implications of reality therapy, then understanding this point was critical. Glasser, sensing this importance, further explained: "An adult who is crazy, withdrawn, and hallucinatory did not choose this behavior out of the clear blue sky. He began developing it years before with short periods of voluntary detachment, withdrawal, and involvement with his own thoughts. His symptoms were kept under control until a severe stress, an extreme rejection, or a long period of loneliness and failure occurred, causing him to grasp and elaborate his previous mild symptoms into a complete withdrawal from reality, a withdrawal we call psychosis."

Glasser had described this process in his very first book more than 10 years earlier when he talked about how the ego, over time, can become thickened, completely surrounding the person and separating him from the world. "A completely psychotic person," he wrote, "is not able to fill any of his needs in the world because of the wall thrown up by his ego. This does not mean, however, that his needs go unfulfilled—it means that they go unfulfilled in the world. Actually they are partially or completely fulfilled within the thick-walled confines of his own ego. We call this method of satisfying needs 'crazy' because, according to reality, or our conception of reality, his needs are not satisfied." In effect, the crazy person creates a world in which, "He is sufficient in himself."[20] Although this description might have been clear to a therapist or someone in the field of psychology, terms like ego thickness made it less appealing to the general public. Now, though, in *The Identity Society*, Glasser was taking the concepts of reality therapy to the masses, and he was explaining some of the most profound implications of the theory in a way that "any interested person could understand."

As noted earlier, when Glasser was writing *The Identity Society* in the late '60s and early '70s, brain drugs that affected mood had already made huge inroads into American households. And, of course, besides the legal mood "affecters" like prescription drugs and alcohol, there were also many illegal drug choices available. He allowed that, "Probably some pills are necessary for failures who are doing little to get involved," and at times the use of a tranquilizer might be wise. (His use of the word "failures" here is consistent with terminology he used throughout the book. In *Reality Therapy* he used the terms "stronger" and "weaker" to describe people's behavior; now he was using the terms "success-oriented" and "failure-oriented.") These statements, however, do not mean Glasser was ambivalent about brain drugs. On an institutional level, drugs might make patients easier to deal with, but he said that did not justify their use. Medical practice was based on relieving pain, but doctors did not understand that some behaviors are actually psychological companions and prescribed medication focusing on the symptom. Because of this connection— the connection between psychological symptoms and doctors prescribing mood-altering drugs—pharmaceutical companies were in a frenetic search to fill the demand.

Glasser agreed that success-identity people could occasionally use alcohol, aspirin, or a sleeping pill without harm. However, failure-identity people enter a danger zone with the same behavior, even though it seemed reasonable. This was one of the reasons why the concept of identity was so important. "Drugs are harmful for people with failure identities," he wrote, "because they make the loneliness, the failure, and the self-involvement tolerable. They allow us to sit on the hot stove and not feel the pain." Rather than viewing loneliness and frustration and pain as symptoms to be eliminated, Glasser saw them as mechanisms built into our brains that alerted us to make a change. He added, "The more ingenious our society is at finding pain relievers, the less progress we will make toward helping failing people find the success that will produce pleasure." Drugs might have their place, but he reminded us, "A pill can never replace a friend."

He so much wanted to emphasize the importance of this internal journey and the power of personal responsibility. "In a survival society, powerful people use punishment to keep control. In the identity society, however, internal control is needed instead of external control." Glasser believed understanding reality therapy would bring people into this place of internal control. And it could be used by anyone. "Reality therapy is not exclusively for the 'mentally ill,' incompetent, disturbed, or emotionally upset. It is a system of ideas designed to help those who identify with failure learn to gain a successful identity and to help those already successful to maintain their competence and help others become successful." The concepts were clear and without the usual psychological jargon, he felt, and could be applied by anyone to the circumstances of his or her life. "The principles of reality therapy," he assured, "may be used by parents with children, teachers with students, ministers with parishioners, and employers with employees. One of the best ways to gain a successful identity for oneself is to use these principles in everyday life; as you try to live a better and happier life yourself, you will help those around you." Glasser was extending a challenge and an invitation all at the same time. *Reality Therapy* had gone from a gleam in the eye of *Mental Health or Mental Illness?* to the psychiatric wards of the veteran's hospital and then to the schools-without-failure classrooms. Now it was being offered to anyone who wanted to know how to live a happier, self-controlled life.

Two other topics are especially noteworthy in *The Identity Society*. The first was Glasser's early insights into the effects of television viewing on young children and its connection to what was then referred to as hyperactivity syndrome. The second topic centered on the correctional system and its strategies regarding incarceration. In both cases his views turned out to be prophetic.

"I consider television a danger to children between ages 2 and 5," he explained, "because they should then be learning by playing with each other, to socialize and communicate. Children need many social experiences to gain confidence in their ability to be involved. The greatest obstacle to a child's socialization, an obstacle probably as harmful to success in the Identity Society as being malnourished was dangerous to life in the Survival Society, is excessive viewing of television." The concept of involvement, the importance of being connected to life, and connected to other people, was as critical for children as it was for adults, probably more so. "Television," he continued, "is a passive, nonsocial medium that stimulates a child's nervous system enough to make him feel comfortable, but does not fulfill his nervous system's need for involvement because it deprives him of social play with others." Drawing on the significant time he spent in elementary and secondary classrooms, Glasser had a clear picture of students who seemed to have no social responsibility and who overwhelmed teachers with their senseless, erratic activity. When asked to read or to complete an assignment they were unable to put forth the needed effort. Glasser noted the "popular explanation for the hyperactivity seen in children is that they have a brain abnormality that has suddenly become almost epidemic." Remember that he wrote this in 1972. "No reason is given for this abnormality," he continued, "in which the brain seems to stimulate the child with bursts of erratic, nervous energy that cause the hyperactivity. Once this diagnosis in made, drugs (amphetamines) are prescribed to calm the abnormal brain activity and make the child less active." Glasser felt strongly that there was nothing wrong with the child's brain that less television viewing and more intellectually stimulating classrooms wouldn't help.

Forty years later we have come to suspect excessive television viewing and video games are a factor in what is now referred to as Attention Deficit/Hyperactivity Disorder. Glasser was on the right track there. The importance of the concept of involvement, though, has not been appreciated, due in part to the belief that children really do have something wrong with their brain and drugs are the only answer. In 2002 it was reported that of the 50 million school-age children in the U.S., 4-6 million are on stimulant drugs.[21] Studies also showed that 15-20 percent of fourth and fifth-grade boys are receiving drugs.[22] We will consider the effects of brain drugs on people, and especially children, later in the biography, but for now we can see Glasser was on the right track here, too. While he emphasized the importance of involvement with other children, he may have underemphasized the vital importance of involvement between children with parents. In the chapter entitled, The Family in the Identity Society, he did describe how parents could be reasonable and humane, and how difficult it was for parents to limit television viewing when the TV was such a good mechanical companion, but you don't get a sense he appreciated the need for a very close, intimate connection between child and parent. It is possible this lack of emphasis on child/parent involvement may have been due to the more distant, almost business-like relationship he had with his own mother.

Glasser was not unique in bringing up the problems within our correctional system, but he was one of only a few voices who saw the concept of punishment for what it was. "Correctional reform does not occur," he explained, "primarily because we do not accept that crime is almost always a product of failure, that in our correctional system we punish failure, and that the punishment of those who fail only drives them further into failure. If we can view criminals as failures more than as people who must be punished, we can change the system to give them a chance for success, an option that our present system denies." His experience at the Ventura School for Girls and the talks he gave to many administrators and staff within the California correctional system gave him a front row seat to the results of a traditional punishment focus. If the correctional system was truly going to correct dysfunctional and destructive behavior, then a much different focus was needed. Glasser resonated with the National Committee on Violence's evaluation that: "Programs of rehabilitation are shallow and dominated by greater concern for punishment and custody than for correction." And he agreed with law professor, Norval Morris, and criminologist, Gordon Hawkins, when they suggested, "We quit attempting to use criminal law as an instrument to coerce men toward virtue. The law is not suitable for such a task." Rather than correct criminal behavior, the President's Crime Commission noted, "The conditions in which they live are the poorest preparation for their successful re-entry into society and often merely reinforce in them a pattern of manipulation or destructiveness." Forty years later U.S. prisons are significantly overcrowded and there seems no reason to think that trend will change. Glasser desired to teach people what it meant to be responsible for their thinking and their behavior, and in the process to develop a success identity that contributed to their happiness, as well as to the happiness of others. People gaining and maintaining a success, more than anything else, would prevent the destructive behaviors that led to incarceration and help those already behind bars to prepare for their release back into society.

    Glasser felt this personal responsibility must be taken into account when determining guilt during a trial. While he advocated for more effective responses to criminal behavior, he did not advocate a *laissez-faire* attitude toward crime, nor did he want to accept excuses for criminal behavior. Much publicized court cases, based on insanity defenses, had gained acquittals for the accused or helped the convicted to gain a more lenient sentence. Glasser, though, did not agree with the basis for these decisions. "I discount almost all of the arguments," he explained, "that criminal behavior should be excused on the basis of insanity, the influence of drugs, or other psychological circumstances." Brian Lennon talked with Glasser about the insanity defense and he thought Glasser's reply was interesting. "When I hear of a man," Glasser began, "repeatedly raping a tree, I will begin to believe in the insanity plea." Ultimately, Glasser believed that rather than accept excuses for bad behavior, people needed to be helped toward developing a success identity, and in the process a success plan for life.

Glasser concluded *The Identity Society* by describing a community approach to mental health. He called it the Community Involvement Center. "The concept of the CIC," he offered, "is that each community would have its own organization to help its failing people, no matter what symptoms they exhibit." Glasser believed such centers, with staff members who understood the principles of reality therapy, could be developed and that they could make a difference.

It is impossible to capture the importance of *The Identity Society* in this brief space. Glasser wanted it to convey the ideas of *Reality Therapy* in a bigger and better way than he had ever done before. His previous books were critically acclaimed and even though they were written for specific professional markets they were also significant financial successes. *The Identity Society* was meant to take the concepts of reality therapy even higher than his other books. It was going to be the crown jewel in an impressive publishing run. *Reality Therapy* and *Schools Without Failure* were significant publishing successes. Glasser thought *The Identity Society* would be even better. As it turned out the sales of *The Identity Society* were more modest.

Glasser later admitted: "[I] thought identity was an important thing, but apparently more important than other people thought. I thought I was making a critical and even crucial observation, and that it was going to be a big seller, but people couldn't relate to it well. I really thought *Identity Society* was going to get everyone excited. Well, it didn't, you know, although," he added, "it's still a heckuva good book." *The Identity Society* was an important step along the way, not only summarizing reality therapy up to that point, but also, as Glasser pointed out later, it "was the start of a lot of ideas that continued into choice theory."

There may be several explanations for its pedestrian performance. One thing to keep in mind is that it probably wasn't fair to compare it to the success of his earlier books. Two grand slams in the psychology market is a good run by any standard. A second thing to consider is the possibility that the beginning of the book may have put some readers off, or at least not grabbed their attention. Glasser believed he had to set up the book by describing a social evolutionary process that spanned millions of years. The big article in *The Saturday Review* just prior to the book coming out really emphasized the evolution aspect. It may not have been the most effective way to hook the casual reader. A final reason the book was less successful revolves around the possibility that people were not ready to accept responsibility for their moods and their behaviors and ultimately, their mental health. Society was already firmly attached to tranquilizers and other brain drugs in the belief that mental problems were diseases, caused by agencies outside of a person's control, similar to any other biological illness or disease. Hence, if the cause was outside of us, or external to us, the solution was also external to us. A book describing how people were internally responsible for their own mental health and how they could, through new insight and disciplined choices, affect positive change in their lives would not be a big seller in such a society. As Glasser himself wrote in the book, "It is much easier for everyone to believe that the person just got 'sick' and that no one has any responsibility for what happened."

Even though *The Identity Society* was not a bestseller, Glasser's professional life did not slow down at all. In fact, the mid to late '70s may have been the busiest time of his life. The Institute for Reality Therapy struggled to keep up with requests for Glasser to make presentations, as well as for materials and training sessions, while the Educator Training Center was at full throttle, with multiple trainers crisscrossing the country. It was a hectic schedule, but Glasser seemed to thrive on it. In 1973, Joe, Glasser's eldest child, was 22 and completing his student teaching at a Glasser model school in Palo Alto; Alice, his middle child, was 18 and at UCLA studying for a degree in public health; and Martin, his youngest, was 15 and attending a local high school.[23] Glasser was especially close to Martin. More than one of his close friends confided to me that Martin was to Glasser what Glasser was to his father. Of the three, though, it was Joe who was most attuned to his father's success and influence, and Joe who most wanted to follow in his father's footsteps. This was unfortunate because of the three, Joe was the least capable of pulling that off. He was very friendly and lovable, but at times he seemed to lack common sense or discipline. Later it would even become difficult for him to hold down a job.

Glasser talked about two events he felt revealed these tendencies in Joe, both occurring in 1974, yet in some ways these events seem to be more of a comment on the lens Glasser was looking through, rather than an indictment of Joe. The first event had to do with responsibility; the second event was almost tragic beyond words. For much of his life in California, Glasser owned a sailboat, and Joe wanted to sail the boat to Catalina Island, 22 miles across open ocean, by himself, at night. Apparently, Glasser gave his okay for this adventure, but emphasized that Joe had to call home when he got there and let them know he was safe. He didn't call, though, as this was before cell phones, so it created a lot of worry and fear. It is true that calling right away after completing a solo trip across open ocean would be the responsible thing to do, but should not calling overshadow the fact that your son just accomplished something that very few would even have the courage to try?

The second event involved Martin and one of Martin's friends. Confronted in a parking lot in San Diego, Martin and his friend were stabbed and seriously wounded. When asked if he knew what caused this terrible incident Glasser responded that he most certainly did. "I know exactly what caused it," he began. "My son, Joe, who really did a lot of senseless things, took him to an amusement park in San Diego, and afterward they were walking to the car. Martin's friend was along, too. His father was a big shot television producer. I can't remember his name. But anyway, they were approached by some Mexican kid and asked for a quarter. Martin was going to give him the quarter. He reached into his pocket to give him the quarter when both Martin and his friend were stabbed. And Martin's intestines fell out on the ground. The other kid was stabbed in the liver. Joe took them to Scripps hospital, but it was a mistake because they had no idea how to deal with trauma."

It may be Glasser knew about details surrounding this event that he didn't share with me, details that were more incriminating as far as

Joe was concerned, however from what we know it seems like a stretch to blame Joe for the attack. On the surface it appears that big brother was taking little brother and his friend out to do something fun when tragedy struck. Colleagues of Glasser who knew his family described Joe in the same way Glasser described him—lovable, big ideas, but couldn't carry through—which confirmed he didn't relate to Joe from a perspective of unfair bias. Glasser loved Joe and was committed to supporting him for as long as was needed, yet he was also frustrated with him. These events, which on the surface don't seem to be good examples of Joe's irresponsibility, might be better examples of a father's struggle to know what to do.

Martin's status worsened in the hospital. Glasser, due to his medical degree, recognized that Martin needed to be moved to a different hospital. Bob Wubbolding remembers being at a training in L.A. when the stabbing took place. "I was at an Intensive week, which Glasser was teaching since he did all of the Intensive weeks. And he would go down to see Martin in the evening and then come back to teach in the morning. People were wondering why he was going down there. Well, Martin was stabbed! His favorite son is stabbed. He's coming back to teach and driving back down there. We never would have known anything was wrong. It wasn't like he was upset or anything, at least visibly. I'm sure he was, but he has this amazing ability to not let things bother him." Glasser's matter-of-fact response to this frightening event, rather than being professionally impressive, can also be interpreted as emotional detachment. People may have wondered how he could go on like nothing happened with his son's life hanging in the balance. Martin recovered, though, and life went on.

Glasser continued traveling and speaking and writing. An important theme that emerged during this time centered on his belief that America's medical system was not set up to care for most of the cases it handled. "More and more people are choosing to become sick," he explained, "which is overburdening the medical profession who are generally trained to deal with people who have something wrong with them and are not trained to deal with people who are making the choice of illness because they don't know what else to do. Too much of our money is being spent in an attempt to deliver medical care to people who really aren't medically ill. We could easily afford to deal with only the people who have true disease."[24] In the years that followed this 1973 statement, healthcare in the U.S. would head in the exact opposite direction from that which Glasser was trying to warn. In 2009, more money per person was spent on healthcare in the U.S. than in any other nation in the world, even though over 50 million Americans did not have medical insurance. Over 17% of our Gross Domestic Product (GDP) is spent on healthcare. A 2001 study found 46% of personal bankruptcies were due to medical debt, a figure that rose to 62% in 2007. To make matters even more frustrating, our high medical costs do not translate into better results. In 2010, the U.S. ranked 49th among other countries for life expectancy rates and 44th for infant mortality rates. The system we have isn't working, which might in itself inspire one to take another look at Glasser's approach.

The Identity Society may have been less successful than his previous books, but it did not dissuade Glasser from writing his next one, *Positive Addiction,* which was published in 1976. He got the idea of positive addiction while reading *The Boys of Summer* (1972), by Roger Kahn.[25] James Michener called Kahn's contribution America's finest book on sports, and a *Sports Illustrated* panel acclaimed it as the greatest of all American books on baseball. While we don't know if

Glasser similarly recognized the book's deeper literary value, what we do know is that he was drawn to the story of George "Shotgun" Shuba, one of the players on the Brooklyn Dodgers championship team of 1953. Shuba, wanting to improve his swing as a 16-year-old boy, decided that he would swing a bat through an imaginary strike zone 600 times a day, a practice he continued through the minor leagues and into the majors. Glasser thought about this for a long time and began to realize that willpower alone could not explain this incredible commitment. No, Glasser thought, Shuba was addicted to swinging a bat. And, rather than this "addiction" weakening him and making him dysfunctional, it actually made him stronger, not just physically, but mentally. Intrigued by this possibility, Glasser began to stop some of the runners who constantly ran by his office on San Vincente Blvd. They would pass by day or night, sometimes even very late. When he asked them if they were addicted to running, after thinking about it they admitted that they probably were. Glasser concluded people could become addicted to activities that, instead of trapping them in a destructive spiral, actually added strength to their lives and freed them to achieve a higher level of creativity, a state he would come to call the PA (Positive Addiction) state of mind.

As an outline became clear in his mind Glasser began to write, on a computer for the first time, the words that would become his next book. Also, for the first time, he conducted research in an effort to collect data for the manuscript. The very first sentence in the book—"Very few of us realize how much we choose the misery in our lives."[26] —signaled its link to all of Glasser's writing up to that time. As to the book's audience, Glasser wrote: "In between the very strong, who are mostly happy, and the miserably weak, are the partially strong or the almost strong enough. It is here that most of us exist, strong enough to get along fairly well but not strong enough to live without a lot of unnecessary suffering. It is mostly to this majority group in our society that this book is aimed." *Positive Addiction* was unique, although Glasser couldn't resist using it as a springboard for his familiar themes. For instance, he reiterated: "Many experts in my field behave as if it (depression) came from the outside, beyond the patient's control, that he 'caught it' as if it were some sort of psychiatric chicken pox. I believe this position is wrong. Depression, no more than acting out, does not come from the outside. We don't catch it like chicken pox. It is out of our weakness we choose to be depressed because we have discovered that not making this choice is even more painful." To Glasser, a real depression was the imprint your couch makes in the carpet.

Glasser wanted people to realize they were not born with a stamp on their foreheads that designated them as either weak or strong. Our destinies are not predetermined. People can learn to become stronger or they can make choices that lead to weakness. What separates the strong from the rest of us, he concluded, is "their ability to find love and worth when most of us would give up and settle for less." He explained that achieving the PA state through positive addiction took initiative, self-discipline, and commitment. It had to be a personal choice and the activity had to have inherent value. Running and meditating are two of the activities described in the book, but there are many more. For instance, Glasser talked about his almost-addiction to public speaking. Self-criticism and competition were two elements that he felt effectively defeated the PA state. He knew this from personal experience and admitted how sensitive he has been throughout his life, an interesting revelation from someone who has been willing to give unrehearsed demonstrations in front of packed gymnasiums, or who consistently debated his fellow psychiatrists, and who has been accused of being matter-of-fact to a fault. If people were consistent in the activity, though, and if they devoted enough time to it, and if they were relaxed in this process, he discovered they could enter a trance-like, transcendental mental state.

His research confirmed this as well. Eliciting the help of Joe Henderson, the editor of *Runner's World,* ran a questionnaire in the October 1974 issue entitled Help Wanted. The questionnaire sought responses to 22 questions related to the activity of running. From a subscription list of 20,000, Glasser was pleasantly shocked when he received 700 responses. The data clearly indicated positive addiction was indeed a reality, although it rarely happened until the runner had built up enough endurance to run effortlessly for an hour. The book wasn't just about running, though.

Glasser wanted people to understand how they could add strength and quality to their lives. Whether it was the catchy title or the content of the book inside, more than a 100,000 copies were sold, and it put the concept of positive addiction into the literature, something which pleased Glasser. He dedicated the book to his parents, yet when we talked about that he admitted that they really didn't know a lot about what he did or the ideas he championed. His parents had moved to Florida in 1949 and remained there until both passed away. His father was 89 when he died. His mother never told the family when she was born, but Glasser figured she was a couple of years older than his father. The school districts in Sarasota, where his parents lived, were actively pursuing the *Schools Without Failure* model and Glasser would go to Sarasota to speak and give trainings. His parents both attended several of those presentations. Glasser's sister also settled in Sarasota. The Glasser sibling who least got along with their mother would be the one to live the closest to her the last 35 years of her life.

When Glasser was finished with the *Positive Addiction* manuscript he called his cousin, Bob. As mentioned, Bob Glasser had edited Glasser's first four books and he thought he would be working on *Positive Addiction*. As it turned out, Bob didn't edit Glasser's fifth book. "Why did you stop at four?" I asked him.

"I stopped at four," Bob said without emotion, "because his children had grown and Naomi thought she could do it and they didn't want to have money going out of the family. I remember very well when he had written the fifth book, which I expected to work on, and Bill talked to me and said, 'Naomi and I would like to come over in the evening.' Well, Marie and I knew something was going on. And they came over, and he said, 'Well, this book doesn't really need much editing, so I'm not gonna have any editing done.' So, I told you what I think was going on, which would not have been appropriate for him to say. It could well be that it needed less. Some people told me that maybe it made me feel good that those books didn't read as well as the ones I did, but that would be self-serving to say that. Harper Brothers, and then Harper and Row, and now Harper Collins, they also edit, so the smoothness of the reading can also be due to their editing. If Naomi did less, maybe they did more. I don't know. I'm sure the real reason was financial. He started off giving me 10%. I think after *Reality Therapy* did so well I asked him for 15%, which he gave me and that's what I then got from then on, of course, of his share." Naomi Glasser was, in fact, a very good editor. More than anyone, she knew what Glasser was trying to say. Now that the children were older, besides having the skill to edit, she had the time as well. It made sense to involve her in this way.

Glasser made it clear later that *Positive Addiction* was not a little sideshow, but an important part of the journey. One reviewer of the book felt the book made the same basic assumptions as *Reality Therapy* and that Glasser presented an interesting conjecture, but provided no scientific data to back it up. This criticism is interesting in that *Positive Addiction* actually had data on which it was based.

Throughout the late 1960s and '70s Glasser maintained a busy schedule that kept him traveling and speaking and demonstrating. One of these talks was given to a large group of teachers at Lynwood High School in Los Angeles. The group was, in general, suspicious of outside experts and felt that only a teacher could understand the challenges of teachers. Yet as he talked, the dynamic and the energy in the room changed. Sue Reilly observed this as it took place and later wrote: "They have become our students and Glasser has established himself as a guy with his own marbles who knows a better way to play the game." This audience—indifferent, skeptical, and even suspicious—represented those who had not given reality therapy ideas a chance, but they also came to represent those who, after listening to Glasser and considering his approach, recognized there was a lot in his ideas that made sense. He had entered a hostile environment, but the power of his approach won them over.

More and more people were being won over, but it was a slow, individual process. Glasser and his team had found their stride. The Institute for Reality Therapy and the Educator Training Center had evolved and developed into successful organizations, both spreading the good news about the principles of reality therapy. An effective working system was in place. Imagine his colleagues' response when Glasser informed them he was planning to change things a bit. And we're not talking about the "color of the carpet" kind of change. Just when everything seemed to be in place and working well, Glasser decided to make significant alterations to his basic beliefs. The year 1976 was an important one for Glasser's ideas.

Notes

1. Norden, E. (1969, March). The Playboy Interview: Marshall McLuhan. *Playboy Magazine.*
2. Norden, E. (1969, March). The Playboy Interview: Marshall McLuhan. *Playboy Magazine.*
3. Glasser, W. (1960). *Mental health or mental illness?* Harper & Row, p. 13
4. Norden, E. (1969, March). The Playboy Interview: Marshall McLuhan. *Playboy Magazine.*
5. Billy Joel featured the song We Didn't Start the Fire on his *Storm Front* album, which came out in 1989. The song went to #1 in the United States and the album won the Grammy for best album of the year.
6. Menand, L. (2010, March 1). Head case: Can psychiatry be a science? *The New Yorker.*
7. Dokoupil, T. (2009, January 23). America's long love affair with anti-anxiety drugs. *Newsweek.*
8. Menand, L. (2010, March 1). Head case: Can psychiatry be a science? *The New Yorker.*
9. Barber, C. (2008). *Comfortably numb: How psychiatry is medicating a nation.* New York: Pantheon Books.
10. From a talk Glasser gave at a workshop at the University of Kansas Medical Center on the health of children. Reproductions of the talk can be found in *The Roots of Responsibility: A Solution to Community Intervention for the Health of Children and Youth,* edited by Wynona Hartley and published in 1973, and in *The Reality Therapy Reader: A Survey of the Works of William Glasser,* edited by Alexander Bassin and published in 1976.
11. Glasser, W. (1960). *Mental Health or Mental Illness?* New York: Harper and Row.
12. Reilly, S. (1973, May). Dr. Glasser without failure. *Human Behavior Magazine.*
13. Reilly, S. (1973, May). Dr. Glasser without failure. *Human Behavior Magazine.*
14. Glasser, W. (1972). *The identity society.* New York: Harper & Row.
15. *Ibid,* p.2

16 Society descriptions are summarized from *The Identity Society* and from Glasser's article in the Saturday Review entitled *The Civilized Identity Society: Mankind Enters Phase Four*, which can be found in the February 19, 1972 edition.
17 Glasser, W. (1970, April 27). Youth in rebellion—why?: An interview with top psychiatrist. *U. S. News & World Report.*
18 Glasser, W. (1971, March). Reaching the unmotivated. *The Science Teacher, 38(3)*, 18-22.
19 Glasser, W. (1972). *The identity society.* New York: Harper and Row. p. 7
20 Glasser, W. (1960). *Mental health or mental illness?* New York: Harper & Row. p.114.
21 Breggin, P. (2002). *The Ritalin fact book: What your doctor won't tell you about ADHD and stimulant drugs.* Cambridge, MA: Perseus Publishing.
22 Marshall, E. (2000, August 4). Duke study faults overuse of stimulants for children. Science, 289:721.
23 Reilly, S. (1973, May). Dr. Glasser without failure. *Human Behavior Magazine.*
24 Hartley, W. *editor* (1973). The roots of responsibility: A solution to community intervention for the health of children and youth. From a talk given by William Glasser for a workshop at the University of Kansas Medical Center. This article can also be found in the *Reality Therapy Reader*, which was edited by Alexander Bassin.
25 Glasser, W. (1977, July). Promoting client strength through positive addiction. *Canadian Guidance and Counseling Association, (4)11*
26 Glasser, W. (1976). *Positive addiction.* New York: Harper & Row.

8
Trip to Chicago

"I was desperate for a theory when Powers came along."
—*William Glasser*

"There's a package for you on your desk." Glasser heard his wife's voice from the kitchen. He was just getting home after a long day and was putting his briefcase down after coming in the front door.

"What was that?" he replied.

"A package came for you today. It's on your desk."

"What is it?"

"It looks like it might be a book," Naomi suggested. "It's from Sam."

As he entered his office, Glasser glanced at his desk and saw the package, which was wrapped in brown parcel paper. He remembered Sam telling him about a book that he should read. Curious, Glasser sat down at his desk and began to take the wrapping off. Naomi was probably right, he thought to himself. It felt like a book. Big things can come in small packages, but Glasser could not have appreciated, as he removed the wrapping, just how much this book would affect him for the next 20 years of his life.

WG

Very soon after *Reality Therapy* (1965) was published, Glasser began to make presentations and give workshops in New York City. To a great extent, Glasser's East Coast presence was due to the efforts of Alexander Bassin. Bassin was the Chief Researcher for the Kings County Supreme Court Probation Department, which in simple terms means he worked within the Brooklyn court system. More important, Bassin "was perturbed by the disheartening results of turnstile sentences given to addicts."[1] The Brooklyn courts were jammed full of the same people being processed by the system in an endless cycle of dysfunction and crime. Bassin's frustration inspired him to co-found Daytop Village, a treatment facility for those struggling with drug and alcohol addiction. His frustration also led him to *Reality Therapy* and the belief that RT approaches would be helpful for those dealing with addiction, whether they were at Daytop Village or being processed within the courts. Bassin arranged for Glasser to come to Brooklyn and speak to people who worked within the court system, especially those involved with the probation and treatment of addicts. One of the people who attended and became involved was Sam Buchholz, a Brooklyn attorney who, like Bassin, was interested in helping to rehabilitate people who seemed trapped in the criminal court system, especially those with mental problems. Similar to Bassin, Buchholz was impressed with the concepts of *Reality Therapy* and he and Glasser became good friends. "I used to talk a lot to Sam Buchholz in those days. We would talk about my ideas and I would tell him that I was looking for a theory that would put my ideas together." During one of these talks Buchholz responded he had just gotten a book Glasser ought to read. He said it was called *Behavior: The Control of Perception*[2] and was written by a fellow named William Powers. Glasser had never heard of either the book or its author, but he expressed interest in what Buchholz was describing, enough interest that Buchholz went out and bought another copy of the book and sent it to him. This was the package that Glasser opened on his desk.

Glasser's desire to find a supporting framework for his ideas was more than a casual hope. In fact, Glasser recalled: "I was desperate for a theory when Powers came along." Al Katz, one of his early colleagues, felt that *The Identity Society* marked the beginning of Glasser's search for a theory to explain reality therapy. Fitzgeorge Peters, another colleague, explained how Glasser knew that he needed a philosophical base. "He knew what to do, but didn't know why he was doing it." By this time Glasser was aware of the criticisms of his ideas—that he did not base his positions on research, that his ideas were not in line with the current literature, and that they did not reflect the accepted practices of his field—and this may have spurred his desire for a theoretical underpinning. He knew the ideas worked. He had seen firsthand how a reality therapy approach could strengthen people, even people who had been institutionalized because of mental dysfunction. For him, the efficacy of the approach was not the problem. For others, though, for people who were not aware of how well the approach worked or for fellow professionals who questioned or even rejected the approach, Glasser wanted to bring his theory into alignment with a supporting philosophical framework. He wanted to create not only a compelling counseling package, but also a compelling approach to life from which anyone could benefit.

Glasser has been a reader of books, magazines, and journals throughout his life, so it was no chore to begin to read *Behavior: The*

Control of Perception, especially since it was recommended by a close friend. However, as a writer who liked to make ideas as easy to understand as possible, Glasser soon found *Behavior: The Control of Perception* slow going, and even a struggle. Still, something held Glasser's attention.

Powers alerted readers at the outset that *Behavior: The Control of Perception* "represented a break with traditional psychologies,"[3] a position that would have piqued Glasser's interest, and that the book "presents a model of the brain's internal organization,"[4] which sounds straightforward enough. For much of the rest of the book, though, Powers introduces and explains what he calls the orders of perception, or control systems of increasing complexity. He uses terms such as feedback, compensator effect, purposive behavior, time scales, intensity, line of command, gamma reference signal, vector control, disturbance, thalamic third order systems, and reorganization, to name a few. Carefully and methodically, Powers makes his case for how the brain works. There are many charts in the book, each of which was meant to visually clarify the model that Powers is proposing, but these charts, which are based on the complicated nature of the book, are complicated themselves. One can imagine Glasser sensing something important in this section of the book, yet struggling nonetheless.

Toward the end of the book, however, the tone changes from complex theory to more understandable application. Given that he has made his case for the science of the brain, Powers begins to talk about the implications for human behavior. And it is here that Glasser would have been drawn into greater focus. Whatever the concept was, according to Powers, be it the concept of the existing social order, or the concept of monetary structure, or the concept of the family, or the concept of sport, "no matter how such concepts arise, what governs a person's behavior is his own structure of system-concept perceptions, and his own set of reference levels for those concepts."[5] Powers was describing a personal internal world, a world in which control was a very important issue. He knew that he was on to something, but he also recognized his own limitations. "To many readers," Powers wrote, "the implications of this theory of conflict for psychotherapy will be obvious and I hope exciting. I will not, however, try to develop a therapeutic approach in this book." As he read this, Glasser must have felt that a therapeutic approach based on this way of thinking already existed. "Instead," Powers continued, "I will close by applying the theory of conflict to show the impracticality of one of the most common modes of human action and interaction: self-control and mutual control of behavior. I think it can be shown that the idea of controlling behavior—one's own or that of other people—stems from an old but incorrect concept of human nature, incorrect because it fails to recognize the control-system properties of human nature. What we commonly think of as control is not control at all but conflict. Intrapersonal and interpersonal conflict thus result directly from our misunderstanding of the feedback control process in ourselves and in others."[6] For Powers, a person was "in conflict" when he wanted two incompatible goals to be realized at the same time. This situation, he pointed out, led to anxiety, depression, hostility, unrealistic fantasies, delusion, and hallucinations. "I have become more and more convinced," he wrote, "that conflict itself, not any particular kind of conflict, represents the most serious kind of malfunction of the brain short of physical damage, and the most common even among 'normal' people."[7]

As Powers described how attempts to control behavior arbitrarily—one's own or that of other people—accomplishes nothing in the long run but to produce conflict and pathology, you can almost feel the momentum gaining speed in Glasser's mind. According to Powers, even the way we attempt to control ourselves, through sheer force of will, is misguided and counterproductive. "Through social custom and the use of reward and punishment," he began, "we have perpetuated the teaching of self-control and have thus all but guaranteed that essentially everyone will reach adulthood suffering severe inner conflict. Self-control is a mistake because it pits one control system against another, to the detriment of both. Exactly the same reasoning applies if the two control systems are in separate human beings. Arbitrary control of the behavior of one person to suit the goals of another person ignores the goals that are already governing the behavior of the other person, and inevitably creates conflict."[8] Powers recognized the ineffective, and even destructive, results to both those being controlled and those doing the controlling. Unfortunately, he pointed out, the history of civilization is a history of people attempting to control other people.

It was significant to Powers that society had for millennia perpetuated distrust, prejudice, hatred, and crime, even as people tried to come up with more forceful ways to punish and control those who misbehaved. "I think we have missed something vital," he wrote with a sincere pleading in his tone. "The model I propose here is not necessarily the one that will solve our problems, but I am convinced that what we need is to be found in this general area." He allowed that he may not have had it all perfectly figured out, but he was sure he was in the right neighborhood. Glasser was pretty sure Powers was in the right neighborhood, too. "Control theory," Powers continued, "shows how our methods of teaching principles and system concepts are themselves the roots of violence."[9] When we attempt to control another person it creates an intrinsic error that urges that person to seek another direction. Our efforts to modify our control tactics only produce corresponding creativity in the person being controlled to circumvent our tactics.

These descriptions from Powers begin to give us a sense of his thesis. The ideas Glasser would embrace and articulate so effectively slowly appear out of the mist. As a person, Powers seemed to possess a unique blend of humility and thoroughness and passion. The earlier sections of the book, which are more technical, mask this passion. However, by the end of the book his humble, yet strong, feelings come through. "If I seem reluctant to get to my final point," he wrote, "it is because I cannot really believe that the answer is so simple, nor can I see any reason why I should be the one to point it out. There is quite literally nothing special about me; indeed I know less about human beings than most of the human beings I meet, which is not a great number. I can invoke no authority of my own, no long string of past accomplishments to lend credence to this thesis. I must rely on each reader confronting these theoretical notions directly, out of sheer curiosity or good will, making an effort to understand that I cannot force or even influence. I, too, was raised in a society in which control of behavior is accepted as natural and necessary. I cannot help feeling anxious about the thought of leaving so important a concept, having such enormous potential importance, open to each individual's private decision to consider or not consider, to believe or not believe. But my own theory tells me that I can do nothing else!"[10] Such language was the beginning of a gentle call to arms, for Glasser even more so.

Powers was convinced no person could control the behavior of other people without causing what he called "intrinsic error," and the only error a person could successfully correct was his or her own. The future of society virtually depended on this paradigm of personal responsibility. "There is only one way I can see for fallible, ignorant beings to live in accord with their own real natures," he challenged, "and that is to discard forever the principle of controlling each other's behavior, dropping even the desire to control other people, and seeing at every level the fallacy in the logic that leads to such a desire. Whatever system concept we adopt in the effort to reach the conflict-free society, it must contain one primary fact about human beings: they cannot be arbitrarily controlled by any means without creating suffering, violence, and revolution. The major premise of civilization has, I submit, been proven wrong."[11] Those familiar with Glasser's writing will see a deep connection and respect for passages such as these.

"Let me clarify this," Powers continued. "In our American society there is a widespread belief in the rule of law (enforced by physical punishment) and in the use of incentives tied directly to our ability to stay warm, well fed, and otherwise happy. There is a stubborn insistence that our worsening social problems can only be solved by strengthening the punishing force behind the law and by sternly withholding necessities from those who will not behave properly. Even further, there is a strong belief that these methods are all that are preventing total collapse of our system, and that increasing social tension is traceable to insufficiently vigorous and consistent use of reward and punishment. If we are to trust the theory in this book, however, we must conclude the exact opposite. The more faithfully we adhere to the system of incentives and the rule of law, the closer must the country approach a state of open revolt. What our leaders (and we ourselves) are doing in an effort to save the country from dissenters, revolutionaries, and malcontents is the direct cause of the increase in numbers of such persons."[12] Powers' theory was challenging deep, core beliefs of society.

He admitted there were pieces in his theory that might be wrong and some of the details in his charts would, through experimentation, be improved. But in closing, he added, "I would, however, be exceedingly surprised if the basic idea behind this theory failed to hold up to test: the concept of behavior as a feedback process organized around the control of perception, and reorganized as a way of maintaining ourselves in a peculiarly human condition defined by intrinsic reference levels. That much is all we need in order to see the fallacy of interpersonal control; the rest is dispensable detail. In order to avoid self-destruction, I think that all we need do is consider openly and very carefully the implications of this basic concept of human nature. That one concept, so antithetical in its implications to the ways in which people have always thought about each other and themselves, gives us a place to stand from which we can move the world."[13] *Behavior: The Control of Perception* began with a series of complicated descriptions and explanations, yet concluded in a deeply human tone that was part invitation, part inspiration, and part persuasion. It was a gentle and hopeful warning.

I have included these longer passages from *Behavior: The Control of Perception,* several in their entirety, because it is important for readers to get a sense of what Glasser was experiencing as he read these same passages. It was these passages toward the end of the book that fueled Glasser's desire to understand the technical sections at the beginning of the book. It was the passages at the end, the ones in which Powers explained the implications of his theory, that caused Glasser to feel a growing kindred spirit with a fellow author. He and Powers were basically saying the same things, although each in a different way and from a different perspective. As much as Glasser appreciated another voice crying in the wilderness, though, what he was after was the theory that explained the success of his reality therapy approach. And that meant he would need to understand the material in the front sections of *Behavior: The Control of Perception,* the technical details and charts. During one of our conversations, after I had described how I was struggling with the book, Glasser pointed out he wasn't willing to put the kind of work into it I apparently was putting into it, but I came to believe this really wasn't accurate. He read the book multiple times, each time hoping for and seeking a breakthrough. When the breakthrough didn't come, however, Glasser recalled how he said to himself, "It's too hard. Why don't I go talk to the guy and have him explain it?"

WG

William Powers lived in Chicago, so it wasn't like a drive across town for Glasser to sit down with him and talk about the concepts in *Behavior: The Control of Perception*. Glasser was committed to discovering a theoretical framework for reality therapy, though, and he was becoming increasingly sure Powers and this concept called control theory held the key. He contacted Powers and explained he had read the book several times; he felt Powers was on to something very significant; he was struggling to really understand the technical elements in control theory; and that he wondered if it would be possible for the two of them to get together and talk about the book. Glasser added he would be willing to fly to Chicago if Powers would be willing to visit with him.

It would have been interesting to know what Powers was thinking as he agreed to meet with Glasser, as well as in the days leading up to Glasser's arrival. Even though by 1977, when he first met with Powers, Glasser had published five books, Powers at first did not know very much about this West Coast psychiatrist who called him out of the blue. Glasser chuckled as he recalled how Powers and his wife, Mary, felt some research was in order. Mary was a librarian and she looked Glasser up. Referring to Glasser, she told her husband, "He's done some stuff and he'd be worth talking to."

At one point in *Behavior: The Control of Perception*, Powers attempts to describe what it is like to act without conflict. Such a person feels effortless and free from the need to force himself to behave in a certain way. At the end of this passage Powers shared something that really caught my eye. "The late Abraham Maslow described the unconflicted person far better than I can," he admitted. "I wish he could read this chapter."[14] Maslow died in 1970, but in a way Powers was still about to get his wish. A famous psychologist[15] did read that chapter and now he wanted to have Powers explain the concepts to him in even greater detail.

As agreed, the two Williams—William Glasser and William Powers—got together and discussed the science of behavior. Glasser flew to Chicago and met with Powers in his home. For two days over which the talks took place, Glasser stayed with the couple as their guest. Powers was a year or so younger than Glasser.[16] The kindred spirit Glasser sensed while reading *Behavior: The Control of Perception* turned out to be true. He remembered Powers as being a very nice, warm person. It would be ideal if their talks were recorded, but they weren't and the closest thing we have to a record of their conversation is the product that came out of their collaboration. Glasser was matter-of-fact, yet appreciative, regarding their time together. "I went there and he explained it to me. It wasn't an hour-long visit, it was like two or three days, a long time, and I left with the feeling that I understood it enough to rewrite it in a more understandable form."

Glasser had stated in his first book he wanted to write in such a way "that any interested person could easily gain a basic understanding of psychology."[17] Now as the ideas began to take shape in his mind for another manuscript, his sixth book, this same goal, that people could easily gain insights into their own behavior, was as strong as ever. Some in his field criticized him or ignored him for what they considered to be his elementary emphasis, but Glasser was firm in sticking to this goal. The mystery needed to be taken out of psychology. Powers had admitted in the preface to *Behavior: The Control of Perception* that "I once felt that it was my duty to supply the model with content as well as form, but I am wiser now, and much more impressed with my ignorance. What is up to me is in this book. What I do best is in this book. Others who know more about behavior and many other subjects are the ones to put the content in."[18] Glasser certainly would have seen this statement beckoning to him as an invitation. "I did see that," Glasser affirmed, "and Powers and I talked about it. I told him I want to take your ideas, giving you full credit, and make them more available to people, people like myself who are counseling and working in schools and that kind of thing. He applauded it. He thought it was wonderful."

Making Powers' ideas more available meant that people would better understand the control theory concepts. The technical concepts in *Behavior: The Control of Perception* would be like a foreign language to many readers. Glasser pointed out that although Powers' book was praiseworthy and respected in behavioral science circles, "no one had taken his theoretical ideas and attempted to translate them into usable psychological theory and practice."[19] During our interviews Glasser confirmed: "I was trying to translate Powers because his book was very, very hard to understand. I worked at it, went to see him, and I was still having trouble understanding it, especially the levels or orders of perception."

Some might say Powers, rather than needing a translator, simply needed a bigger megaphone. His ideas were clear, some might argue, but very few people had heard of him or were aware of his work. As one of the most widely read authors of books dealing with psychology and human behavior, Glasser was now offering Powers a larger platform. In Glasser's own words: "After reading his book four times and thinking about it almost constantly for six months, I contacted Powers and asked him if he would work with me and help me to write this book, which should be usable by the layman. He read my earlier books, felt we had much in common, and agreed to act as consultant to the project. *Stations of the Mind* is the result of this collaboration."[20]

Once again Glasser embarked on a writing project with another person as an important resource. Powers became the new Harrington. G. L. Harrington had been the supervisory muse who inspired the creation of *Reality Therapy;* now William Powers was given that mantle in the creation of Glasser's version of control theory. As with Harrington, Glasser quickly and consistently gave credit to Powers for the concepts he was writing about. "I gave Powers full credit for what I was doing," Glasser emphasized. "I don't pretend that it was my idea." Readers of *Stations of the Mind* are reminded of Powers' importance through Glasser's use of the pronoun "we," rather than using the singularly personal pronoun "I." In the preface to Stations of the Mind, Glasser explained, "At times on my own and often with his help Powers and I have moved the ideas in his book beyond the basic concepts of his more theoretical volume. If, as you read, you notice that I use the term we on most occasions, I do this because the thinking was mostly a collaborative effort. The writing I must take responsibility for alone."[21] As in the preface, Glasser emphasized in chapter one: "I will call extensively upon William Powers' sensible theory of how our brain works."[22] With all of these examples of Glasser according so much credit to Powers, it is interesting this would later become an issue in the minds of some.

And so, Glasser wrote, with the help of William Powers, another book, his sixth, which was titled *Stations of the Mind,* and like his previous books was published by Harper & Row. Powers wrote the foreword for the book in which he noted, "Bill Glasser has invented an unusual method for learning a new theory: write a book about it."²³ In control theory, Glasser had found a theoretical framework that explained how human beings were motivated to behave primarily by internal, rather than external forces, and he became driven to present the principles of reality therapy within the new control theory concepts. Besides the visit to Chicago, Glasser phoned Powers on a regular basis for a year, comparing the details of their individual beliefs and seeking to accurately represent control theory in the process. The process of their work together must have been effective, since Powers wrote, "Glasser has been scrupulously careful to check his understanding of control theory with me every step of the way. If there are any differences between his concepts and mine as the book now reaches its final stages, they are unimportant, and tend to be in areas where the theory itself needs work. As far as the main concepts in this book are concerned, you can be sure that Bill has checked his translation against my understanding, and that in the background there is a solid scientific foundation for what he asserts about systems that control their own input."²⁴

At the beginning of *Stations of the Mind,* Glasser proposed: "Throughout this book, as we explain how our brains work, we will make clear that because we are living creatures we are moved by inside forces. While outside forces affect what we may choose to do, they do not cause us to behave in any particular or consistent way."²⁵ The elements of reality therapy were based on a belief in personal responsibility and in the personal power individuals have to make better choices. Control theory provided the science on which reality therapy was based, and as a result, Glasser pursued a careful understanding of how the science worked. If Glasser was going to be a translator, he would have to know the language of control theory as well as he knew the language of reality therapy.

Much of *Behavior: The Control of Perception* was complicated, and Glasser's version of it, *Stations of the Mind* also turned out to be somewhat complicated. *Stations of the Mind* was much more readable than *Behavior: The Control of Perception,* but it was still more complicated than anything Glasser had written. In spite of this, *Stations of the Mind* introduced new terms and concepts that would remain with Glasser and appear frequently in his writing for the rest of his career. For instance, Powers helped Glasser more clearly see that the only person we can control is ourselves, a belief statement that would later become the first in a list of Glasser's control theory axioms. From Powers' concept of redirection and reorganization, Glasser developed his view of organized and creative behaviors. The famous "stopping at a stoplight" and "answering a telephone" scenarios as examples of our freedom to choose were from Powers, as was the idea of a thermostat as an example of our personal inner control mechanism. It was Powers who came up with the idea of an internal world, which Glasser later defined as our quality world. The significance of this internal world led Glasser to embrace verbs more fully—for instance, a person is depressing or choosing to depress, rather than a person is depressed. And because of BCP's charts and diagrams depicting brain activity and human behavior, it was Powers who inspired Glasser to develop his own chart on how the brain works. To be sure, William Powers had a significant influence on William Glasser.

Powers' model was based on what he called the 10 orders of perception, which were 10 different levels or ways from which people made sense of the world around them. The orders were listed in a hierarchy that began with simple levels of perception, then moved to higher or complex levels. Glasser wanted to capture the details of the orders of perception in *Stations of the Mind,* yet he struggled with how to convey them in a way that mattered to people. Even though Glasser would eventually move away from an emphasis on the orders of perception, the chapter he devoted to the orders in *Stations of the Mind* contained further examples of Powers' influence. "All we ever know of the real or external world or outside world," Glasser explained in this chapter, "is the energy that comes from the world and strikes the sensory receptors of our perceptual system." Those familiar with the present Glasser chart on how we behave, an understanding of "the chart" being one of the learning cornerstones of the Glasser Basic and Advanced workshops, will recognize this way of describing our relationship to the real world. "Everything else," he continues, "that we claim is the real world is in fact our own perceptions of that world, perceptions which we constantly try to change so that they coincide with the world in our head."[26]

Glasser wove the beliefs of reality therapy with the science of BCP and besides introducing new ways of looking at behavior and mental health, he also renewed his emphasis of already familiar themes—themes such as rewards and punishment having only a temporary and almost always a negative effect; choosing our misery in an attempt to stabilize our lives; the potential of severe misery and unhappiness ultimately leading to neurosis and even psychosis as a person seeks to create a reality that satisfies his/her needs; severe misery also possibly leading to physical symptoms or what Glasser called "diseases of reorganization,"[27] which is another way of describing the body's creative response to continual stress. Regarding diseases of reorganization he explained further "those who reorganize with sickness would, albeit unknowingly, rather lose physical than mental control of their lives."[28] His beliefs surrounding psychosomatic illnesses were not new, however BCP psychology added greater support to those beliefs. He included a chapter on addiction and the effects of drugs on people. (Given his then recent book entitled *Positive Addiction,* he made sure to refer to it as negative addiction in *Stations of the Mind.*) Once again, he came back to the bedrock foundation of the book—that being that our behavior is about our attempts to control for our perceptions. Similar to a person setting a thermostat for a certain temperature, people also set or create expectations in their heads for how they want the world to respond to them. Because of this dynamic, drugs and alcohol can be especially dangerous, in that these substances "reduce our ability to sense a perceptual error."[29] In other words, as Glasser explained, it would be like a pilot setting the plane on autopilot to fly at 10,000 feet, but as the plane drops to 5,000 feet there being no error signal. "This is why," he says to get our attention, "when counseling alcoholics we must at times be brutal enough to break through and cause the alcoholic enough error so that he/she senses something is wrong. This is hard to do because this rough, forceful counseling causes error in the 'caring' counselor, but it is the only approach which will work."[30]

He included in the chapter on drugs and alcohol several of the then famous prescription drugs, such as Thorazine, Haldol, Prolixin, and Ritalin. Glasser flat out stated that hyperactive is a misnomer and that hypo-behaviored was a better diagnosis for what appeared to be a growing epidemic in children's behavior. Their pressing, demanding behavior was a cry for attention, a long, drawn-out tantrum. Referring to drugs like Ritalin he allowed that "used for a short while and coupled with attention, firmness, teaching, and minimal TV watching, these drugs can help us to deal with difficult children, but we must not be misled by the initial calming to believe that needed behaviors can be learned from a drug."[31] Brain drugs were well established by 1979 and 1980, when Glasser was writing *Stations of the Mind,* and his comments to his own field of psychiatry were similar to his comments regarding Ritalin to the physicians, educators, and parents who were seeking help. "Too many psychiatrists believe that we must tranquilize away the delusions and hallucinations no matter how much drug we have to use. But getting rid of the delusions and hallucinations," he reminded, "only stops reorganization; it does not provide the behaviors needed to resolve the conflict that started the process."[32] He kept bringing people back, ultimately, to responsibility and self-control.

Glasser admitted something in *Stations of the Mind* that would be good for those wanting to lead lives based on the principles of reality therapy to consider. He wrote, "William Powers says it takes about two years of hard work to change from seeing the world in stimulus-response terms to BCP, and in my experience his estimate was very close. It has taken me two full years to get to the point where, at least, I now see almost everything this way. I still can't behave this way as much as I would like to, but I'm working very hard to reduce the amount of ineffective SR that I still use."[33] Glasser was the author of *Reality Therapy* and an expert on internal control theory, yet when he met Powers he still hadn't come to grips with just how much stimulus-response thinking affected his own life. Rather than this being discouraging to the rest of us, I believe others can actually take hope in this. If William Glasser struggled with the SR to BCP transition, then maybe it's all right if others on the journey struggle, too. When we talked about this very thing during one of the interviews, I said, "If even *you* have to go through this transition time, then maybe the rest of us shouldn't be frustrated if it takes us a while to get it." He responded quickly "Yah, that's possible. I didn't want to make it sound like it's simple."

Powers had warned readers in the foreword of *Stations of the Mind* about such a time frame. "I've found that most people take about two years to reach the point where they suddenly realize that they understand the basic concepts of control theory. It takes about a week for them to think they understand it."[34] He also reminded readers, "Just keep returning to one basic principle: we control what we perceive, not what actually exists, and not what we do."[35] This was the key to Powers' control theory thinking and Glasser tried to stay true to this maxim throughout the book.

Years later, even after further tweaks and changes to his theory of human behavior, Glasser felt *Stations of the Mind* was a good book. It was too complicated for his liking, even arcane, as he put it, but it represented a significant evolution in his ideas. There was one statement in the book with which he later disagreed. It read, "It seems that for people to be able to become psychotic, that is, to undergo long-term, sometimes continuous reorganization and live their life directed by this system, they must have not only a large error but also some genetic predisposition. We seem to need some genetic psychochemical propensity for at least one or more of our major neuro-transmitter systems to be pathologically involved in this disruptive reorganization."[36] After I shared that with him, he shrugged and said, "I would never say any of that now." When I pressed him a bit he replied, "Well, that's just where I was." Overall, though, throughout his career, Glasser stayed true to the main ideas in *Stations of the Mind* and to the principles of Powers' version of Control Theory. This doesn't mean he didn't modify its details to better fit his approach. He did make changes, and they would come sooner rather than later, but the bigger picture stayed in focus.

Glasser remembered Powers being the last person, other than Glasser himself, to write an introduction or foreword for one of his books. "I don't think anyone else ever did that," he said thinking back. "I got to the point where I felt others were not as far along in their thinking as me, and I still think that way." Glasser actually liked what Powers wrote in the foreword; the same cannot be said of the book's introduction, which was written by Hans Selye, who had done so much research and writing on the existence and effects of biological stress. Nominated for a Nobel Prize in 1949, Selye was very well known throughout the 1960s and '70s as the psychological expert on stress. When I mentioned that Selye had written the introduction for *Stations of the Mind* and how that must have been a big deal, Glasser disagreed. "No, it wasn't a big deal," he candidly shared. "It was a mistake, actually." Why was it a mistake, I asked? "Because," he continued, "Selye was supposed to read the book and write the introduction after that, but he never read the book. He just wrote a standard thing that was more about him than the book. My publisher sent him some money, but it was hard to get him to write it. I wanted to cancel him doing it. I was looking for verification and I thought I would get it from him. It was a big disappointment."

Glasser first read *Behavior: The Control of Perception* in 1976, the same year *that Positive Addiction* was published. He went to Chicago to meet Powers at the beginning of 1977, probably February or March of that year. While the Institute for Reality Therapy and the Educator Training Center carried on with training and mentoring support, which Glasser himself was still very much involved with, his real creative focus was directed toward understanding control theory. He was writing the manuscript for *Stations of the Mind* in earnest by 1978. The year in which *Stations of the Mind* was published, 1981, turned out to be significant for Glasser both professionally and personally. The first Reality Therapy convention was held in Illinois during the summer of 1981. Further, it was decided the Institute would benefit from having an Advisory Board of Directors, a structural support piece that has continued ever since. Not done yet, 1981 was also the year in which the *International Journal of Reality Therapy* was launched. This valuable resource has served as a communication tool for philosophical viewpoints to be shared and practice strategies to be explained. On a personal level, Glasser's father, Ben Glasser, passed away at 89 years of age.

Glasser is convinced his father died as a result of injuries from being beaten up by his mother. Glasser's nephew, who is a physician and lived in the area, was pretty certain Glasser's mother had a stroke and that during the stroke she somehow believed that Glasser's father was attacking her. "She," in Glasser's words, "went after my father and damn near killed him." His father never recovered from the attack. "He couldn't deal with it," Glasser explained. Glasser's nephew shared with Glasser the last thing his father said. Ben Glasser was weak, he was talking very softly, but he motioned to the nephew to come close and he said, barely above a whisper, "I want you to know I always paid my own way." Glasser affirmed, "And that was true. I never picked up a check for my father. None of the children ever did. My father built this house for me. He did all these things. He wasn't a rich man, but he always paid his own way." When Glasser's father passed away his parents had been married for over 60 years. Glasser, who was 56 himself, had always loved his father deeply and his passing must have affected Glasser on a deep, emotional level. As in the past, though, his matter-of-fact way of processing life kicked into gear.

Glasser's career can be divided into three distinct eras. His trip to Chicago to meet and work with William Powers represents the bridge between the first two eras. When Glasser got on the plane in Los Angeles to travel to Chicago in 1977 he was still in the first era, the Era of Reality Therapy. Getting on the plane in Chicago to return to Los Angeles, after spending time with Powers, marked the beginning of the second era, the Era of Control Theory. It would be more than three years from the time of that trip back to Los Angeles until *Stations of the Mind* was published, but the book being published was simply the fruit of what began with that plane trip. As with most worthwhile journeys there were setbacks ahead for Glasser, some of them sooner than he wanted. He chuckled as he shared with me how on the train ride from Powers' neighborhood back to O'Hare airport he fell asleep and missed the airport stop completely. He remembers waking and getting his wits about him. The train had continued on to a yard area or what felt like, as Glasser described it, the "end of the line." He got out of the car he was in and carefully and gingerly walked across multiple electrified tracks, suitcase in hand, on a search for transportation back to O'Hare. Setback or not, Glasser had found what he believed to be the theoretical framework on which reality therapy could be based. Powers had made a compelling case for the science of internal motivation. Now Glasser just needed to explain it so more people understood it. More setbacks than electrified tracks lay ahead, but at that moment, on that plane ride back to Los Angeles, his mission was clear.

NOTES

1. From the Our History section of the Daytop Village website at http://www.daytop.org/history.html.
2. Powers, W. (1973). *Behavior: The control of perception.* Hawthorne, New York: Aldine de Gruyter.
3. Powers, W. (1973). *Behavior: The control of perception.* p. 1
4. *ibid.*, p. 18
5. *ibid.*, p. 172
6. *ibid.*, p. 251
7. *ibid.*, p. 253
8. *ibid.*, p. 260
9. *ibid.*, p.264
10. *ibid.*, p.266
11. *ibid.*, p.270
12. *ibid.*, p. 270
13. *ibid.*, p. 272
14. Powers, W. (1973). *Behavior: The control of perception.* p.260
15. Glasser's masters degree and almost doctorate were in psychology. He ultimately completed his medical degree and specialized in psychiatry.
16. In 1977 Glasser would have been 52.
17. Glasser, W. (1960). *Mental health or mental illness?* New York: Harper & Row.
18. Powers, W. (1973). *Behavior: The control of perception.* p. xi.
19. Glasser, W. (1981). *Stations of the mind: New directions for reality therapy.* New York: Harper & Row, Publishers, p. xx.
20. *ibid.*, p. xx.
21. *ibid.*, p. xx.
22. *ibid*, p. 9
23. *ibid*, p. ix.
24. Glasser, W. (1981). *Stations of the mind: New directions for reality therapy.* New York: Harper & Row, Publishers, p. x-xi.
25. *ibid*, p. 2

26 Glasser, W. (1981). *Stations of the mind: New directions for reality therapy.* New York: Harper & Row, Publishers, p. 90.
27 Glasser, W. (1981). *Stations of the mind: New directions for reality therapy.* New York: Harper & Row, Publishers, p. x-xi., p.171.
28 *ibid*, p.198.
29 *ibid*, p.209.
30 Glasser, W. (1981). *Stations of the mind: New directions for reality therapy.* New York: Harper & Row, Publishers, p.212, 213.
31 *ibid*, p.220
32 *ibid*, p.220.
33 Glasser, W. (1981). *Stations of the mind: New directions for reality therapy.* New York: Harper & Row, Publishers, p. 234.
34 *ibid*, p.xiii.
35 *ibid*, p.xiii.
36 Glasser, W. (1981). *Stations of the mind: New directions for reality therapy.* New York: Harper & Row, Publishers, p.270.

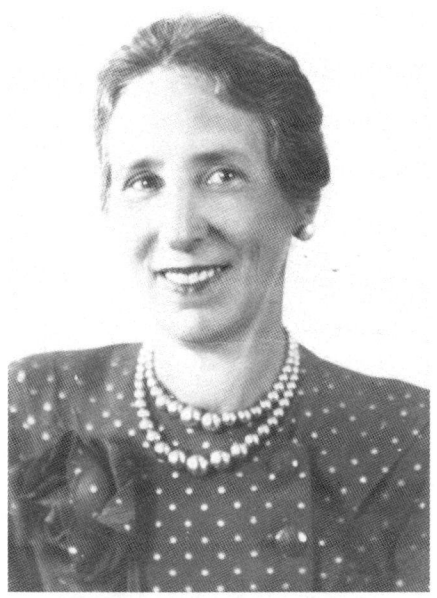
Glasser's mother, Betty

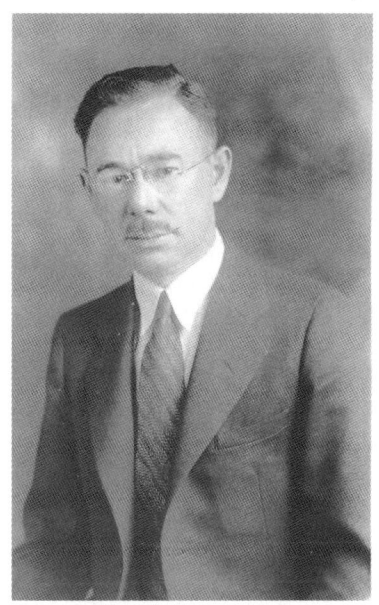
Glasser's father, Ben

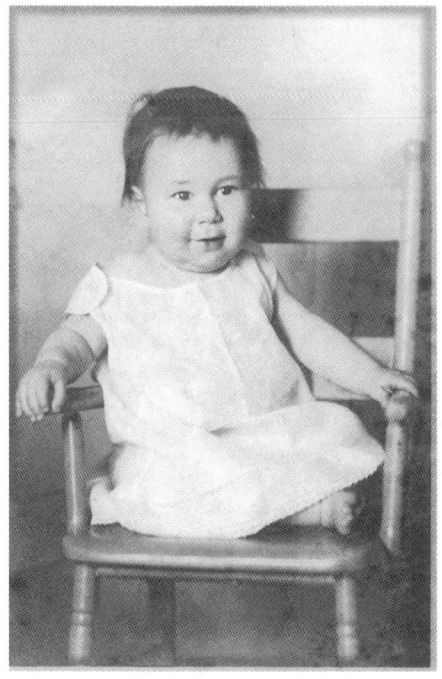
Glasser as a baby

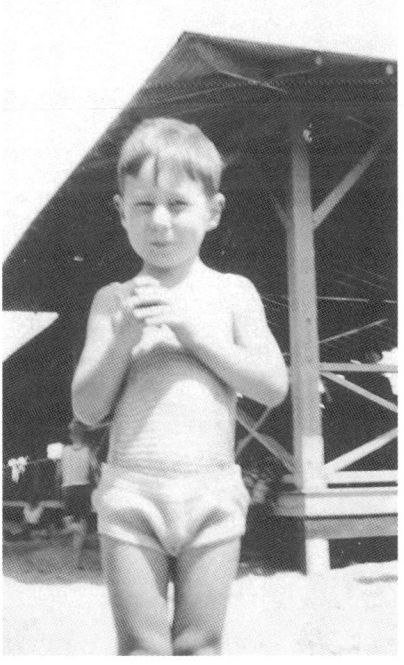
Glasser as a young boy

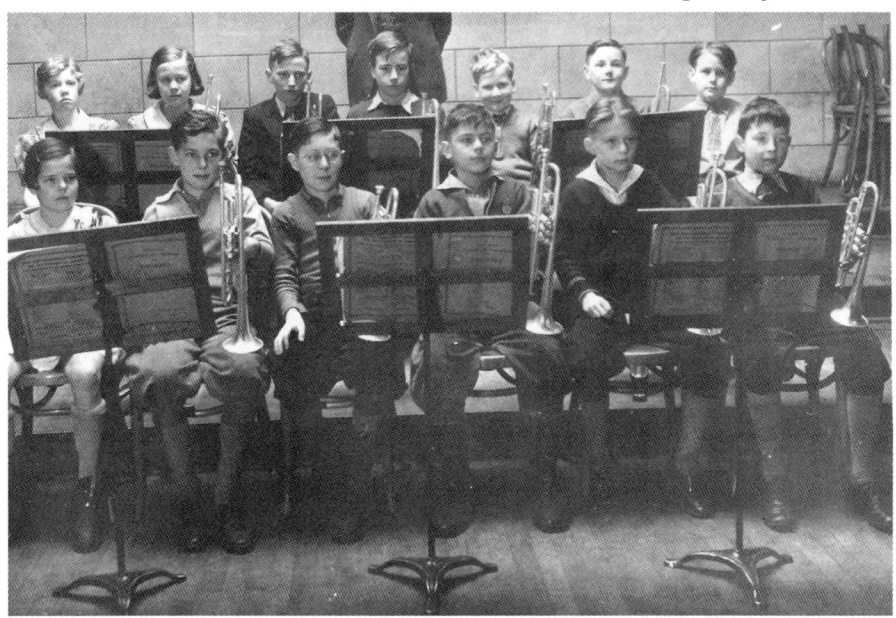

Billy Glasser playing trumpet in a small elementary school band. Glasser is third from the left in the front row.

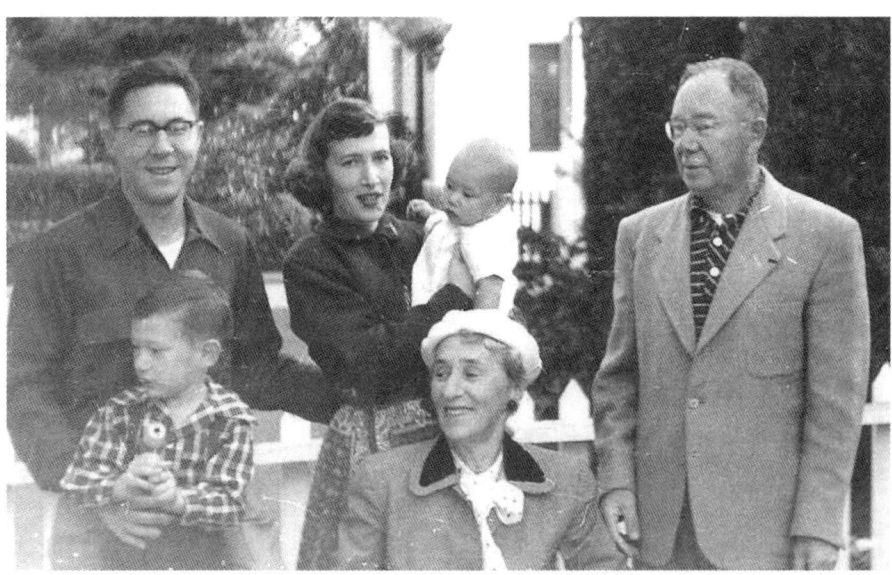

Glasser with wife Naomi, children Joe and Alice, and parents Betty and Ben.

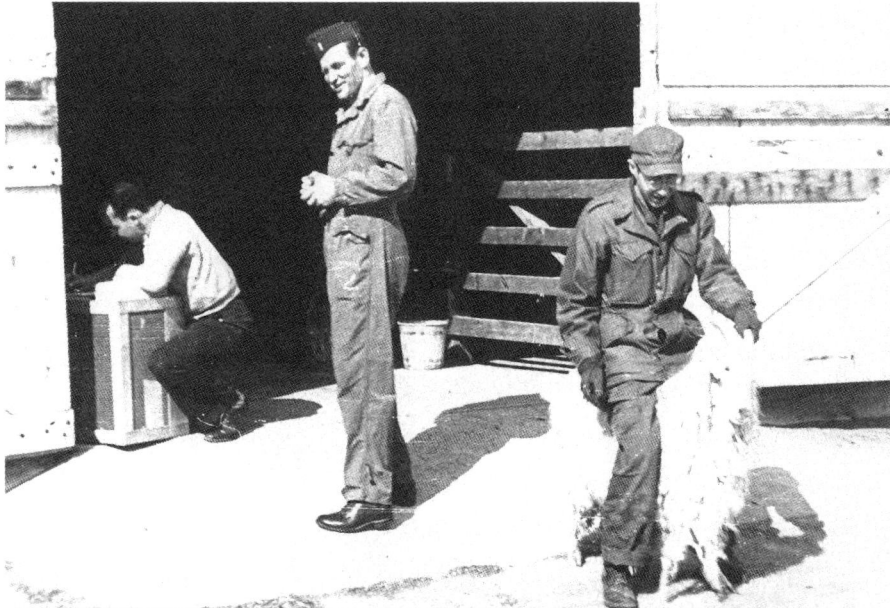

This represents the only known picture of William Glasser riding on a goat. Taken while he was serving in the chemical corps at Dugway Proving Ground in Utah, *circa 1946*

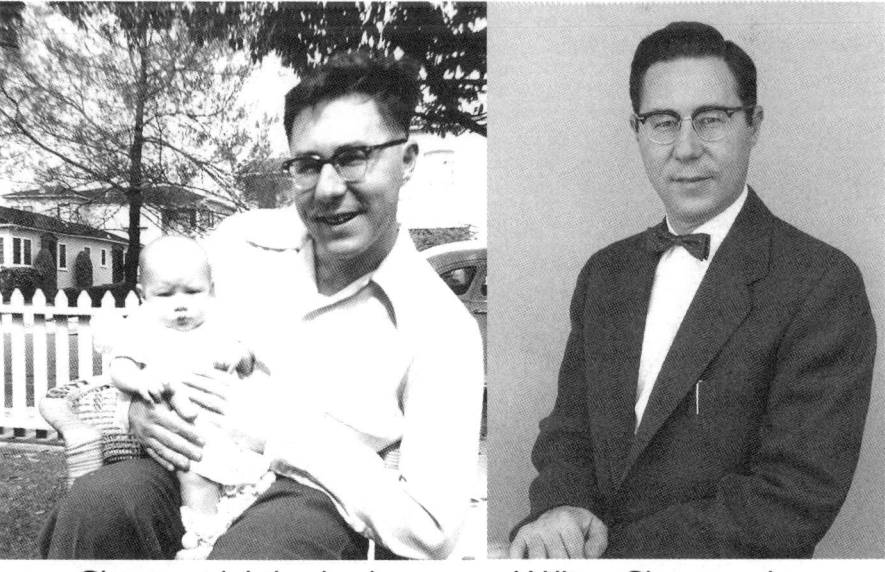

Glasser with baby daughter in 1954.

William Glasser at the start of his career.

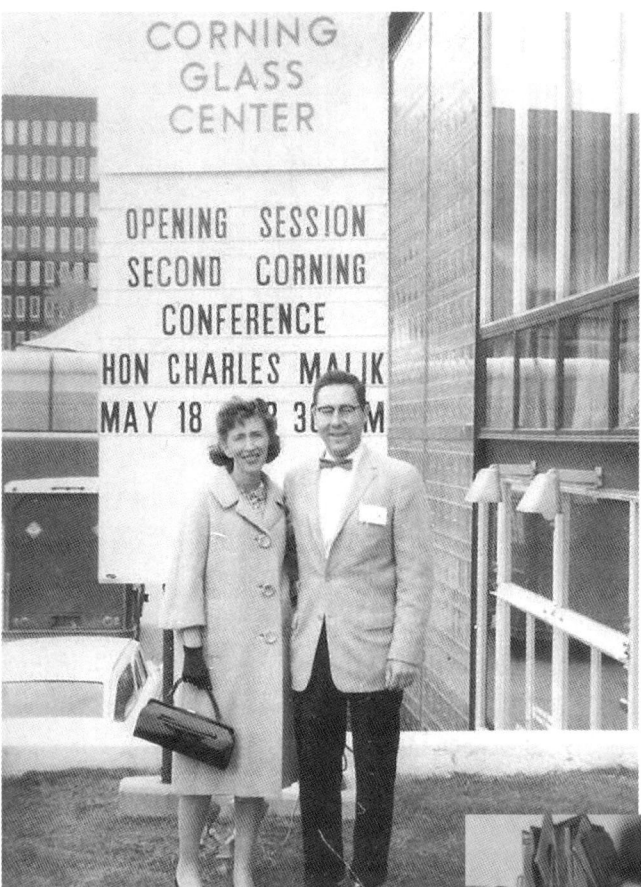

Glasser with wife Naomi as an invitee to the Second Corning Conference in 1961.

William Glasser 1977

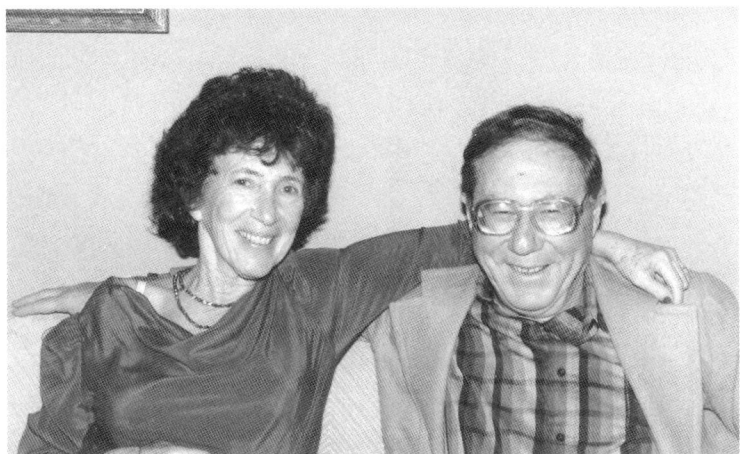

Bill and Naomi Glasser 1985

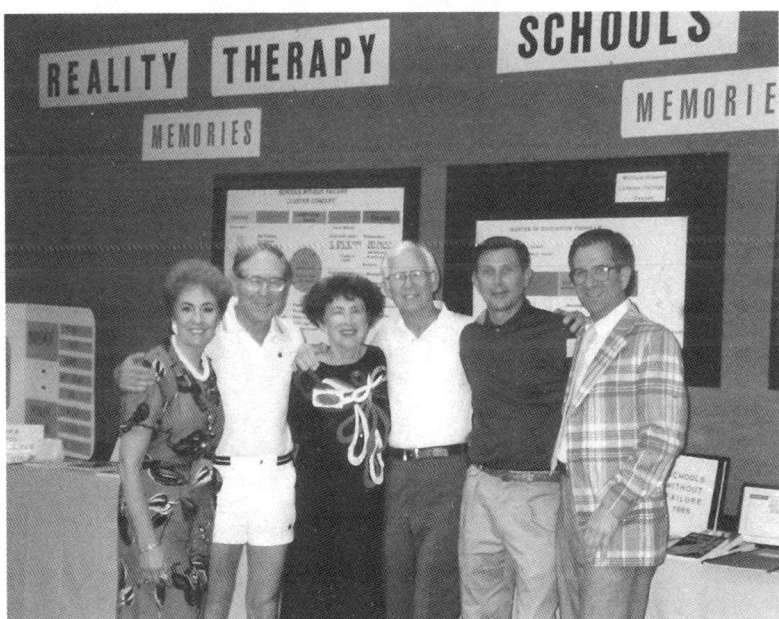

From l. to r. — Carleen Floyd, William Glasser, Naomi Glasser, Donald O'Donnell, O'Donnell's assistant, and Bob Wubbolding. The picture was taken at the start of the 1990 Glasser convention in Cincinnati. Glasser had just finished playing tennis and the group wanted him to see the Institute history and memorabilia room. Carleen was chairperson for the room's content and set-up. After Naomi passed away from cancer, Glasser married Carleen in 1995. Glasser and O'Donnell eventually had a falling out over the Institute history displays. Bob Wubbolding and his wife Sandie were co-chairs of the 1990 convention.

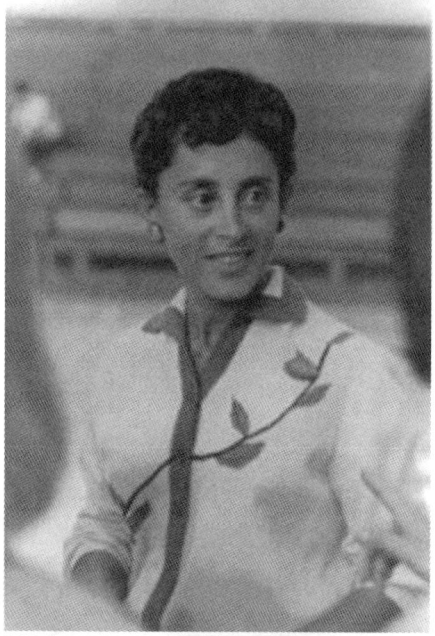

Adrienne Nater, a school vice-principal, lost her job in the mid-60s because she was using Glasser's ideas in her work with student offenders.

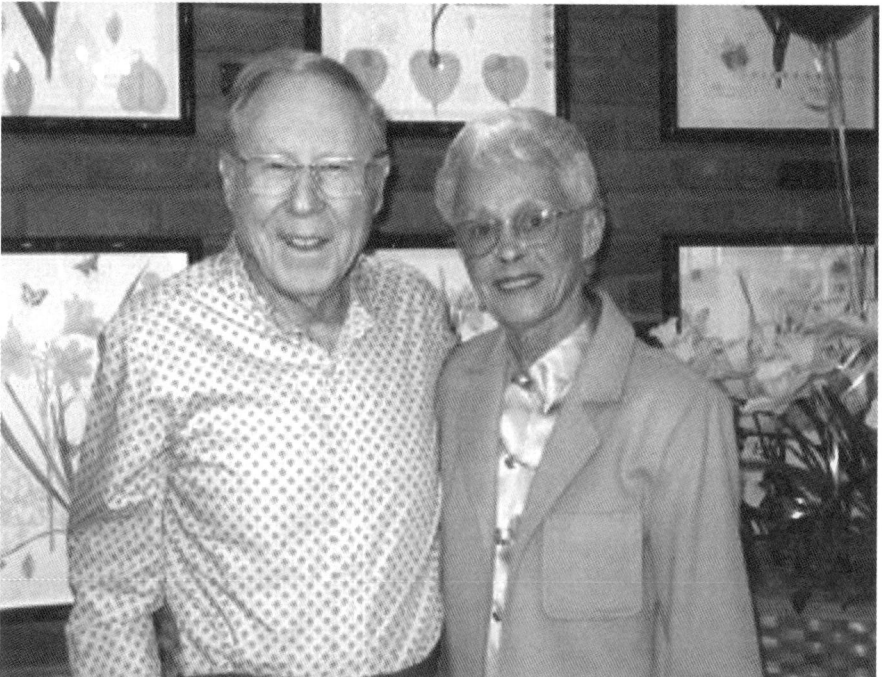

Adrienne Nater meets William Glasser, 40 years later.

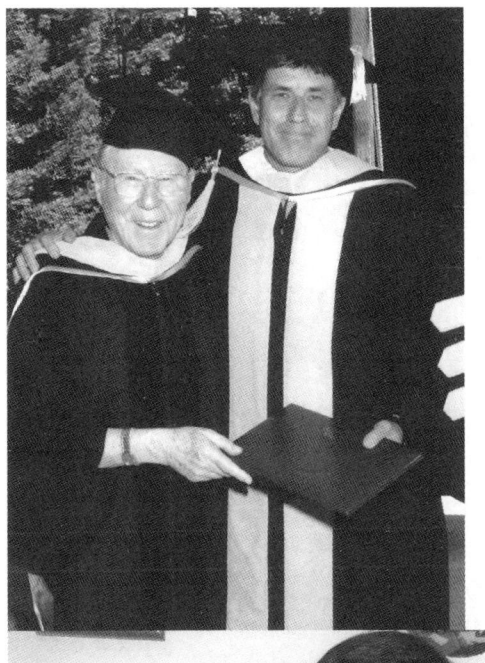

Glasser and the author. Roy received his doctoral degree based on his biographical study of William Glasser, while Glasser received an honorary doctorate from Pacific Union College. (2006)

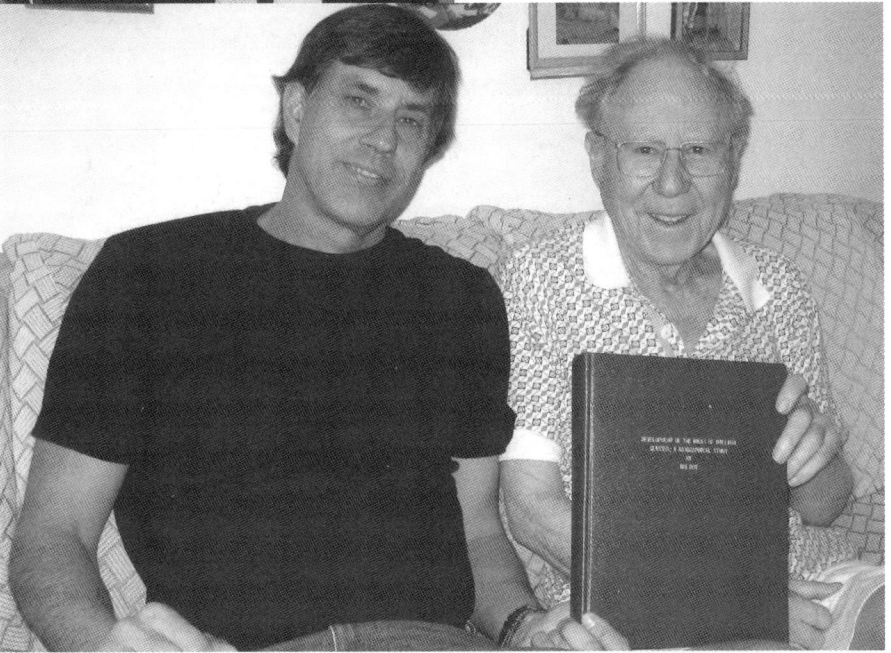

The author presents Glasser with a copy of his dissertation, which was titled *Development of the Ideas of William Glasser: A Biographical Study*.

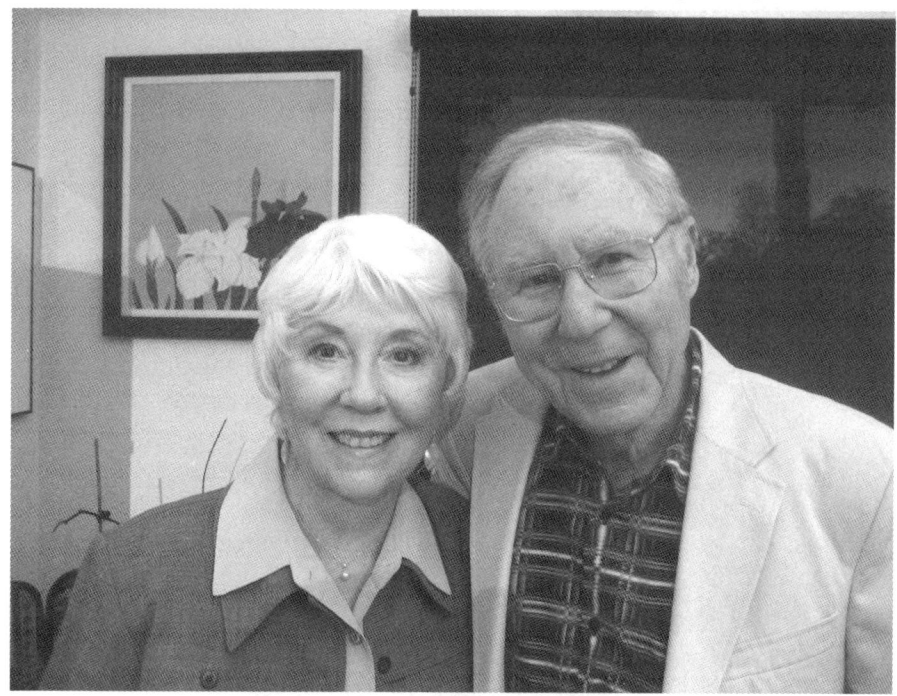
Bill and Carleen Glasser 2007

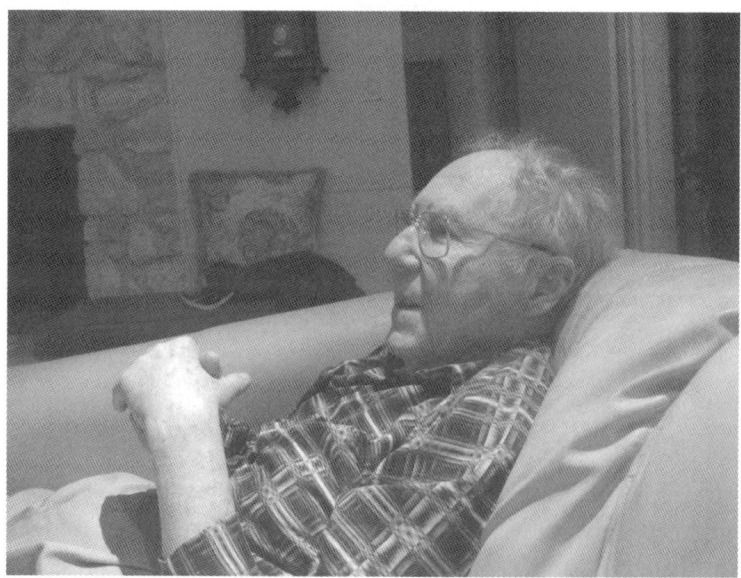
Bill Glasser 2007

9
MAKING IT HIS OWN

*"Everything we do—good or bad, effective or ineffective,
painful or pleasurable, crazy or sane, sick or well, drunk or sober
—is to satisfy powerful forces within ourselves."*
—William Glasser

In the movie, *Butch Cassidy and the Sundance Kid*[1], Butch (Paul Newman) and Sundance (Robert Redford) are two old-West train robbers who rob one too many Union Pacific trains and end up receiving the full attention of E.H. Harriman, the owner of Union Pacific, who hires a special team to track down the bandits and kill them. Butch and Sundance elude the trackers for a short time, but soon realize they need to get out of town, maybe even out of the country. Butch, ever the schemer, decides that Bolivia is the place to go and the pair arrive in South America ready to begin a new life. After marginal success at bank robbing they decide to go straight and live by the law, rather than against it. A local mining company is hiring and they head there to seek employment. An old codger, a fellow American actually, who runs the mining company talks with them about the company and about how difficult it is to pay his workers, since bandits keep stealing his payroll money. He then begins the interview.

"Can you shoot?" the codger asks as he moves out into the sun and tosses a small palm-sized box onto the dirt about 40 or 50 feet away. He had asked to see Sundance's gun a few moments before and now he nods for one of them to take the gun and shoot the box.

Sundance, a dead shot with a pistol, slowly walks out to stand by the interviewer and looks at the box lying in the dirt. He takes the gun back from the codger and spins it a few times before expertly inserting it back into his holster. The codger interrupts him, though, when he sees the spinning pistol.

"I don't want all the fancy stuff," he explains. "I just want you to hit it," whereupon he places Sundance's hand on his own gun and begins to guide it up to the aiming position. Sundance cooperates, albeit uncomfortably, and brings the gun up to eye level. He aims, steadies his gun, and pulls the trigger. The bullet misses the target by six inches. Butch walks out into the sun, too, and stares at the untouched box still lying in the dirt, incredulous that Sundance could have missed. The codger lingers for a moment, but then heads off to another duty. As far as he is concerned the interview is over.

When the codger is about 10 feet away Sundance asks, "Can I move?"

The codger stops and turns. "What?"

"Can I move?" Sundance asks again.

"Can you move?" the codger asks back, frustration in his voice. "Now what the hell . . ."

But before the codger can finish the sentence Sundance quick draws his pistol and, never bringing the gun higher than his waist, fans the hammer releasing three bullets in fast succession, each of them blasting the box into ever smaller pieces.

The codger lingers for another moment, the box in shreds 50 feet away, and matter-of-factly says, "You're hired," before turning and heading off to the next item on his to-do list.

WG

The concepts of control theory had provided Glasser with the framework he had been looking for and he was excited as *Stations of the Mind* began to take form, and especially so when it was published. However, not everyone shared his excitement. Up to that point, all of the Institute members had been trained in reality therapy. His trainers were skilled in teaching the beliefs and details of reality therapy. Many of the trainers had been involved in the reality therapy concepts for years. Some of them had become a part of the reality therapy movement in 1965 (a few even before that), which was 16 years earlier than the publication of *Stations of the Mind*. For those who had, over a period of years, come to an understanding of reality therapy, this new thing called control theory was not something to be particularly excited about.

Al Katz, one of reality therapy's earliest converts, remembered: "To us, the jargon, the concepts, were difficult to understand. The concepts were out in the ozone. He was making sense of it, be we weren't. I can remember walking down the street in Montreal, Canada, with a colleague, and turning to him and saying that we need an English translation of *Stations of the Mind.*" It shouldn't be overlooked how significant the shift to control theory was for a lot of people. The principles of reality therapy explained the most important elements of what it meant to be human and people made sense of the principles at a deeply personal level. To those who had embraced reality therapy and now depended on the principles of reality therapy from which to operate their lives and make sense of the world around them, it felt as if Glasser was asking them to re-tool or remake themselves at a foundational level. Such shifts, either personally or corporately, are not easily done. Those who had studied reality therapy since the late 1960s and who were now reality therapy trainers, had come to their understanding and expertise over a long period of time. They had attended workshops and certification classes, often at great expense when you add the travel and lodging costs, and had then developed teaching materials they could use in their own workshops. The epicenter of reality therapy was southern California, an area that was familiar with the earth trembling and shifting, and now Glasser's colleagues felt the ideological underpinnings of their most cherished beliefs shifting beneath them.

One writer recalled, "These changes occurred even when colleagues within his organization balked at the idea of new directions." Glasser was aware of their concerns and discomfort, but he was convinced of the need to join the reality therapy approach with the framework of control theory. Colleagues expressed their discomfort regarding control theory and the fact that it appeared they were now going to head into uncharted territory, however for Glasser, control theory represented a solution to be embraced, rather than a problem to be avoided. This shift in his theoretical framework, this change that affected his entire organization, led another writer to note, "Unlike many counseling theorists, William Glasser has never been content to allow his theories to be taught or used without constant scrutiny, addition and sometimes even major changes."[2] It is one thing to respond to an earthquake, to react to the circumstances around you; it is quite another thing to be the earthquake creator, to be the cause of the shift. This moment in Glasser's journey is noteworthy for the courage and commitment it took to lead in this change. After so much effort and so many resources had been devoted to the details of reality therapy, this shift was a big deal.

It was also significant for Glasser personally, since he is not a creature of change by nature. He is a contradiction in this way. He is known for being a creative genius, not just for his ability to crank out well-written books and journal articles year after year, but also for his ability to facilitate on-the-spot demonstrations of counseling role-plays and classroom meetings. Yet, for all this creative ability he clings to sameness in many ways. He would live in the same house his entire married life, even after his first wife passed away and he remarried. He has a very small circle of close friends, a few of them since college. He likes going to the same restaurant in Santa Monica, the Versailles, and he gets the same dish, roast tongue, each time he goes. When he discovered something he liked and with which he felt comfortable, Glasser stayed with that person or place or idea. He's never been the type to pursue change for the sake of change.

When *Stations of the Mind* was published in 1981 it proclaimed a new context for reality therapy, not a new direction *per se,* but a new context from which to understand reality therapy's effectiveness. What began when a friend recommended a little-known book to Glasser in 1976 led to a significant new emphasis in his beliefs. It was a discovery in Glasser's mind, like finding a missing puzzle piece or unlocking a secret passageway, and *Stations of the Mind* described the discovery in detail. Maybe, actually, too much detail. For anyone else, the reviews of the book would have been positive and affirming; for Glasser, however, one review in particular, even though worded supportively, was a death knell for the book it was trying to affirm. The reviewer said *Stations of the Mind* "represented an ambitious attempt to tie together reality therapy, control theory, and elements of brain research into a detailed approach to a theory of perception," and the book "made a useful new contribution."[3] It continued, "The book illustrates clearly how an internally motivated psychology contrasts with many of the commonly accepted ideas of behavior psychology." So far so good, but then the review closed with, "In general, the book makes a valuable contribution to the literature. Although more difficult to follow than some of his previous work, it could serve as a valuable resource in learning courses that often emphasize behaviorism." It was frustrating to Glasser to have produced something that was in any way "difficult to follow." His career had been about helping to make the complex understandable to anyone who wanted to understand. He did not write *Stations of the Mind* to serve as a "valuable resource" hidden away on a university library shelf. He was convinced that the combination of control theory with reality therapy was life-changing and ultimately, world-changing. *Stations of the Mind* was meant to sound the alarm for change.

In spite of his initial intentions, Glasser came to see *Stations of the Mind* as too arcane, too cumbersome, and too complicated. He had so much wanted to take Powers' ideas and make them more accessible to more people, but the complexity of Powers' model was still quite present. Glasser acknowledged he had wanted to mollify Powers and to please him and this was one of the reasons that too much complexity remained. He had a deep respect for Powers and recognized how much work Powers had put into the control theory model, however he began to believe he had to change the control theory ideas even more if readers were going to understand them and be able to apply them to their lives.

Glasser, like the Sundance Kid before him, needed to do it his way. He needed to describe control theory in a way that made sense to him and to others. When reminded how he became less concerned about pleasing Powers and more concerned about saying it how he wanted to say it, Glasser replied, "Right, right. Because certain things of Powers, like the levels of perception, they might be accurate, but to me they're meaningless." During another interview he explained as time went on he "pretty much gave up on the levels of perception." Glasser acknowledged the levels of perception were very much Powers

Making It His Own

and that Powers still felt they were important. "He (Powers) still teaches that. He doesn't fault me for not teaching it. I just told him, it's just too complicated and people don't understand it, and I don't understand it well enough to explain it well." Glasser could have retreated into the confines of reality therapy. Certainly there were colleagues who would have welcomed that decision. But he recognized key elements in control theory that, rather than retreating from, needed to be emphasized, and the elements needed to be emphasized in language with which Glasser was comfortable. He may not have been enamored with the package of explanations Powers had put together, but Glasser was enamored with control theory.

Given Glasser's obvious commitment to control theory in the months that followed the publication of *Stations of the Mind*, colleagues scrambled to understand the new framework and even to be a part of the framework's continuing development. Meetings in which people came together to talk about control theory took place in Glasser's living room. Besides Glasser and his wife, others in attendance included William and Mary Powers, Bob Wubbolding, Gary Applegate, Perry Good, Ron Harshman, and Dick Hawes. Wubbolding remembers the meetings at times being marked by excitement and enthusiasm, while at other times they were marked by withdrawal and a feeling of futility. In general, though, he recalls the excitement of being a part of the ground floor development of Glasser's version of control theory. One of the things the group worked on was a visual or graphic representation of the elements of control theory and reality therapy. As mentioned, Powers had included a significant number of models and charts in his book, and it seemed to have inspired Glasser to graphically capture reality therapy as well.

A chart was published in 1983 that revealed their progress, but also showed early signs of what would become an uneasy truce of separate models. A brochure was developed by the Institute for Reality Therapy that actually had two charts. On one page is a chart entitled A Diagram of the Brain as a Control System. Still part of the title, but in smaller letters, it read A Control System* Acts Upon the World to Attempt to Get for Itself the Perception (Picture) that it Wants. The asterisk acknowledges William Powers as the author of *Behavior: The Control of Perception*. The chart resembles the charts in Stations of the Mind and, indeed, it lists William Glasser as the creator of the chart. On another page of the brochure is another chart that is titled The Basic Concepts of Reality Therapy. This chart emphasizes failure identity versus success identity and responsibility versus irresponsibility; it also describes the journey of a person moving from negative addictions and symptoms to being a secure, fulfilled person. The details on these charts are less important than the separateness between them. Rather than a graphic that combined the important elements of each of their approaches, there were two charts, one for Powers' control theory model and one for Glasser's reality therapy model.

In spite of the separateness, some very important elements came out of meetings like these. One of these elements is the car as a metaphor for what came to be known as the concept of total behavior. Wubbolding remembered that at one point after a discussion on total behavior, Glasser remarked, "The car has got to go!" Wubbolding continued, "I left the meeting believing that he was not going to use a car as a symbol of total behavior. As I remember, the discussion centered on the fact that a car is too mechanical to represent the complexities of human behavior. As it turned out the car remained and is now enshrined in the pantheon!"[4] Wubbolding also remembered coming to

Making It His Own

the conclusion that nothing is written in stone and that things can change very quickly. He wondered then if this was a plus—as in the ability to think creatively and act quickly—or a minus—as in the tendency to act on a whim and lacking a steady purpose. Glasser's thinking, and as a result the thinking of those within his organization, was in transition. Time would tell if it was a plus or a minus. For now, his colleagues were entering the world of control theory and comparing it to the world of reality therapy they knew so well.

Glasser, convinced of control theory's worth and further convinced he needed to describe its essential elements differently than he had in *Stations of the Mind,* began to write another book. It would be his version of control theory. Like the Sundance Kid shooting his gun in the way he was comfortable, Glasser would describe control theory in the way in which he was comfortable. "Since 1977," he began the new book, "when I was introduced to control theory through William Powers' highly theoretical book *Behavior: The Control of Perception* (1973), I have been fascinated with the possibilities of using this theory to add strength to our lives. This book is my attempt to put these possibilities into practice, but it is a book of ideas, not research."[5] Rather than trudging through the topic and seeking to prove every point based on scientific evidence or based on what others had said before him, he would simply explain how our brains worked and why we behave the way we do. He would explain how to begin to gain control over our own life, even if that life is out of control at the moment.

Take Effective Control of Your Life, which was published in 1984, was Glasser's clearest description of human behavior up to that point, and for me personally, it remains one of the clearest and best-written descriptions of human motivation and behavior that he ever wrote. Other books, like *Reality Therapy* (1965) and *Schools Without Failure* (1969), made a significant impact on the fields of psychology and education, but they left you wanting more. *The Identity Society* (1972) was his attempt to alert everyone, not just counselors and teachers, of the importance of the principles of reality therapy, but again it left you wanting more. Glasser himself recognized this "more" vacancy and continued to seek the connecting piece or pieces. The principles of control theory represented this piece and he now wrote with a special confidence and clarity.

So many of Glasser's essential elements, elements that continued into the Quality School approach in 1990 and then the choice theory model in 1998, can be traced to *Take Effective Control of Your Life*. It is true, to a great extent, the book corralled previously stated ideas and concepts, yet these concepts were now presented in a new package that was clearer than ever before. "Driven by our genes," he began, "we are captive to these pictures, but what we need to learn is that we are not captive to how we attempt to satisfy them."[6] A person's behavior is made up of not only action or a specific movement, but also of thinking, feeling, and even our internal physiology. Most important, Glasser claimed our behavior, including even our misery, is always something we choose.

"Everything we think, do, and feel," Glasser asserted, "is generated by what happens inside of us." This "inside" emphasis was not new, but his recent control theory insights helped him explain it more clearly. "If I believe that the motivation for all I do, good or bad, comes from within me, not from the outside world, when I am miserable, I cannot claim that any misery is caused by uncaring parents, a boorish spouse, an ungrateful child, or a miserable job. If I were a machine this claim might be valid. I could be programmed to feel good only if those I needed treated me well. What I will explain," he continued, "is that, regardless of our circumstances, all any of us do, think, and feel, effective or ineffective, is always our best attempt at the time to satisfy the forces within us."7

Take Effective Control of Your Life contributed to or clarified many of Glasser's key points, points that recalled reality therapy elements and combined with control theory elements. Key points:

- Outlined the basic needs, now five in number—survival, love and belonging, power, freedom, and fun;
- explained every person has a personal picture album in his or her head in which he or she stored pictures of the people, things, activities, ideas, and places that helped him or her to meet one or more of the basic needs;
- clarified how our personal picture albums act as a thermostat and that when our reality doesn't match those pictures, a signal or urge is sent for us to behave in a way we think will bring our reality and the pictures in our head closer together;
- likened our behavioral choice process to that of rummaging through a storeroom of potential behaviors and then choosing the one that would most likely work the best;
- described how humans are internal control systems who desire to be in control, but not controlled;
- introduced the concept of total behavior and its four separate parts—doing, thinking, feeling, and physiology—and explained we have direct control over our doing and our thinking;
- explained why it sometimes makes sense to choose to be miserable;
- warned that our valuing system, the labels we so quickly apply to the pictures of the world as we want it to be, often lead to the restriction of freedom;
- detailed the concepts of creativity, reorganization, and organized behaviors, and how even craziness can become an organized behavior; and
- makes a case for physiological creativity being the cause of most chronic illnesses.

These key areas represent essential Glasser elements and would set the agenda for presentations and trainings for years to come. Several of these areas are of special interest. For instance, he settled on the five basic needs—survival, love and belonging, power, freedom, and fun—which expanded on the original two—love and worth. He would later become rather inflexible regarding the needs, but he didn't come across that way when he first introduced them. "There may be other needs," he wrote, "but these are the ones I find in my head, and most people I talk to find the same ones."[8] He even stated, "It is not important to the thesis of this book that I establish with any certainty what the basic needs are that drive us. To gain effective control of our lives, we have to satisfy what we believe is basic to us and learn to respect and not frustrate others in fulfilling what is basic to them."[9]

During one of our interview sessions I ventured to say that maybe a basic need was missing from his list. It seemed to me, I explained, people had a deep need to understand the mystery of their existence, where they come from and where they are going, and to come into an awareness of their purpose in life. At the time I referred to it as the existential need,[10] which is a secular term, even though the basis for this need seemed to be of a spiritual nature. Human beings from the dawn of recorded history have sought and prioritized a connection with a deity. Entire cultures embrace the journey of the soul, so it would seem that a need for spirituality or purpose, as I would come to refer to it, could be included on the list. Glasser admitted that throughout his career he has been approached about how spirituality and religion fit into his model. This didn't surprise me. I have no hard data on how many people within Glasser's organization or on how many people who are interested in Glasser's ideas, in general, who consider themselves to be personally spiritual or corporately involved with a religion, but I have a sense the percentage might be significant. The number was significant enough that Glasser wrote:

Others argue that religion, or the holy spirit inside us all, is the single need from which all others are derived. This may be, but there is no hard evidence that this is the case for many people. Iraqis and Iranians are fighting as I write this, killing and dying for the same Moslem faith. I don't dispute their beliefs, but it seems to me that despite their strong religious claims, they are fighting for power. It is inconceivable that any religion would advocate killing as a holy function, but there are plenty of religions that advocate and encourage their followers to struggle for power the same way many politicians do.[11]

Years later he would categorize religion as a quality world issue.[12] People put religion in their quality worlds in the same way they put sports into their quality worlds. Years later, it would also become very conceivable how people could kill one another as a holy function. After 9/11, news reports regularly updated the world on terrorist attacks and suicide bombings, most of them motivated or supported by religious beliefs.

One of the changes that occurred in *Take Effective Control of Your Life* was Glasser's use of the term "pictures" rather than "perceptions." "I like to think," he began, "that all our senses combine into an extraordinary camera that can take visual pictures, auditory pictures, gustatory pictures, tactile pictures, and so forth. In simple terms, this sensory camera can take a picture of anything we can perceive through any of our senses. I like to use the word pictures rather than the technically correct term, perceptions, because pictures are easier to understand."[13] While the term was easier to understand, the effect of these mental pictures should not be underestimated. "The power of the pictures is total," he continued. "In our relentless efforts to satisfy them, we may go so far as to choose behaviors that endanger our lives, as with anorexia."[14] When our reality seems to match these pictures in our head we feel a degree of satisfaction. The less our perceived reality matches these pictures the greater the urge is to change our behavior so that our reality and our pictures become more alike.

As good as *Take Effective Control of Your Life* was as an explanation of how our brains work and our own role in what motivates us, it didn't really sell. Glasser admitted he was surprised when it didn't sell that well. The book had so much of importance to say, and he didn't want to watch it just ride off into some publishing sunset. As he thought about the situation, he began to wonder if maybe the title of the book was the problem. When asked if Harper Collins had come up with that title he shook his head and said, "No, it was my title, and I thought it was a good title." However, something wasn't working. Now, instead of the longer Take Effective Control title he was drawn to the phrase Control Theory. He remembers thinking right in the middle of a talk he was giving: "If I could just say control theory, instead of take effective control of your life, that it would be a theory. Take effective control is not a theory."

It is interesting how such moments in time can turn out to be so significant; a crossroads moment that sets a new course. Somewhat like side view mirrors that read Objects May Be Closer Than They Appear, this was a moment for Glasser that was much larger than it appeared. The term control theory was not a trademarked term. It had been around before Powers or Glasser had pondered it, studied it, and eventually wrote about it. Glasser became aware of the idea of control theory through the writing of William Powers, and Powers was led to the concepts of control theory through others before him, most notably Norbert Wiener. Glasser didn't feel he would be taking the term "control theory" from Powers. Ever since learning about control theory, Glasser had wanted to give it a bigger stage with a top billing. Renaming his most recent book to *Control Theory* would do just that. A final nudge for change might have come from an experience Glasser had in Ireland. Right around this time, Glasser was giving the very first Basic Week training in Ireland. Brian Lennon, who attended the training, remembers buying *Taking Effective Control of Your Life* and bringing it home. "My wife got a hold of it and started reading it right way. I shared with Glasser, though, that she was having a hard time reading the book on the train on the way to work. People were watching her to see if there was any change each day! Glasser laughed," Lennon recalled, "and said that he didn't really like the title and would change it." Such is the process of change.

And so the hardcover *Take Effective Control of Your Life,* a year after it was published, became the paperback *Control Theory.* Glasser meant no harm by the change. He just felt the term control theory was in the public domain and therefore useable by anyone. The Era of Control Theory, which had begun on the plane ride back to Los Angeles after visiting with Powers in Chicago, was now fully christened. The Control Theory Era would last for 19 years—from 1977 to 1996— yet in the end it would produce mixed blessings. Of the label change initially to *Control Theory,* Glasser simply said, "I was right about that. *Control Theory* sold quite a few books."[5] He would write more books and articles based on the control theory themes and would come to be known as the expert in control theory, yet as the years went by he became less and less attached to the label of Control Theory. In 1996, he would ultimately go with a different title, *Choice Theory,* and even requested that Harper Collins not only stop printing more copies of *Control Theory,* one of the best books he ever wrote, but that they also shred any existing copies still on hand.

In the early '80s, though, Glasser was excited about control theory and the ways in which it supported and expanded the ideas of reality therapy. His creativity and energy, rarely in short supply, were cranked up a notch even for him as he considered the possibilities. As he was writing the manuscript for *Take Effective Control of Your Life*, it occurred to him that seminars could be developed in which people were taught the principles of control theory. The book and a companion seminar would be a powerful learning combination. He remembered, "I had the idea that we could teach *Take Effective Control of Your Life* and that we could take it to everybody!" Plans were laid and money was spent to put the plan into motion. There was a feeling the seminars could be a moneymaking venture. An advertisement for the seminars read:

> A Glasser TEC Seminar is taught in two full days, 9:30 to 4:30, always separated by an interval of one, two, or three weeks. The separation is to allow time to practice what has been taught so that feedback can be obtained on the final day. Seminars are limited to 100 participants who are divided into small working groups of no more than ten. Besides the seminar leader who lectures and circulates, the small groups are assisted by TEC trained facilitators. Dr. Glasser will personally conduct some of these seminars but most will be led by long-term personally trained associates. At present, the fee for the two days is $135.

Confidence in the idea of the seminars was high and more people than just Glasser invested in it. Unfortunately, the seminars did not take hold and money was lost in the process. Was the $135 fee too high for the 1983 economy? At any rate, it was at this point that a schism developed between Powers and Glasser. Glasser recalled the enthusiasm for the seminars, the planning, and the early efforts to get the seminars started. For him it was fairly simple. They tried and it didn't work. While money was lost in the process, Glasser emphasized the only money lost was his. "Nobody lost any money. I refunded all the money." Powers and his wife weren't so sure, especially Mrs. Powers, who was apparently frustrated by more than just the failure of the

TEC seminars. "She got the idea," Glasser continued, "that I had taken her husband's ideas and was going to make millions off of them without giving him any money."

William Powers and William Glasser both put a great deal of energy into understanding and writing about control theory. It shouldn't come as a surprise that in the process they each came to be partial to their own views and explanations, a partiality that in itself created the potential for schism. Glasser was a successful and well-known author when he learned about control theory and began to work with Powers. William Powers was a careful and thorough author, but worked in relative obscurity. It had to have been bittersweet for Powers when Glasser came along with his bigger pulpit, and his publishing connections, and his professional network to share the concepts of control theory. Part of Powers must have wanted control theory to take off and have a great impact on the world, however that was going to happen, and part of him must have wanted to be the person who did the sharing. He was the one who had done the deep analysis. He was the one who had recognized control theory's importance and explained it in greater detail than anyone before him. Yet now with the publishing of *Stations of the Mind* and then *Control Theory*, William Glasser was viewed as the theory's creator and expert. Yes, Glasser had at every turn given Powers credit for his analysis and his writing. Still it wasn't the same. Glasser's name was plastered on the cover of these books and that is the name people came to associate with control theory. Whatever misunderstandings there may have been over the Taking Effective Control seminars, those misunderstandings were more like the final straw in a situation that was ripe for fracture.

Fifteen years later, Larry Litwack, the longtime editor of the *Journal for Reality Therapy* and a faculty member at Northeastern University, organized a panel discussion in Boston that included Albert Ellis,

Alfie Kohn, William Powers, and William Glasser. Glasser remembers Ellis, who had written a 25-page critique on Choice Theory, speaking very positively about choice theory, which was noteworthy since, in Glasser's words, "People don't hear very many positive words come out of Albert Ellis's mouth where other people are concerned." Glasser himself reemphasized his position regarding Powers' control theory views. "I said I believe in *Behavior: The Control of Perception,* but that you have to go further than that to make it usable in counseling or teaching." Glasser went on to remind me that Powers had said in his preface that the BCP book represented what he knew and what he does best. "Others," Powers admitted, "who know more about behavior and many other subjects are the ones to put the content in."[16] Like Powers, Glasser recognized something very significant in the elements of control theory and once again, on the stage in Boston, he affirmed those elements, along with the book's author and book from which he first learned about them. On the day of the Boston panel presentation, Glasser remembered that during a private moment Powers told him that it was his wife who had gotten angry, not him. Powers added that his wife was also upset about Glasser changing the label he used from Control Theory to Choice Theory, which was surprising since one might have guessed she would have been glad that Glasser was done with the Control Theory label.

Judging from their beliefs and their writing, one can surmise that Powers and Glasser were gentlemen who were not in the habit of spoiling for fights. They were passionate about their beliefs, but not obstinate; they wanted to look good, but didn't want to make others look bad in the process. In the years following the publishing of Glasser's book *Control Theory* the two of them, in spite of the schism, regarded one another with admiration and respect, even if from a distance. Glasser continued overseeing the outreach and training of The

Institute for Reality Therapy (a short time it later would become The Institute for Control Theory, Reality Therapy, and Quality Schools) and the Educator Training Center, and Powers founded the Control Systems Group (CSG), which emphasized the concepts of Perceptual Control Theory (PCT). Ultimately, the Control Systems Group would come to take exception with Glasser's view of control theory. Emails between CSG members and Powers reveal they felt strongly that their version of Perceptual Control Theory was the only accurate version available.

It is interesting, actually, how intensely people within the CSG family feel about Glasser. One email describes Glasser as one of PCT's (Perceptual Control Theory) most faithless suitors since in his opinion, Glasser wanted to keep PCT as a mistress while maintaining his marriage to another theory, in this case reality therapy. "I think we all know who gets the shaft," the writer lamented, "when the day of reckoning comes." Another email bemoaned, "We also think that his [Glasser's] ethics stink when he portrays himself as the guru on control theory." Mary Powers wrote, "Glasser is convinced that what he has done is expand and clarify control theory—he hasn't." And William Powers himself, who so completely endorsed Glasser's understanding of control theory earlier, according to his wife, said in reference to Glasser's level of understanding, "I thought he knew more than he did." In Powers' view, Glasser simplified the concepts too much.

Stations of the Mind was marked by many "we" pronouns; *Take Effective Control of Your Life* was marked by "I" pronouns. It's not that simple, of course, but it seems inevitable that Glasser and Powers would head in different directions. What began as a team effort shifted toward two conceptual heavyweights continuing to forge their own trail. People within the Control Systems Group felt Glasser misunderstood and misinterpreted the principles of control theory, something with which he disagreed. "The setting of the control is what you're controlling for, and then the behavior makes sure you can do the control. It gets back to *Behavior: The Control of Perception*. I've never, never argued that." In 1987 Glasser sat for an interview with Pauline Gough, then the editor of the *Kappan Journal*, who asked him how he arrived at control theory. "In the course of my research," he began, "I came across a book, *Behavior: The Control of Perception*, written by William Powers and published by Aldine Press in 1973. I found the book obscure and difficult to understand, but Powers was one of the first to give the concepts of control theory (which, at that time, were engineering concepts) a biological application. Working a little bit with Powers and a great deal on my own, I refined those ideas and applied them to human behavior."[17] Again, the "we" had become an "I."

The hardcover jacket of *Take Effective Control of Your Life* has an endorsement written by Norman Cousins, a journalist and editor who became famous with the publication of his book, *Anatomy of an Illness* in 1979. His ideas got the attention of the UCLA medical school and they invited him to become a professor in their program. When I asked Glasser if he knew Norman Cousins he quickly replied: "I made it my business to know him. I had people in town who knew him and invited us to dinner and introduced us. We played tennis a few times, and we gave a joint presentation at UCLA, although he didn't stick around to hear my part of it. As far as the endorsement, he regretted that he wrote it because they had put tremendous pressure on him because of my hassles with the UCLA department of psychiatry. We didn't maintain the friendship."

Glasser's dealings with Cousins, as well as his dealings with Powers, are examples of things happening behind the scenes that most people don't see or hear about. The price of success for the very successful is steeper than most understand. There are big obstacles to overcome, to be sure, but it is the myriad smaller obstacles, the constant little feuds and distractions that, at times, seem even more impressive when they are overcome. Feuds and distractions are almost always people problems, often involving the people closest to us. They are the small things caused by differing views, perceptions, habits, needs, and preferences. We are each totally unique, each seeking to arrange the world toward our personal fulfillment. Glasser was and is in the same social waters as everyone else, although as a widely read author and speaker, the pond he was in was a bit larger than most. His unique insights and abilities contributed to his being able to navigate the complex world in which he lived and worked, although he had his foibles, too. When I traveled with him and attended many of his presentations during our interviews I began to notice something that at first I couldn't even put my finger on. Later though, I began to conclude he was more comfortable speaking in front of hundreds of people, even thousands of people, than he was with just a few people in a more intimate setting. In a 1982 interview, which would have been at the same time that *Take Effective Control* was being written, the interviewer noted: "Glasser is a fascinating lecturer who can hold the attention of large numbers of people for very long times when he speaks from the stage. One to one I found him shy, usually not very talkative, and hesitant to talk about himself. The vivacious, outgoing member of the team is Naomi Glasser." The interviewer admitted that as the time approached for their visit she had a "fear that Glasser would choose that hour to be his shy self and not talk."[8] Bob Wubbolding, a longtime associate of Glasser's and for many years the Director of Training for The Glasser Institute, saw this tendency, too. "He has this amazing ability to connect with a large group of people in his lectures. We've always said that he is more comfortable with a group of 500 people than he is with one person." For him, as with the rest of us, some of his personal traits and abilities helped him a great deal, others less so.

And so Glasser pushed ahead into the Era of Control Theory, convinced that people could be strengthened to literally take effective control of their own lives. The energy and passion that fueled his efforts through the decades of the 1960s and '70s to teach people about reality therapy and to help schools become schools without failure now, in the 1980s, took on a greater energy and focus as he sought to improve his ideas through the framework of control theory. Like the Sundance Kid, Glasser had decided to follow his instincts. "Once I wrote the book *Control Theory*," he declared later, "I felt I was really on to what was going on."

NOTES

1. Hill, George Roy. (Director). (1969). *Butch Cassidy and the Sundance Kid.* [Film]. Los Angeles: 20th Century Fox.
2. Cockrum, R. (1989). Reality therapy: Interviews with Dr. William Glasser. *Psychology: A Journal of Human Behavior,* 26 (1), 13.
3. Hardy, C. (1981). Stations of the mind (Review of the book Stations of the mind). *Educational Studies,* 339-340.
4. Bob Wubbolding email, January 27, 2005.
5. Glasser, W. (1984). *Take effective control of your life.* New York: Harper & Row, Publishers.
6. Glasser, W. (1984*). Take effective control of your life.* p. xiii.
7. Glasser, W. (1984). *How to take effective control of your life.* p. 2, 3
8. Glasser, W. (1984). *How to take effective control of your life.* p 16
9. *Ibid.,* p. 16
10. I now refer to it as the need for Purpose.
11. Glasser, W. (1984). *Take Effective Control,* p.17
12. Glasser's model of how the brain works includes several components, with each of the components affecting all of the other components. These components or concepts included the *basic needs,* the quality world, the *perceived world,* the *comparing place,* the *behavioral station,* and *total behavior.* The *quality world* was a label used to describe a kind of unique mental picture album in which a person stores the sights, sounds, smells, tastes, and touches that are need-satisfying to one or more of the *basic needs.* At the time he wrote *Take Effective Control,* Glasser was using the term picture album, rather than the term *quality world,* which he later developed.
13. Glasser, W. (1984). *Take Effective Control,* p.21
14. *ibid.,* p.23
15. The hardcover of *Take Effective Control of Your Life* sold 42,000 copies, whereas the paperback version, newly titled as *Control Theory,* sold 273,000 copies.

16 Powers, W. (1973). *Behavior: The control of perception*. New York: Aldine de Gruyter, p.xi.
17 Gough, P. (1987). The key to improving schools: An interview with William Glasser. *Phi Delta Kappan, 68*(9), 658.
18 Evans, D. (1982). What are you doing?: An interview with William Glasser. *The Personnel and Guidance Journal, 60*, 460.

10
Back to School

"The ultimate use of power should be to empower others."
—*William Glasser*

The low drone of the jet engines kept inviting him to take a nap, but Glasser looked out the small window next to his seat at the panorama that stretched out below him. At an altitude of over 30,000 feet very few details could be discerned. He could see mountains and valleys and plains. Basically, all he could see was the big picture. It was a view with which he had become comfortable. He was good at seeing the big picture. Unfortunately, this trip wasn't about the big picture. This trip was about details in the life of his son, Joe, who at the time was in a doctoral program at Florida State University in Tallahassee, Florida. The details were that Joe was on the verge of flunking out of the program and Glasser was heading there to see if he could help Joe get around the impasse or through whatever it was that was blocking him. Joe was 35 years old at the time, yet he still hadn't found his niche. He had a problem with follow-through and seemed to lack the ability to bring a task to its completion. He had big ideas, even good ideas, but making them happen was something else. He had been unable to hold down a job and Glasser was hopeful that the doctoral program would provide structure and a clear goal. Alex Bassin, who more than 20 years before had promoted *Reality Therapy* and partnered with Glasser within the New York City correctional system, was now a professor at Florida State and was supporting Joe as best he could, but it appeared it wasn't going to be enough. Once again, it seemed, something was going to thwart Joe reaching his goal. As Glasser headed to Tallahassee it wasn't lost on him that almost 50 years earlier his mother had headed across the country, with him and his sister in tow, to make sure that Glasser's older brother, Hank, successfully completed his undergraduate program at Stanford. Glasser chuckled as he continued to look out the window and thought about this comparison between him and his mother. He wondered if he had the same look of determination on his face that he could still picture on his mother's face as they drove from Cleveland to Palo Alto.

The year 1986 was significant for Glasser. Besides the trip to Tallahassee, which did help Joe successfully complete the degree, Glasser was involved with a number of key decisions. He began a scholarship fund to help provide reality therapy training for those who would not be able to get the training otherwise, which was an easy decision, even though he donated a significant amount of his personal money into the fund. Another decision—the decision to close his private practice office—was much harder. Ending his private practice may have been influenced by his starting to drive out to Simi Valley at least once a week. Again he was driving up highway 101 to try and make a difference in a school. Each time he drove to Apollo High School he was going right by the off-ramp he used to for the Ventura School for Girls more than 20 years earlier. He was 61 years old now and as busy as ever. With his next book being published, he was about to become even busier. The new book, *Control Theory in the Classroom*,[1] marked a shift back to the educational setting. Dating from his early years at the Ventura School, his work at the elementary schools in East Los Angeles, his work at Pershing Elementary School with Donald O'Don-

BACK TO SCHOOL   241

nell, and to his writing of *Schools Without Failure*[2] to that moment in 1986, Glasser had always been interested in the potential of schools. The Educator Training Center was still fully engaged in providing training and support for educators across the country. Yet, since 1978 his focus had been so much on understanding and implementing control theory that he had not been involved in the schools to the same degree he had before. In 1986, Glasser was, to use a well-known phrase, back to school.

"I returned to working in the schools," he explained in an interview a few years later, "after I learned control theory. I kind of left the schools for about 10 years because it seemed to me there wasn't a great deal that I could add to the concepts of *Schools Without Failure*. Then, when I became aware of control theory, and worked hard to understand and expand it—and make it applicable to people—especially to those who manage people like teachers and administrators—it seemed to me that the time was ripe to begin to apply this theory to the schools."[3] Even as he was working through the challenges of getting *Take Effective Control of Your Life* published, and then changing a year later to *Control Theory;* even as he was introducing his own organization to this new approach called control theory; and even as he was working through misunderstandings with Bill and Mary Powers, Glasser was still writing for schools. An article he wrote in the fall of 1985, which was titled "Discipline Has Never Been the Problem and Isn't the Problem Now," outlined how control theory informs us that a "lack of discipline is not the problem; the problem is our unwillingness to accept the biologic fact that we cannot be externally motivated to act in the interest of anyone except ourselves."[4] Glasser's articles had a way of predicting where he was going next and this article was especially predictive, in that at the same time he was writing the article he was also writing *Control Theory in the Class-*

room, which would alert teachers and principals to the concepts of control theory and the idea that schools must become places where students want to learn. Glasser especially emphasized students needed to work together in learning teams.

Glasser had heard of the Johnson brothers before meeting them in person at Disney headquarters in Los Angeles. Few educators then had not heard of them. By the mid-1980s, David and Roger Johnson were known as two of the primary leaders in the field of cooperative learning, and teachers across the country were flocking to their four-day workshops to learn how to bring this learning strategy into their classrooms. To help them plan for a new model community that would be built adjacent to their Epcot and Disney World properties, Disney called in thought leaders from various fields to help them create this perfect town[5]. As a result, William Glasser, who at the time was up to his neck in control theory writing and speaking, and the Johnson brothers, who were up to their necks in teaching classes at the University of Minnesota, writing cooperative learning books and giving cooperative learning trainings, found themselves sitting across the Disney table from one another. Glasser remembers Ron Goleman, the author of *Emotional Intelligence,* and Howard Gardiner, the multiple intelligence guru, also being a part of the brainstorming. While exciting in concept, Glasser doesn't have fond memories of the Disney process. "It felt like they were just trying to get a big name," he stated somewhat cynically, "so that they could say Glasser or the Johnsons were involved." In an even more cynical tone he groused "everything Hollywood touches turns to shit." His tone wasn't improved as he also recalled how hard it was to get reimbursed for his expenses with them. Something good did come out of the meetings, though, as Glasser and the Johnsons became friends.

One can almost see the wheels turning in Glasser's head as he sat at that table listening to David and Roger talk about their favorite topic. He had been sold on the value of cooperative learning prior to meeting them, and had used forms of it throughout his career, but hearing their confidence and their joy in person—Roger with his direct, convincing manner and David with his dry wit and quiet insight—would easily have connected new dots for Glasser. What if, he wondered, the Johnsons would in some way partner with him on the *Control Theory in the Classroom* manuscript? During a break he approached David about this possibility, hoping they would be interested in participating.

Two things are noteworthy. Again, here is Glasser's tendency to team up with people, either real partners who actually contribute to the project in some way, as with George Harrington in *Reality Therapy* (1965), Donald O'Donnell in *Schools Without Failure* (1969), and William Powers in *Stations of the Mind* (1981), or figurative partners who have mapped out a unique, but well-known territory, as with Marshall McCluhan in *The Identity Society* (1972), and W. Edwards Deming in *The Quality School* (1990). This time he seemed to be motivated by the idea that the Johnson's involvement would add credibility or value to what he was doing. Or possibly their involvement would serve as an endorsement of the project.

The second thing was his lack of recognition of his own status. Glasser knew, at some level, that he was a big deal, but more often this realization seemed to be lost on him. He didn't see, for instance, that at these same Disney meetings the Johnsons were looking across the table thinking, that's William Glasser. Early in his career, David Johnson had worked with tough inner city kids in New York City, and the book *Reality Therapy*, according to him, "laid out a clearer road map than anything else." Johnson saw Glasser's ideas as groundbreaking, especially for people who worked with children and teenagers, and over the years he stayed in touch with Glasser.

When asked in 2004 how Glasser was viewed by the field of psychology, Johnson answered, "You know, I'm a very poor person to ask that question to, but I will give you my impression. The field of psychology has splintered. The cognitive researchers and theorists probably pay no attention to Bill. Most social psychologists probably don't follow Bill's work. It's in the personality area and treatment area that he would be known. Except that whenever you work directly with schools, and you see who's had an impact, you would have to include Bill. That's where you run into Bill's work. There are other school programs—Goodlad, Sizer, and Project Zero at Harvard—but when you run into a Glasser school things are different. His work really affects every day life in the classroom. Teachers who have taken Bill's work seriously will be different their whole career. Once you see the principles in action you just can't go back. It just works better."

Few people really appreciate the professional price Glasser paid for forging the Reality Therapy and Control Theory trail. And few people are aware of the attitudes within the field of psychology. "Leaders in this field are highly competitive people," Johnson continued. "Ellis[6] and Perls[7] would get together and ask, How many people came to your last workshop? I'm charging $10,000. What are you getting? I never saw Bill mixed up in that at all. Bill was always centered on how do you improve the world. How do you help people? These other guys were on huge ego trips." Glasser was criticized for not having research to back up his claims, but Johnson had an opinion on that as well. "From a hardcore point of view, there isn't good research on Bill's work. But you can see the impact on the field, so even as a hardcore researcher I've always had a lot of respect for Bill and what he is doing. He doesn't have the data or the research that should be there, but he has practical procedures so that when you see it in action you know it works. He doesn't come out of a social science background. He comes out of helping kids. He can't be faulted for missing research."

When Glasser reached out to David Johnson, maybe hesitantly, maybe wondering if the Johnsons would care about the *Control Theory in the Classroom* book, he didn't realize the esteem with which David Johnson held him. "I was honored to work with Bill on the control theory book," Johnson emphasized. "He asked me to get him a set of cooperative learning lesson plans and I was very pleased to be a part of the project."

Control Theory in the Classroom[8] introduced educators to Glasser's new focus on the ideas of control theory. Higher standards and longer school hours were not the answer, and focusing on discipline ignored the real problem. In his opinion, less than half the students were doing any work at all, and most students did not like school. The growing disparity between the haves and the have-nots combined with traditional teacher-centered methods were killing even the desire to learn. In response to the competitive atmosphere in schools, he suggested students often collaborate in learning teams. It was also important that teachers become knowledgeable in the principles and strategies of control theory. Teaching in the same ways, but doing it for longer hours, was not the answer. There must be a fundamental shift in instructional practice.

Glasser explained the key components of control theory—that our motivation comes from within ourselves; that our behavior is our constant attempt to satisfy one or more of the five basic needs; and that everything we do is initiated by a satisfying picture of an activity we store as a pleasant memory. Teachers have the challenge of taking into account the pictures students have in their heads. Students are motivated by reasons that are personally important to them, rather than by external manipulations imposed on them. The constant focus by schools seemed to be on student discipline, but Glasser explained: "When we talk about better discipline with no attempt to create a more satisfying school, what we are really talking about is getting disruptive students to turn off a biological control system that they cannot turn off."[9] As humans, whether teacher or student, our behavior is always our best attempt to meet our needs and gain more control over our lives. Students have no interest in superficial busywork that has no relevance to their lives. There is no power in boredom and get-tough discipline approaches would not solve that. The set-up must be changed. "It will take time," Glasser wrote, "to realize that teaching is not doing things to or for students. Teaching is structuring your whole approach in a way that they want to work to learn."[10]

During the two decades that led up to his writing *Control Theory in the Classroom*, Glasser had already given his voice toward increasing the element of caring in schools. Reality Therapy from the beginning had emphasized the idea of involvement or personal connection and those elements continued to be emphasized as he transferred his focus to schools. Now he wanted to combine the elements of cooperative learning with the principles of control theory, and in the process improve the relationships in classrooms. It is important students have positive relationships with their teachers, but it is even more important students have positive relationships with each other. Cooperative learning strategies were effective because they strengthened the learning outcomes and student relationships all at the same time. Glasser pointed out the response to *A Nation at Risk*[11] emphasized more schoolwork and less caring. Almost three decades later *No Child Left Behind*[12] would seek again to cure low student performance with more schoolwork through higher standards and high stakes standardized testing. Unless classes became more satisfying and caring, though, no amount of longer school hours or high stakes testing would improve student performance.

Glasser felt teachers were a type of manager and students were a type of worker, with the key question being how to get students to produce competent schoolwork. He talked about the approach of modern managers versus the approach of traditional managers and began to refer to the ideas of W. Edwards Deming, a very prominent author, speaker, and business consultant throughout the 1970s and '80s. Glasser appreciated very much Deming's focus on improving the system rather than on fixing underperforming individuals. Deming also emphasized the goal must always focus on quality and every part of the organization should be involved with the evaluation of quality indicators. In other words, quality isn't something we test for at the end of the production line; quality is something we evaluate every step of the way. Self-evaluation, according to Deming and Glasser, was the most important form of evaluation. As Glasser concluded, "When students figure out some of their own education, they are involved in the most powerful of all learning processes."[13]

"What's this I hear about some talk you attended yesterday?" Glasser asked one of the Institute interns. He had heard from Linda Harshman, then the executive director of the Institute, that several of the interns were talking about a presentation they had attended.

"Yah, it was good." The intern was busy sorting through some files when Glasser came by.

"Where was it?" Glasser wondered.

"It was at Woodland Hills High." The intern was answering the questions, but not much more.

"What made it good?" Glasser pursued the subject further.

"Well, I think you would have really liked it too. The guy was a good speaker, but not flashy. Kind of like you. Anyway, he is a principal of a special high school in Simi Valley and talked about what kids really need in school, you know, what they really respond to. He's on some special self-esteem task force for the state. He seemed to know what he was talking about."

"Sounds interesting. Do you remember his name?"

"His name was . . . his name was . . . Brad . . . something." The intern closed her eyes as she tried to think of the speaker's name. "His name was . . . Brad . . . Greene. Yah, Brad Greene."

Brad Greene was the principal of Apollo High School in Simi Valley, California. Already in the district as a middle school teacher, Simi Valley High School hired him to begin an alternative secondary school program. His innovative spirit stretched the comfort zones of some of the district administrators, but the new school quickly grew to eight classrooms. The students themselves named it after the Apollo space program. They were into every detail, including designing new stationary for the school. Just as the intern had related to Glasser, at the time of the talk, Greene was a member of the California Task Force on Self-Esteem. Glasser remembers the task force having quite a bit of success in instituting new approaches, including smaller class sizes and a more caring learning environment.

Glasser followed up on his chat with the intern and gave Brad Greene a call. He asked Greene questions about the school and wondered if he could come out to the school for a visit. What Glasser found at Apollo was a strong, relational, effective principal guiding an alternative high school with 26 certified staff and 350 students. The students came from several area high schools and represented all kinds of academic, social, physical, and emotional abilities. Many of them were very bright, but not performing well in a traditional high school setting. Others were at Apollo because of drug-related issues or because they had gotten into some other trouble with the law and were now involved with the juvenile justice system. The school had a longer year, evening classes, and basically did everything they could to cater the program to the needs of the students. Compared to the Ventura School for Girls, Apollo High School was closer to functioning like a real high school. Glasser liked the feel of what he saw and asked Greene if he could work at the school to help it do an even better job. Greene and Glasser related well to each other and Greene asked his teachers if they would be open to Glasser coming to the school on a regular basis and working with those teachers who wanted to work with him. Many of the teachers said yes, and Glasser began coming to the school at least once a week; during some months he came to the school several times a week. Glasser had a clear goal: "What I wanted to do at Apollo was produce the first quality school. And I wanted to do it with students who would ordinarily be considered very hard to teach."

The idea of a quality school was a picture in Glasser's head even as *Control Theory in the Classroom* was hitting bookstore shelves. Glasser had thought a lot about Deming's management ideas[14] and was convinced that his focus on quality and his views on the way workers should be treated was right on target. He had read what others had written about Deming and had read Deming's book, *Out of the Crisis*,[15] but as with Powers' book almost 10 years earlier, he found the material unreadable. Instead of traveling to see Deming, though, he was able on his own to make a strong connection between the elements of quality and the elements of control theory. Looking back Glasser remembers: "I just wanted to make all this stuff readable and accessible to people." Deming's work served to confirm the direction

Glasser was already heading in. When asked if Deming's ideas on self-evaluation turned a lightbulb on in his head, Glasser replied, "No, no, I had been thinking that way since *Reality Therapy*. Evaluating your own behavior was one of the fundamental points of *Reality Therapy*. There was a lot in Deming's 14 Points that was complementary to control theory, especially the one about driving out all fear. Driving out fear is all about external control. That was a point that kind of led me to write *The Quality School*."

Convinced that a different school environment and different kind of teacher/manager were needed, the manuscript for Glasser's next book, *The Quality School,* had been brewing in his head. Piece by piece, idea by idea, an outline for the manuscript was taking shape. Quality needed to be the goal and the only way to reach quality was by building schools on and around the concepts of control theory. As Glasser sought to clarify the essential points in the new book, help came from an unexpected source. Glasser had written a small booklet that in a preliminary way described his view of what a school would be like when control theory elements were put into place. In response to this booklet, a man by the name of Jim Grimes, who at the time was an elementary school principal in Illinois, sent Glasser a "rigorous, 16-page critique." Glasser described that "[Grimes] was highly supportive and, at the same time, extremely skeptical. He suggested flatly that, in the early form in which he read them, many of the ideas just would not work. But the tenor of his input was right on! Please show us how to make the ideas work."[16] Glasser acknowledged Grimes probably had no idea how much his critique helped to clarify his thinking. *The Quality School* would be Glasser's attempt to answer Jim Grimes' plea to show folks how to make it work.

To be able to show teachers how to make control theory work is what motivated Glasser to begin driving to Simi Valley and volunteer his time at Apollo High School. Greene remembers Glasser wanting to be in every classroom, getting to know the students and the teachers, so that at the first staff meeting he could ask the teachers: "Do you want to work with me for the next four years?" The teachers responded they would like that very much, and Glasser began to become a part of the school fabric. "He would go into a classroom," Greene explained, "and spend time just watching and observing. He might ask a teacher if it would be all right if he visited with the kids the following day and find out why they were doing what they were doing. He would talk to the kids directly." This process became a regular fixture at Apollo. "Bill would visit a classroom for as long as it took for him to feel connected, or as long as it took him to feel he understood what was going on. He would then go to another class, and so on. Then the staff meeting that day was comprised of him meeting with those teachers, as well as some of the students from those classes. He would dialogue with these teachers and students in front of the rest of the staff." Greene described how significant this practice was for the staff. "Glasser did a couple of things that were turning points for the staff. When he interviewed difficult kids and handled it really, really well, it showed us how it could be done. He interviewed the kids in front of the staff, and then after the interview was over he would visit with staff some more." Slowly, the teachers were learning what to ask and what not to ask students during a problem-solving conference, as well as the best tone of voice and facial expressions to use when doing the asking.

Greene remembers Glasser would often say, "I have no idea. It's really a puzzle," but then he would go about discovering the answer. "Whenever he came for one of his visits Glasser didn't leave without giving us homework. I always had something to do before Glasser came back the next time. And he never forgot what the previous assignment had been. At one point we were having a bit of a problem with fighting. So Glasser says that when kids fight over the next couple of weeks to write down what they say, word for word. He comes back and looks at what we documented and acts like the mystery is now solved. 'Now we know what to do. The kids are saying in a variety of ways that they are only fighting when they have an audience. We're dealing with the wrong people. We're dealing with the fighters when we need to be dealing with the watchers.' I then followed Glasser as he went to four classrooms and talked with students about how in a quality school we don't hurt each other or speak cruelly to each other. He asked them if they wanted to be a quality school, and if not, he would leave. He asked them if others were, to some extent, encouraging the fighting and the students said yes, that was happening. It became clear that sure enough it wasn't just the fighters who were involved."

Attendance was another problem facing Apollo High School. "They only had a 65% attendance rate," Glasser remembers. "So I talked with the students about why they were coming to school. They said they needed an education. When I pointed out that they needed to attend classes more often and do more school work than they were doing to get a diploma, they responded that they did more work in some classes. When I asked them why in some classes, they explained that certain teachers really work with them. 'They don't punish us. They give us chances to do the work until we learn it.' So I said, 'If we can start changing the school in the direction you just described, would you be willing to become part of a group of students who comes to school a bit earlier in the morning and calls those students who are having attendance problems and tell them, please come to school, we need you here?' And they said, yes, they'd do it. And so an attendance team was developed, we called it the A-Team, and we would even go to a kid's house who hadn't come to school. Five or six students would pile into a station wagon and we would go to see the kid. And they would tell the kid, face-to-face, we need you at school. And the kid would come. We went from a 65% attendance rate to 92%, which is about as high as you are going to get in any public school."

Apollo High School served as a laboratory as Glasser homed in on traits that would be present in a quality school. Several journal interviews during this time period, the late 1980s, alerted educators to what such a school would look like. He was convinced that the need for power was at the core of almost all school problems. Instead of engaging in the struggle to force or manipulate students into learning, teachers needed to focus on "teaching in a way that makes students want to learn."[17] Glasser didn't like the word "motivate," because to him it implied an external force or pressure. For him the teacher's job was to facilitate. In an interview with Ron Brandt, who at the time was the editor of the *ASCD Journal*, Glasser captured what should be the goal of every school when he stated: "The ultimate use of power should be to empower others."[18] This empowering included teaching students, in the same way that teachers were in-serviced, the fundamentals of control theory. For Glasser, "not teaching students how we function is like asking them to play a game without teaching them the rules."[19]

Of interest in the Brandt interview is evidence of Glasser continuing to search for the right labels. For instance, he hadn't come up with the term "quality world" yet. Instead, he described how "each of us builds inside our head a kind of hypothetical world—I call it an 'all-you-want-world.' Starting at birth and throughout our whole lives we store pictures in it, pictures of what we have found to be need-satisfying for us."[20] Like a potter slowly forming a pot on a turning wheel, Glasser was shaping the package of his ideas. The quality world would become part of the pantheon in his next book. While such details were clarified over time, what was consistent throughout was the idea that "control theory teaches that we can't force people to do what they don't want to do."[21] This element needed to be at the core of any exemplary school.

And so, drawing from his own all-you-want-world, drawing from *Reality Therapy, Schools Without Failure,* and *Control Theory,* drawing from his years of experience in classrooms at the Ventura School for Girls and the East Los Angeles elementary schools, drawing from thousands of class meetings he conducted in schools across the country, drawing from the ideas of W. Edwards Deming, and now drawing from his ongoing experience at Apollo High School, Glasser began to write his description of a school of quality. The book ultimately would be aptly titled, *The Quality School: Managing Students Without Coercion.*[22] *The Quality School,* fueled by word-of-mouth testimonies from fellow teachers, sold well[23] and once again brought Glasser onto the educational stage. It ranks as one of his best-written books, and it struck a chord with many educators looking for a better approach. One result of this interest was the formation of The Quality School Consortium, a group of over 200 schools that desired to exemplify The Quality School elements. It would be impossible to include all the points the book described, but the following list will begin to give an idea of the elements Glasser was emphasizing.

The key goals and ideas in a Quality School:
Eliminate coercion.
Incorporate self-evaluation.
Relationships are highly valued—especially among students.
Staff and students like coming to school.
No student will be able to say, "No one cares about me."
Cooperative learning is a common instructional format.
The focus is on quality; low-quality work is not accepted.
There is no busy work.

> There are no bad grades; B's are required to receive credit.
> To receive an A, students would have to produce something beyond competence.
> Grades can be improved.
> No nonsense is taught or tested; no objective tests, all tests are open book.
> There is no compulsory homework.
> There is no elitism.
> Rules are kept to a minimum.
> There is no punishment.
> Parents are not asked to fix problems that occur at school.
> When students get into trouble and need to be suspended, there is no set suspension time. The suspension lasts as long as needed for the student to address the mistake.
> If they are making it hard for a teacher to teach or for fellow classmates to learn, students may be asked to leave class.
> A loving, flexible environment is more valued than a rigid, threatening one.
> Focus is on changing the system, rather than on changing students.

This list is certainly not exhaustive, but each entry, in its own specific area, supports the belief that students must be managed in a way that convinces them the work they are asked to do will satisfy their needs. It was in *The Quality School* that Glasser first used the term "lead manager" as a way of describing a manager, in this case a teacher, who recognized that people are internally motivated for personal reasons that are important to them, and tapping into this internal motivation reality was the only way to foster sustained quality effort. Boss managers, on the other hand, believed people could and should be controlled through pain or pleasure, punishments or rewards. Boss managers had tradition on their side, as managers have been trying for decades, centuries even, to manipulate or coerce people into preferred behaviors. Glasser identified this traditional management tendency as part of the core of the problem. "Unless we can get rid of coercion," he emphasized, "we will not make even a dent in the problems of education."[24]

Consistently, slowly, and without fanfare, Glasser coached staff members and students at Apollo High School so that it might become a quality school. In the process, which was something Glasser had in mind all along, he learned a lot about the needed elements of a quality school and the ways to reach them. Greene remembered, "Glasser was very respectful, very open, like he seemed aware that he was on our territory. He never insisted on his way. He accepted when I said things like 'Maybe we aren't ready for that' or 'Let me talk with the teacher about that.' He didn't come to graduation and he declined an award the kids wanted to give him. He never charged a dime, although I did have to buy him lunch at his favorite Simi Valley deli." A year after *The Quality School* was published, Glasser asked Brad Greene to work for the Institute. An appreciation for each other and a trust between them had developed over the years and Glasser recognized the depth of his colleague's school administration experience and the expertise he had gained in implementing control theory. On top of that, with the success of *The Quality School,* Greene and Apollo High had taken on educational celebrity status. Principals and teachers were interested in hearing what Brad Greene had to say.

The Quality School Consortium and its accompanying Quality School Training Program, while very successful at first, went by the wayside after a few years, which I was curious about. The Educator Training Center was dissolved in 1997, as all of the training programs were brought under one Institute roof. It wasn't just this restructuring that led to the consortium's demise. Glasser explained that, at first, school administrators had to sign a contract to become a part of the consortium, but that they were then thinking if they signed this contract they would now have Glasser Quality School. He remembered a similar phenomenon in the *Schools Without Failure* training. "Schools were like if we buy the book and do it—presto! They didn't understand the difficulty of giving up external control. Schools really struggling with managing without punishing."

Glasser and the Institute trainers came to realize just how important the principal was in the process of school improvement. "An effective principal is really important," Glasser offered. "Initially, the program is too fragile to make it on its own." He recalled two very effective school leaders from his own past—Beatrice Dolan at the Ventura School for Girls and Dean Caughey at Western Reserve University Medical School—who wanted to run schools where people were successful and where they enjoyed school. "Schools need to have joy!" Glasser proclaimed. Principals are a key piece in the journey toward this kind of quality. Principals who were committed to the principles of control theory, first at a personal level and then at a professional level, and who gently and persuasively kept these principles in front of colleagues could guide schools toward non-coercive quality. Kaye Mentley, a principal in Michigan, read *The Quality School* and what the book described resonated deeply with her, so much so that she called Glasser and said she wanted her school to be like the school he had described. After a process of staff support and training, Mentley's school, Huntington Woods Elementary School in Wyoming, Michigan, became the first Glasser Quality School. It was a special school and many visitors toured the school to see and hear control theory principles in action. Kaye Mentley wanted to start another quality school in Grand Traverse, Michigan, and after mentoring a principal to take over at Huntington Woods, she headed north where she oversaw the opening of Grand Traverse Academy, a 12-grade Glasser Quality School. Mentley's story is significant for several reasons. The first is that effective leadership makes a difference. Achieving a non-coercive model school is possible under the leadership of an empowering principal. The second reason is that while good schools can rise up out of effective leadership, also they can sink back into mediocrity when effective leadership isn't present. For a combination of reasons this took place at Huntington Woods. Glasser described how it also took place at the Quality School in Texas he wrote about in *Every Student Can Succeed*.[25] When the principal left the school, the Quality School program went with him. Glasser also recalled that his wife, Naomi, had wanted to write a book about the schools in Johnson City, New York, which had become well known for cutting-edge success in outcome-based education. "She flew back there to look them over, but came back saying there was nothing there that had anything to do with a Quality School. A change of leadership was a part of that deterioration." Creating quality schools can be done, though, and individuals like Bea Dolan, Brad Greene, and Kaye Mentley are examples of the kind of leaders needed to do it.

So much good can come out of an environment that is friendly and caring. "My own life was turned around," Glasser recalled, "by a teacher in graduate school who asked me what plans I had for the future. This brief conversation was the first time that anyone in any school had taken a personal interest in me, and from it I was empowered to try to enter medical school. Between a teacher and a student, a little interest goes a long way."[26] When friendship and caring aren't present and when, on top of that, students are asked to complete meaningless or boring busy work the situation is ripe for students to resist and even rebel against this arrangement. Traditional schools blame students for this misbehavior and rely on sanctions or punishment to bring the students back into line. Such schools depend on the students' parents to be a part of the punishment process. When sanctions and punishments do not work it is not unusual for frustrated educators and parents to turn to drugs to solve the student behavior problem. Glasser desired that Quality Schools have drug-free campuses, and this included Ritalin and other prescription stimulant drugs. In the past, he had suggested brain drugs like Ritalin might be an option, but he later changed his mind completely on this topic. "I would never suggest that now. I was trying to come across as having an open mind, but my mind has closed up, especially since 1996." One reason his mind changed was the way kids were misdiagnosed in the first place. "So what does a child do who comes to school and doesn't like school; doesn't believe he is succeeding there; and doesn't believe anyone cares about him? He shows his disapproval in a variety of ways and the school calls it ADHD. But it's just his way of expressing his unhappiness at the situation." Another reason his mind changed was the data on neuroleptics (brain drugs) indicated they were dangerous for the health of the brain, especially so for children.[27] His goal was for schools to teach in a way that medicating students would not even be a temptation.

What is well known is for many educators The Quality School approach became a journey. What is less well known is for Glasser himself, the author of *The Quality School*, the approach became a journey as well. One of the most significant developments that came out of this journey was Glasser beginning to disassociate himself from school discipline plans. He remembers the shift taking place right after he finished writing *The Quality School*, but the process probably began with his study of control theory. The more he understood how ineffective and even destructive external control was, the more he wanted to stay away from it. And with this in mind, the more he considered school discipline approaches, the more he became uncomfortable with them. Many were surprised when this discomfort was directed even at his own discipline approach. In 1974, Glasser had published a small booklet entitled *Glasser's Approach to Discipline*,[28] in which he outlined and described a 10-Step Approach to School Discipline based on the concepts of reality therapy. None of the 10 steps contained even a shred of coercion, yet Glasser began to distance himself from the plan nonetheless. At least three concerns contributed to Glasser's growing discomfort with discipline plans. One of the concerns was not particularly significant, whereas another was very significant. In all, the concerns formed a package that would lead to Glasser formally and publicly rejecting all discipline plans, and that would ultimately lead to a significant schism within the Institute's membership.

The first concern had to do with what could be called the recipe effect. In other words, a list of steps implies that all a teacher or principal needs to do is follow the steps. When it was pointed out to Glasser the 10-Step Plan was non-coercive he quickly answered, "It's non-coercive, but it was still cooky-booky." Glasser didn't want educators to think managing students was as simple as following a recipe. The second concern was that while educators could read his books and receive the control theory training and talk a good non-coercive game, so to speak, implementing a non-coercive approach when they returned to their schools was quite another matter. It was interesting to see well-meaning teachers, who had been steeped in external control their entire lives, yet who wanted to use internal control strategies in their classrooms, actually attempt to use internal control approaches in an externally controlling way. Glasser felt he had to pull back from a discipline emphasis when educators were having such a hard time understanding how a lead manager works. In the early 1970s Glasser was known for being the school discipline expert. Advertisements in school journals touted his "get tough" approach. Now he wanted to firmly distance himself from all of that. A third concern, which would turn out to be the most troubling of the concerns, was that discipline programs, by nature, focused on fixing the kid. The student was viewed as the problem and the discipline strategies were meant to fix him or her. The student as the problem was the focus. Glasser was appreciating more and more that an individual, whether a student or a teacher, was rarely the real problem. Glasser and Deming believed the real problem could almost always be traced to a systemic issue. Therefore, the focus needed to be on the system, rather than on an individual. As he realized how much schools struggled with this, and especially as he actually observed schools reverting to external control strategies, often portraying their actions as being endorsed by Glasser himself, he decided a decisive response was needed.

The publishing of *The Quality School* in 1990 corresponded with the 25th anniversary of the publishing of *Reality Therapy* in 1965. The two books served as appropriate bookends for his career up to that point. Both were groundbreaking summaries of his forward, non-traditional thinking, and invited others to join him on a more effective path. The annual Glasser conference in 1990 was titled a Silver Jubilee and was planned to commemorate this 25-year milestone. The evening program had various individuals paying tribute to Glasser and his contributions, several of these individuals having been with Glasser for all of those 25 years. Bea Dolan was to be a featured guest, but her health would not allow her to come. She was one of the most important people in his life and Glasser was disappointed when she wasn't able to attend. Her letter, a portion of which appeared in the program, meant a great deal to him. "We, at Ventura," she wrote, "started every treatment program the department had—citizens' advisory groups, ward advisory groups, small and large group counseling, off campus services, etc.—and what did we get? We got each other, a reward beyond compare!" Years later when Glasser shared his memory of this with me, his eyes teared up as he recalled her support.

The message written on the inside cover of the Silver Jubilee program indicated others had indeed responded to Glasser's invitation to join him on a more effective path.

> A Message to Dr. Glasser:
>
> It has been said that "a journey of a thousand miles is begun with one step." When you first used the phrase "reality therapy" you took that first step. And when you spoke of eight steps, schools without failure, identity society, positive addiction, control theory, environment, procedures, and quality, your stride increased.
>
> Tonight, as you pause in your journey, we, the Institute for Reality Therapy, wish to say, as best we can, "a thousand thank yous." Thank you for choosing to make the journey. Thank you for your ideas. Thank you for your achievements, for your authenticity, for your support, for your encouragement, for your friendship. Thank you for showing us the way.
>
> Our program tonight is for you and for the Institute for Reality Therapy. We look forward to another 25 years of your journey. Our hope for you and Naomi is a long, happy and healthy life. Our hope for us is that we can keep pace with your journey.

It was a special evening in so many ways. Presenters for the program included Donald O'Donnell, Doug Naylor, Alex Bassin, Richard Hawes, Diane Gossen, Barnes Boffey, Perry Good, Linda Harshman, and Glasser's son, Martin. In the midst of this support and unity it would have been impossible to believe that several of these people, within just a few years, would no longer be a part of the Institute. More important, the expression of hope that Naomi and Bill would live long, healthy and happy lives would prove to not be enough for one of them. Even as she sat there on this special evening taking in the love and support of the entire Institute, a devastating illness was knocking on the door of Naomi Glasser's life. For the time being, though, they were all together. *Reality Therapy* had been having an impact for 25 years and the night, this Silver Jubilee evening, was a night of affirmation and celebration.

NOTES

1. Glasser, W. (1986). *Control theory in the classroom.* New York: Harper & Row, Publishers.
2. Glasser, W. (1969). *Schools without failure.* New York: Harper & Row, Publishers.
3. Chance, E & Bibens, R. (1990) Developing quality middle schools: An interview with William Glasser. *Middle School Journal, 21,* 2.
4. Glasser, W. (1985). Discipline has never been the problem and isn't the problem now. *Theory Into Practice, 24(4),* 241-246.
5. The first phase of Celebration, Florida, was begun in 1996 and as of 2000 had a population of over 2,700 residents. By 2007 that figure rose to over 4,000.
6. Albert Ellis was a pioneer in the field of cognitive behavior therapy.
7. Fritz Perls is known for the creation and development of Gestalt Therapy.
8. Glasser, W. (1986). *Control theory in the classroom.* New York: Harper & Row.
9. Glasser, W. (1986). *Control Theory in the Classroom,* p. 53
10. Glasser, W. (1986). *Control Theory in the Classroom,* p. 79
11. This 1983 report, commissioned by President Ronald Reagan, declared that American schools were not preparing students to become part of a competitive workforce.
12. Proposed by President George Bush, Congress passed the No Child Left Behind Act in 2001. Touted as standards-based education reform the act required states to develop assessments in basic skills. Federal funding was then tied to the results of these tests.
13. Glasser, W. (1986). *Control Theory in the Classroom,* p. 133.
14. W. Edwards Deming (1900-1993) became famous for his work in Japan following WWII where he assisted the Japanese in a workforce turnaround that is still the stuff of legend. Japan went from being viewed as a producer of sub-par products to being respected for producing some of the best products available in the world. "Made in Japan" was no longer a

joke. A hero in Japan, Deming's work in the United States was only beginning to be fully appreciated when he died in 1993. Right up until his death he was a sought-after speaker and business consultant.
15 Deming, W. (1986). *Out of the crisis*. Cambridge, MA: MIT Press.
16 Glasser, W. (1990). *The quality school: Managing students without coercion*. New York: Harper Collins.
17 Gough, P. (1987). The key to improving schools: An interview with William Glasser. *Phi Delta Kappan, 68(9)*, 651.
18 Brandt, R. (1988). On students' needs and team learning: A conversation with William Glasser. *Educational Leadership, 45(6)*, 45.
19 *ibid.*, p. 43
20 *ibid.*, p. 41
21 *ibid.*, p. 43
22 Glasser, W. (1990). *The quality school: Managing students without coercion*. New York: Harper Collins.
23 *The Quality School* has so far sold 114,000 copies.
24 Glasser, W. (1990). *The quality school: Managing students without coercion*. New York: Harper Collins.
25 Glasser, W. (2000). *Every student can succeed*. Chula Vista, CA: Black Forest Press.
26 Glasser, W. (1990). *The quality school: Managing students without coercion*. New York: Harper Collins.
27 Breggin, P. (2002). *The Ritalin fact book: What your doctor won't tell you about ADHD and stimulant drugs*. New York: Perseus Books.
28 Glasser, W. (1974). *Glasser's approach to discipline*. Long Beach, CA: Educator Training Center.

11
Pain and Joy

"A loving man needs a loving woman more than
a loving woman needs a loving man."
—*William Glasser*

The final buzzer had sounded, the game was over, but she remained in her seat and watched as straggling players left the court and the arena around her emptied. A premonition may have urged her to take it in a while longer. She had just watched the final regular season game of her beloved UCLA Bruins, one of the most storied NCAA Division I basketball programs, defeat Arizona State, 85-77, and finish the 1992 season with a record of 28-5. Their record that year was good enough to give them the number one West Region seed for the NCAA men's tournament, but not quite good enough to be compared to the powerhouse UCLA teams of the '60s and '70s. The Bruins did well in the 1992 tournament, making it all the way to the Elite 8 before losing to Bobby Knight and his Indiana University team. They had beaten the Hoosiers earlier in the season, so the loss was harder to swallow than some. And then there was the view, at least for UCLA fans, that any loss was hard to swallow after the standards set by the John Wooden era teams. Unmatched by any program before or since, the John Wooden UCLA teams won 10 national men's basketball championships. From 1967-1973 his Bruins won seven national titles in a row and during those years the team amassed a won/lost record of 205-5. Over a period of seven basketball seasons they lost five games. Five. So the 1992 team record of 28-5 wasn't quite there, but it was very good nonetheless. And she had been there for every one of their home games in 1992. The team would now head off to Albuquerque and March Madness, where the Western regionals would be played, and open the tournament against Robert Morris University, a comparatively small school from Pittsburgh. Not feeling that well, she wouldn't be traveling to Albuquerque. Her rooting for the Bruins in person ended with this, their last regular season game in Pauley Pavilion. And while others may have pushed a little toward the exit and hurried to get to their car in the parking lot, she sat and lingered just a while longer.

Naomi Glasser was a diehard UCLA Bruins fan. It may come as a surprise to some that she was a Bruins' season ticket holder, but why should it be a surprise? During Bruin games Pauley Pavilion was filled to the brim with energy and creativity. The student chants alone made the cost of the season tickets worth it. And the Bruins, for the most part, were a very good basketball team. The arena was not far from the Glasser home and she came to look forward to their games. She looked forward to the college basketball season, in general.

Glasser began dating Naomi Silver in 1945 and they got married on September 20, 1946. Soon thereafter they had their first child, he completed medical school, and they moved to the West Coast where they built and set up a home in the southern California hills overlooking Santa Monica, Brentwood, and the Pacific Ocean. Two more children were born after the move to California and she focused on raising them, as well as on supporting her husband in any way she could.

Glasser was an insightful and talented man, and Naomi was his equal in many ways. One interviewer compared the two of them when she wrote, "Glasser is a fascinating lecturer who can hold the attention of large numbers of people for very long times when he speaks from the stage. One to one I found him shy, usually not very talkative, and hesitant to talk about himself. The vivacious, outgoing member of the team is Naomi Glasser, his wife."[1] Vivacious and outgoing would seem to match nicely with the atmosphere of Pauley Pavilion on game day.

Although her children were her first priority, as Glasser's prominence grew as an author and a speaker, and as a supporting organization took root and grew to support him, Naomi was quick to become the most important piece in that support network. Her strength and her intelligence were focused on his success and the success of the Institute. Al Katz, a longtime friend of the Glassers, noted, "Naomi was a very strong, brilliant woman, a tremendous support. She knew what she wanted and," chuckling as he said it, "she knew what he wanted. She would spare no effort. Her whole life was devoted to him. She must have had other interests, but I didn't know them. She did like UCLA basketball. That's the only thing I knew about her outside of the Glasser efforts." As a result of his books, magazine articles, and speaking appointments, Glasser was receiving a great deal of attention. He frequently found himself in the midst of people, large groups of people, with many of them trying to get to him. For someone so shy this was not comfortable for him and he didn't do that well "schmoozing with people." As one colleague described him, "He's friendly and gracious, but not a schmoozer." Naomi knew this better than anyone and would step in to protect or help him. Linda Harshman, who served for many years as the executive director of The Glasser Institute described: "His social skills, his interacting with people, he's come such a long way from where he started, this little guy with his polyester pants on, looking at the floor as he's talking. Thank God he had Naomi. People who liked his ideas would descend on him and Naomi would perform that protective role and did the piece he couldn't do."

Naomi Glasser also became very involved with planning the international conferences. Bob Wubbolding, longtime colleague of Glasser, recalls Naomi's role in preparing for the conference that was to be held in Ireland during the summer of 1993. "Naomi was a very strong woman, and as a matter of fact, was a good friend of my wife. She used to refer to Sandie as her little sister. And people were somewhat in awe of Naomi. She was very firm about her ideas and expressed them without any shyness. Sandie and I were living in England in 1992 and we went over to Ireland to kind of investigate the university where the conference was going to be held the following year. As it turned out, Naomi had already been there to do the negotiating. I'll never forget the Irishman who said, 'Oh, yes, Naomi has been here, and she is a formidable woman.'" He laughed quietly here. "I've never forgotten that," he continued, "a formidable woman. She was very, very strong, and very supportive of Bill, of course, and a wonderful person. And when she spoke, people listened."

Fitzgeorge Peters, who briefly lived with Glassers when he first moved to Los Angeles, confirmed Naomi's active and supportive role in Glasser's work. "Naomi freed him from all of the minutia. She played a major role in all of the conventions and was a huge support to Bill. I can remember the two of them going off to the side and talking about how he was doing or how he came off in a talk."

When Glasser was asked if Naomi kept him humble at home, he replied it wasn't like that at all. "She was independent and wanted to contribute, but our relationship was very cordial. She looked up to me and was very supportive. If anything she thought I should get more credit instead of less." Naomi probably did feel the way about his success that Glasser described, yet when Laura Lennon, a friend from Ireland, asked her if she was ever overwhelmed at the fame of her husband, Naomi replied, "When I get to feeling that way I ask him to take out the garbage." Regardless of whether or not Glasser was taking out the garbage, his success was important to her and the success of the Institute was important to her too. She threw her strength and her ability, two things she possessed a great deal of, into her husband and the Institute achieving as much success as possible.

"Naomi was not a person besieged by a lot of doubts about things," Glasser began. "She understood what she wanted and she understood what other people around her wanted. She came to Institute board meetings and gave her opinion. She had strong opinions and she stuck with them. She had strong opinions, probably stronger than mine, about how the Institute should be run. I never cared as much about that as she did."

Naomi was such a partner and supporter of her husband that it seems impossible their marriage might have had the usual relationship challenges. Glasser wrote in *Staying Together,* his first book about marriage: "A good marriage is the most difficult of all affiliations to maintain,"[2] something he was aware from personal experience. *Staying Together* was, as the cover of the book stated, a control theory guide to a lasting marriage. Personalizing the book, Glasser shared in some detail similarities and differences between him and Naomi. Applying the basic needs of survival, love and belonging, power, freedom, and fun, Glasser felt that, except in one area, they were compatible. That one exception was his very high need for freedom, which urged him to pursue his career and do all of the traveling necessary for success. "Naomi and I talked about this a lot, especially the conflict between my obligations to her and our family and my desire to pursue my career. We disagreed about my travel and it got to the point where

I would only travel so many nights a month—I think it was seven nights a month."³ Glasser didn't think this was unreasonable and said he tried to live within this number. Yet as one listens you can hear there were deeper frustrations than just the number of nights he was gone.

When is the moment in a marriage when something shifts? Can it be identified as one moment or is it the sum of many smaller moments, moments that could barely be called moments. Many of you now reading this passage have been married or are married right now. Is your marriage everything it needs to be? If not, when was the moment the sparkle of the relationship began to fade? And when the fading begins, even if only slightly, how does the relationship change? Eventually, without love and communicative negotiating, the married partners can become like two strangers living under the same roof. Fortunately, Bill and Naomi Glasser loved and communicated their way through 46 years of marriage, even when they couldn't see eye-to-eye on everything. What they didn't see eye-to-eye on, though, created problems they had to continually work through. The same traits people can be applauded for at work may not be valued as much in a personal or intimate setting at home. Naomi's keen intelligence, her very specific expectations, her strength, and her blunt communication style were all affirmed in her work with the Institute staff and her work planning the conferences, however Glasser wasn't always as enamored with these traits at home. From his perspective Naomi was critical and seemed to "complain about everything." Even the author of *Reality Therapy* and *Control Theory* has to work things out at home.

Nothing can prepare a person for the news that she or a loved one has cancer. So much goes through your mind so quickly. Yet ready or not, this is the news Naomi Glasser was given in 1992. She was diagnosed with colon cancer and it was decided that she would be operated on in July. Glasser was certain the surgery would be successful, and in a way it was. The cancer was removed from her colon, however it was discovered that it had metasticized to her liver. The prognosis was not good. Naomi headed home where she and Bill settled in for this final stage of her journey.

The house was different now from when they first moved in 35 years earlier. Six years after building it they had done a major remodel that added the upstairs living room and the bedrooms underneath it, including the master bedroom in which Naomi spent so many of her final days. Prior to her cancer diagnosis she actually wanted to sell the house and buy a new one. Glasser dragged his feet on this idea, though, partly because a new house would cost a significant amount of money and partly because he was used to their house. "I was really attached to our house. It was a family house. Very few people have a family house anymore."

Glasser stayed with Naomi at home for the six months prior to her passing away. They talked about a lot of things during this time, including even the possibility of ending her life before she deteriorated to the place where no quality of life remained. He even procured the drug to do the job in case she reached that point. Her special strength remained to the end and the drug was never used. "We talked about it. We talked about what we would do. She said, 'I don't think I want to live this way and I want you to get me some medication to kill myself.' The point is, I see people hold onto life when it's past where I'd want to hold onto it. But I'm also not the kind of person that would like to blow my brains out. So I thought of easy ways to do it and I think going to sleep would be one of the easiest ways, cuz I like going to sleep." What a gut-wrenching time for them, yet Glasser, true to his form was once again matter-of-fact, not cavalier, not cold, just matter-of-fact.

The two of them also talked about Glasser's future. Knowing his need for companionship and his need for someone to take care of him, Naomi encouraged him to find the right woman after she was gone. Glasser listened, but he didn't seem to realize how well Naomi had him pegged. He had written in *Staying Together* that "a loving man needs a loving woman more than a loving woman needs a loving man,"[4] but he didn't see himself with that kind of need. He even wrote later in the book, "I am not planning to get married again."[5] He followed that statement, though, with his intention to stay open to the possibility of marrying again, so he was probably already feeling what Naomi had predicted in the aloneness of their bedroom two years earlier.

Robert Glasser, Bill's cousin, remembers "Naomi was ill a very short time. Marie and I had lunch with her about two weeks before she died. She didn't look bad. She walked slowly, but outside of that, you could hardly tell anything was wrong. She wanted to live through Thanksgiving, which she did, but that was about it."

Bob Wubbolding remembered a small, yet key moment during Naomi's illness. "The interesting thing is Naomi never said good-bye on the telephone. She would just end the conversation and hang up. But a few days before she died she called Sandie and at the end of their conversation she said good-bye. My wife said that she knew that was the end."

Naomi Glasser died on December 4, 1992. Glasser was close to publishing a follow-up book to *The Quality School,* which would be titled *The Quality School Teacher,* the UCLA Bruins were gearing up for another varsity basketball season, and her children, all grown up by now, were busy beginning young families of their own, but Naomi Glasser was done. She had been such a strong presence and help for the Institute, and such a strong protector and helper to Glasser, her loss could not have been felt more keenly. Besides the loss of a close companion Glasser also lost her writing support and editing skills. One friend lamented, "Bill just couldn't take it when he found out his wife was dying. She meant so much to him in the sense that he could focus so much on his ideas." One of Glasser's editors at Harper Collins explained, "Bill missed Naomi desperately as an editor. She was a good critic. I met her several times. She was very impressive. They were close, I never saw him without her, and he coveted her input. She was dedicated to what he was doing and seemed to understand exactly what he was saying." Naomi edited the manuscripts for *Positive Addiction* (1976); *Stations of the Mind* (1981); *Take Effective Control of Your Life* (1984) and *Control Theory* (1985); Control Theory in the Classroom (1986); The Quality School (1990); and The Quality School Teacher (1993). Her legacy also includes two books she edited on her own—*What Are You Doing?: How People Are Helped Through Reality Therapy* (1980); and *Control Theory in the Practice of Reality Therapy: Case Studies* (1989). The last book she edited for her husband, *The Quality School Teacher,* she worked on even as she was feeling terrible from the effects of the cancer. The Dedication for *The Quality School Teacher* read:

> For the past fifteen years my wife, Naomi, has edited my books and also two books of her own, *What Are You Doing?* and *Control Theory in the Practice of Reality Therapy.* In all cases, her meticulous editing made what I said concise and crystal clear. If you have had the opportunity to read these books, you may not agree with me, but what she did guarantees that you had no difficulty understanding my meaning.
>
> It is with great sadness that I write these words, as this is the last book she had the chance to edit. She passed away from cancer in December 1992, after a brief but devastating illness. Ill as she was, she insisted on editing and was critical of herself for not being able to do what she thought was her best. I assured her, and I think that you will agree, that her

work was high quality right to the end. I think when she read the final manuscript she was satisfied.

I want to acknowledge here that my work would not have been of the quality that I am told it is without her dedicated help throughout a long and satisfying marriage. Those who knew her—and her friends in the schools and in the counseling profession were numerous—understand what she did and will miss her caring and dedication to the ideas we use, which have helped so many people.

Not long after Naomi's death, just a few weeks actually, Glasser's cousin, Robert, and Robert's wife, Marie, asked Glasser over for an evening meal. They knew he was alone now and wanted to supportive. Robert remembered "a day or so later he called back and asked if he could bring a woman with him to dinner. We were extremely taken aback, you know. What can you say? We said okay, but it was just a few weeks after Naomi had passed away. Marie and I talked about it, the way he was moving on after Naomi had died, and wondered whether moving on so quickly reflected a good marriage or a bad marriage. In our amateur psychology we decided it must reflect a good marriage. If a person feels free to go on, if they didn't have guilt or have to put on some mourning clothes, that seems like a good thing." Did Robert and Marie have this figured correctly? Some might question their amateur psychology and say Glasser moved ahead with other relationships too quickly. It would seem those close to Naomi would especially feel this way. Is this an example of his matter-of-fact behavior taken to an extreme? Glasser responded, "I didn't grieve much after she died; I grieved while she was dying, you know, together with her."

One is led to question here the extent to which Glasser understood grief and the grieving process. During another visit, Glasser explained, "When Naomi passed away, no, I didn't grieve for her, because I thought I had been a reasonably good husband. I never said no to her. But, I don't know about grieving. I don't know, I don't know if I'd even grieve if Carleen passed away. I just, I don't, grieving is not a process which I am really very much personally involved with."

What should we conclude here? Did Glasser actually lack the make-up or the mechanism to grieve or did he somehow not recognize common grieving symptoms? One colleague shared that it was very rare, but occasionally he would see a flash of anger from Glasser that would normally be associated with the grief process. One such moment was after Martin was stabbed and another moment occurred when Joe was accused of child abuse. Martin healed and the charges were dropped against Joe, but as each of the incidents was unfolding Glasser was dealing with some strong feelings. Reportedly, he was extremely angry with the person or persons who had caused the pain or injury to his sons and exclaimed in both cases he could have killed them. "If this sort of thing happens to you," Glasser commented further, "you'll find you have emotions you never even dreamed you had."

Another of these rare moments occurred at one of the Glasser conferences after Naomi had passed away. Bob Wubbolding remembered how he felt that Glasser "would totally deny the stages of grief. Yet I saw him get furious at something that happened at the conference in New Orleans. A person said something along the lines of, 'That never would have happened if Naomi had been here.' He blew up at that, enraged at her, cursed about it, very furious. I think she did him a big favor by triggering some anger, which I took to be a part of his grief. I'm purely guessing at this. If you have someone close to you die, it's only natural to get angry at something or someone. The person actually left the Institute, not realizing that it wasn't personal. She thought it was and was hurt by it." These episodes were rare, maybe telling in some way, but rare.

In the months after Naomi died, Glasser did move ahead with his life both personally and professionally—probably too quickly for family members and close friends, and probably not processing grief in the way that most would. He admitted to answering ads in the social section of the newspaper, but said, "That wasn't real great." He dated a woman for a while, but that went nowhere. He and Naomi had worked on *The Quality School Teacher* book together, which was published in 1993, just a few months after her death. Unabated by his circumstances he continued to write and published *The Control Theory Manager* in 1994. His belief in the principles of reality therapy and control theory, even after losing his life partner, urged him to continue helping people see and experience the value of a loving, non-coercive life. In spite of his continued activity, though, he was beginning to realize Naomi was right about him needing a life partner. He had to admit he was pretty lonesome.

She had placed her purse on the table and was quickly going through the small pile of mail, just to see if there was anything interesting, when her eyes fell on an envelope. Unlike the junk mail and bills, this letter was personal, written in someone's handwriting. Looking to the top left-hand corner she saw the name William Glasser along with his home address. She looked at the center of the envelope and sure enough it was her name, Carleen Floyd, written there. Apparently, this delivery was no mistake. It was exciting to get a letter from Glasser himself, but why, she thought, would he be sending something to me? She was a member of the Institute for Reality Therapy, in fact, an advisory board member of the Institute, so it was within the realm of possibility she would receive a communication from the head of the organization. Except if it was from the Institute, wouldn't it have come in an Institute envelope?

The letter had crossed the country from Los Angeles, California, where Glasser lived, to Cincinnati, Ohio, where Carleen worked as a school counselor. She had attended Xavier University, where Robert Wubbolding, one of the faculty at Xavier, taught her the counseling approach of reality therapy. Attracted to reality therapy she began reading all of Glasser's books. "I was turned on by his ideas," she explained, "because it was such a hopeful message." Drawn further into the concepts of reality therapy, she became a member of the Institute and soon became involved with the organization's regional activities, and ultimately the organization's national and international leadership network. When control theory was introduced to Institute members, as a school counselor she was very positive about it. Seeing the effectiveness of the control theory ideas in the school setting she wrote a book of her own entitled, *My Quality World Workbook*.[6] The *Cincinnati Post* ran an article that highlighted Carleen and her new book. "The activities in the book," she described to the interviewer, "are designed to help children choose behaviors that will help them. It teaches children to find positive alternatives and find ways to get their needs met in a positive way."[7] Shortly after the workbook was published she sent a copy to Naomi and Bill, calling Naomi by phone ahead of its arrival to ask if they would take a look at it and see if maybe they would approve it. "It was thrilling for me when he let me know that he thought it was a very good book." The year her book came out, 1990, was the same year the Institute celebrated the 25th anniversary of Reality Therapy at the annual conference, which was held in Cincinnati. Carleen had helped Naomi get ready for the conference. "She was quite friendly to me," Carleen remembered. "We shared a huge interest in fashion, because we both liked clothes. She was such a lovely, wonderful person and everyone in the Institute really respected her and liked her and cared about her."

Carleen's contact with Glasser had been minimal. He would come to board meetings and since she was on the board and sitting around the same table she figured "he was aware of who I was." And she added, "I was certainly aware of who he was. He was the head of the organization and I literally hung on every word he said. Everything he said that I could use in my teaching, I wrote it down."

At the same time Naomi was struggling with her illness, Carleen was going through a struggle of her own. Her marriage was disintegrating and by 1993 she confided to a friend she did not think the marriage would last. Her then husband confirmed this when he asked for a divorce. This new reality forced her to address what she was going to do with her life and even where she was going to live. So much hurt and frustration, yet she clung to the hope of a better future. In the midst of this time she thought out loud to Kathy Curtiss, a fellow Institute trainer, "Oh, Kathy, if only I could be in a relationship with someone who knows about reality therapy and knows control theory. That would be such a wonderful thing." Later she shared her situation with Linda Harshman, a kindred spirit to her, partly because Linda had gone through her own painful divorce years earlier, and Linda asked Carleen if this news regarding her marriage and impending divorce was confidential. Carleen figured people were going to find out about it and told Linda it didn't matter if she told people. And Linda, who worked so closely with him at the Institute, mentioned it to Glasser.

Carleen had carried the unopened envelope to the living room and sat down, still reviewing in her mind her different contact points with Glasser. The thought even crossed her mind that she may have done something wrong or ill-advised enough that it merited a letter from Glasser himself. Then she thought maybe he had heard of her marriage difficulty and had sent a note of condolence. Finally, she decided to open it and see what it had to say.

September 9, 1993

Dear Carleen,
Linda told me that you are going to get a divorce, that your marriage has not been good for a long time. My question is simple: are you involved with someone else or are you free to spend some time with me? There is no doubt that you care for me professionally and I have the strong feeling that the caring is also personal. Are you open to slowly and carefully exploring a new relationship with me?

I, as you may know, tried hard to get something going here with a woman who seemed compatible but it has not turned out to be workable. What I have learned is that at our age with all our history, you have to go slowly and kind of let what may happen, happen. To let it happen, we have to be willing to enjoy the time we have together and not focus too much too quickly on the future. If the time we can spend together gets better and better, the future will take care of itself. Too much focus on then kills the now and then, with no present, there can be no future.

If, after spending brief periods of time together, we find that we are able to love each other both mentally and physically all the time we are together, we can part happily knowing that there will be another intense reunion soon. We could do things like spend a weekend in New York City going to the theatre and museums or take a week or ten days at my condo in Hawaii. I could come through Cincinnati on weekends as I travel or you could come here once in a while and see both your daughter and me. As busy as we are and with no responsibility other than to please each other, we would find that the times we are together go a long way. It is all the other stuff that makes relationships so difficult. If we grew to love each other, we would find a lot of ways to be together.

I cannot promise to see you exclusively as I live here and I will need some companionship here even though right now I do not have anyone. If your answer to this letter is positive I won't look very hard. At the same time, I don't ask that you be exclusive with me, just don't date any "drug addicts." Basically, I ask that you give what we may have a chance and let it grow from there. If you have any interest in what I suggest, drop me a note and tell me where and when to call you so we can talk a little. I would not venture to write this letter if you were not both mentally and physically attractive to me. If you think I am presumptuous just write and tell me that what I offer is not for you but think it over. Don't say no too quickly.

I realize that what I am asking you to do is not standard but I have never believed that love—and I mean exciting, sharing, sexual, laughing, totally non-boring love—can flourish under the standard conditions. I don't have too much time left and I refuse to spend what I have without pursuing excitement. We could be exciting.

   Love — Bill

She sat there continuing to look at the letter. She was the only person in the room, in the whole house for that matter, but she became aware of the silence. Here, a moment earlier she had wondered if maybe the letter was meant to communicate with her about something she had done wrong or maybe it would offer condolences over her marriage ending, but it was none of that. "It wasn't that at all," Carleen later described. "It was almost a letter of delight or congratulations, and proposed that we see each other. I almost nearly died. I really couldn't believe it." In the stillness of the moment she tried to process what the letter was saying. And was she on her own with this or could she talk to someone about it? "The only person I told about it was Sandie Wubbolding," she continued. 'You're not going to believe what I got,' I tell her. 'Bill is asking if we could see each other.' It sounded just like Bill Glasser. I had read all his stuff. At first I was beyond thrilled and just delighted. But then I began to think and to analyze and to worry. I'm on the Institute board, I'm a respected faculty member. What if I get involved with him and it doesn't work out? I'm a proud person and I was worried about that. I knew my worth, though. I hadn't always known it, but I was coming to know it and I felt I could be an asset to his life." Bruised from her marriage this thought process was no small thing for her. A question that had to be answered in this process and she had thought long and hard about it was, simply put: Can I still love a man? She came to know the answer to that question and to realize she could love a man who loved her and valued her. For a week, though, after receiving the letter she considered these kinds of questions and thought about how to respond.

Glasser had decided to go the snail mail route and for him it must have felt like the letter was truly being carried by a snail across the country. He went to the mailbox every day, but no reply. After two weeks he was beginning to think Carleen didn't want him, but was trying to figure out a way to tell him. Compounding Glasser's problem, Carleen decided to write back using snail mail, rather than calling him. Written by hand, her response mirrored his warmth and directness.

> Dear Bill,
> Your letter was so clear and straightforward – I loved it! Here is my most direct and sincere answer to what you are suggesting:
> First, I am not involved with anyone at this time, nor do I plan to date any "drug addicts." I'm also not interested in any more cold and empty men like the one to whom I've been married for the past fourteen years.
> As for you, I see you as the most complete man I have ever met. I've experienced you in the brief moments I've been able to spend with you, as a very real and whole person and I have been aware of myself wanting to connect with you somehow. I would be very interested in having that opportunity any time after the dissolution of my marriage has become final, which should be near the end of October.
> Your suggestion about moving very slowly, carefully exploring a relationship, is a wise one, especially for me right now. I am in no hurry and I am certainly not ready to even consider the future until I have a present.
> To gently nurture an open and honest relationship with you sounds not only intensely appealing to me, but also a whole lot of fun! I am excited at the prospect, yet it is somewhat frightening at the same time. I really would like to talk with you a little more about it.
> I hope to hear from you soon. Until then I send you my warmest thoughts.
>
> Love,
> Carleen

Carleen remembers being drawn to Glasser's confidence and chivalry that honored a way of being from days gone by. "He just wrote a letter up front and put it out there," she praised. "He was confident. He was asking permission. It was a throwback to an older time." After receiving Carleen's response he called her and they began a telephone friendship that grew to be something much deeper. As a result, almost a year after Naomi passed away, Glasser began to court Carleen in earnest. His creativity and energy, never in short supply, seemed to expand as he focused on this new relationship. He started making frequent trips to Cincinnati and Carleen would travel to Los Angeles, and when they went out everything was first-class. "I think he wanted to sweep me off my feet," she admitted. "I think he sensed what I needed." Comfortable together, excited by one another, both with a passion for control theory, within a few months they knew they were in love.

As wonderful as this was it also created a challenge. He was firmly placed in Los Angeles. His home was there, the Institute for Reality Therapy was there, his colleagues and friends were there, and his tennis buddies were there. She was firmly placed in Cincinnati. Her home was there, her work was there, and her support circle was there. It isn't uncommon for circumstances like this to sabotage a couple's future plans, even if they love each other, if in the end one of them or both of them loves their present life more than the future possibilities with their new partner. And sometimes it just boils down to pride. Who loves whom more? It can be like a high-stakes game of chicken, as when two cars speed toward each other, each driver daring the other to swerve away first. For one partner to leave everything behind and essentially start over requires a great deal of love and faith. Bill and Carleen's love for each other, and the recognition that their relationship was not just a case of casual enjoyment, necessitated this discussion topic be addressed.

Glasser didn't turn his back on Los Angeles, but in the spring of 1994 he moved to Cincinnati. He kept his house and the Institute remained in its southern California location, but he personally relocated to a high-rise that Carleen had always wanted to live in overlooking the Ohio River. She began the process of starting over—selling her home and most everything she had—and he, normally a creature of habit, moved to another state completely—both of them beginning to step into a future that only months before had not seemed possible. In July of that year they left for Ireland and began a tour of Europe that lasted the entire summer.

When they returned to Cincinnati, Carleen learned Schwab Middle School wanted to hire her as a Quality School consultant, which meant she needed to quit her job as a counselor at her old school. Apparently, when it rains change, it pours change. She was very excited about it, though. Interestingly, the school didn't know about her close relationship with the *Quality School* author himself when they hired her. This development brings up several noteworthy items. One of the items is Schwab Middle School basically had William Glasser fall in their laps, yet they did not capitalize on it nearly as much as they could have. As he had at the Ventura School for Girls, the inner city elementary schools in East Lost Angeles, and at Apollo High School, Glasser began observing and assisting in classrooms and working with teachers to change the learning culture. A number of teachers realized what they had, but not all of them. In spite of this, the school made great strides, for which Carleen was thankful, yet she was a bit frustrated that district administrators didn't know what they had and seemed not to care. The lesson here is that each of us may have a "William Glasser" in our lives, whether in our organization, our friendship circle, or even in our home, yet for whatever reason we miss the gift of what this person has to offer. Glasser was not there to make money. He was there because he loved Carleen and wanted to help her in her project to support the school's improvement plans. As with many other times in his life he was working for *gratis* because first and foremost he was motivated by a desire to help people, especially teachers and students. What kept the Schwab district from seeing this and fully tapping into Glasser's expertise? What keeps you and me from seeing and affirming the expertise in a friend or colleague? Another item of note is that Glasser turned 69 years old in the spring of 1994, yet he didn't hesitate to jump into the challenges at Schwab. He was a famous author. People by the thousands would attend his presentations every year. He had a worldwide following. Yet here he was sitting among middle schoolers in an inner city school trying to get to know them, to understand them, and to help the school become a place where each of them, teachers included, wanted to attend every day. When the school year began there needed to be a serious police and security presence in the hallways. Physical safety was an issue. Yet here was Glasser, observing and supporting in classrooms, walking the hallways, and meeting with staff after school. A man motivated by fame and pride would not have left California and moved to Cincinnati, and such a man would certainly not have entered the struggle at Schwab. It should be noted Glasser was not that kind of man, and because of that he modeled what love can inspire us to do.

Several things were coming together and it was beginning to feel to both he and Carleen that decision "crunch" time was upon them. The 94/95 school year was winding down and the question—Los Angeles or Cincinnati?—still needed to be answered. Carleen admitted, "I had made up my mind not to come to California unless I was his wife. I had no intention to pressure, yet I needed to know where I stood with him." Glasser had wanted to wait an appropriate amount of time before he remarried, but two and a half years had gone by since

Naomi had passed away.

At this same time it so happened another of Glasser's books, *Staying Together*,[8] was about to be published. And on this particular day he had stayed home from Schwab to write the jacket flaps for the book. When he finished he called Carleen at work to see what she thought about what he had written. She remembers him saying, "Okay, I finished the end flaps. I want you to hear them." She described how he went on about needing to get it done because it was going to press immediately. "Okay, okay, okay," she replied as she went to shut her office door. "If you have an old copy of the *Staying Together* book," she said, still savoring that moment, "if you read the end flap, somewhere at the end he says Carleen and I will be married in July."

"And he read that to you?" I asked.

"He read that to me."

"Did you pick up on it right away?"

"I did. Are you kidding? I said, 'Read that last part again. Read that last part again,' and he read it, and I said, 'Are you serious?' And he said, 'I sure am, Dolly.' He calls me Dolly. And I said, 'Really?' He said, 'Really,' and I started to cry. He said, 'It's nothing to cry about.' I said they were tears of happiness. We then got to talking about where and when we were going to do it, and that's when he asked me, 'What would you think about having our wedding at the convention?'"

"I thought it was a great idea," Carleen continued.

Glasser was in the room during this point of the interview and chimed in, "I thought it was a great idea because I wouldn't have to pay for it." He chuckled as he finished the story. "At the end of the evening people were saying it was the first time they had gone to a wedding and had to pay for their own dinner. And I said, well then, you know the leader is no fool here."

The international conference was held in Philadelphia that year, and even coincided with the national July 4th celebration. As part of the Saturday evening banquet, with more than 500 people present, William Glasser and his bride, Carleen Floyd, made their vows to one another. Carleen remembers the unity that was there; even with 500 people present you could feel the unity. "There wasn't a ceremony. Bill and I just got up and talked to one another. We expressed our vows to each other. In Pennsylvania, which is a Quaker state, you make a promise to one another, but you have to do it in front of witnesses." Everyone in the banquet hall sang Love Can Build a Bridge together, which was a fitting affirmation and blessing for the new couple.

Mrs. Carleen Glasser now cast her gaze to Los Angeles and began to prepare for her move to the West. They had overcome the challenges of a long-distance relationship, had sorted through which city to ultimately live in, and effectively supported one another through the bumps in the road at Schwab. They found one another later in life, at a time when they both knew more clearly what they wanted and needed in a mate, and they both were very well-versed in the concepts of reality therapy and control theory. This clarity and knowledge contributed to their happiness and their ability to handle the details that hit every relationship eventually.

Carleen explains, "Bill's influence on me is to let certain things go. I tend to be a grinder-away-at-things, a worrier, it's genetic. He's helped me to not be such a worrier. It's not that he's not empathetic. He is there for me on things that merit it."

Glasser adds, "What Carleen does is she senses what I need, whether I need to be left alone or whether I need company. So I always feel comfortable with her. She respects me. There are times when I want to be left alone and she leaves me alone."

"I influence him," she continues, "in ways that are superficial, I guess. His appearance, for instance. I think his taste in fashion has improved, the public appearance side of him. I've also influenced him to be more aware of the touchy-feely aspects of life. He's never been a real shower of affection."

Glasser agrees. "I don't go around kissing strangers."

"He's more of a hugger now." She looks toward Glasser and he shrugs slightly, admitting she's probably right.

"Carleen makes life easy for me. She takes care of the whole house. I do a little bit."

"He takes out the garbage and he unloads the dishwasher," she says matter-of-factly.

This comment opened the door for Glasser to expound on his belief that dishwashers should clean dirty dishes, and you shouldn't have to wash a dish off before you put it in the dishwasher. We smile at his conviction on this point. The most important point of the conversation, though, was made by Carleen.

"We're never at odds with one another's values."

Glasser's productivity during the early 1990s—a period which included Naomi's illness and passing, as well as his courtship and marriage to Carleen—continued at its usual high-speed pace. Along with numerous journal and magazine articles, Glasser had three books published—*The Quality School Teacher*[9] in 1993; *The Control Theory Manager*[10] in 1994; and *Staying Together*[11] in 1995. Another sizeable piece of writing that is less well known, as much of it is confidential, are the letters in which he responded to people's inquiries or comments. If you have read any of Glasser's books you may have noticed one of the last things he writes is an invitation to readers to get in touch with him if they have questions or comments, often with an additional assurance that he will respond to each letter personally. The Institute files are a testimony to him keeping his word regarding that promise. Reviewing much of this correspondence I was amazed at how affirming and detailed his responses were.

In addition to his writing and presenting[12] during this time was the development of the Quality School Consortium, along with an annual Quality School Conference to support the new consortium. Glasser's book, *The Quality School,* resonated with many educators and requests for support and training began to pour in. When Glasser approached Brad Greene, then principal at Apollo High School, about the possibility of coming to work at the Institute it was because of this great wave of interest in the book's ideas. Greene did join the Institute in 1991 as a consultant for the new consortium and later became one of the Institute's most successful faculty members.

A chapter in Glasser's life that began with tragedy ended with a honeymoon. He had survived a difficult life blow and had moved on. As this chapter of his life closed, to use a weather metaphor, the sky was blue with beautiful white clouds drifting overhead. These clouds would soon become more threatening, foretelling a rougher road ahead, but for the moment the blue sky could be savored.

NOTES

1. Evans, D. (1982). What are you doing? An interview with William Glasser. *The Personnel and Guidance Journal, 60*, 460.
2. Glasser, W. (1995). *Staying together*. New York: Harper Collins. p. 5
3. Glasser interviews, May 27, 2004; July 26, 2007
4. Glasser, W. (1995). *Staying together: A control theory guide to a lasting marriage.* p. 74
5. *ibid.*, p. 90
6. Glasser, C. (1990). *My quality world workbook.* Chatsworth, CA: William Glasser, Inc.
7. Wilson, K. (April 3, 1990). Teacher's fun workbook helps children find positives. *The Cincinnati Post.*
8. Glasser, W. (1995). *Staying together: A control theory guide to a lasting marriage.* New York: Harper Collins.
9. Glasser, W. (1993). *The quality school teacher.* New York: Harper Collins.
10. Glasser, W. (1994). *The control theory manager.* New York: Harper Collins.
11. Glasser, W. (1995). *Staying together: A control theory guide to a lasting marriage.* New York: Harper Collins.
12. Institute records show that during 1992, as an example, Glasser had over 60 speaking engagements with an average attendance of 400 people per event.

12
DECISION IN AUSTRALIA

> "In Australia I really became faced with certain things. And these are the things I'm taking a strong stand on. This is something I've never done. Glasser's been known as wishy-washy, and I was really tempted to stay wishy-washy. It took a great, great thing to unwishy-washy me, but I am going to do it."
> —*William Glasser*

It seems hard to imagine how the Glasser convention during the summer of 1995, the one where everyone in attendance stood together and sang *Love Can Build a Bridge*,[1] could have been so different from the annual Glasser convention held just a year later. If the 1995 convention were portrayed in one word, that word would have been "unity;" if the 1996 convention were captured in one word, remarkably that word would have been "schism." But what came to a head in 1996 actually began to take root many years earlier and developed on several fronts simultaneously. Like *The Perfect Storm*,[2] Sebastian Junger's best-selling non-fiction book that describes what happened when three separate weather fronts, each coming from a different direction, slammed into one another off the coast of New England, Glasser, too, was dealing, from multiple directions, with the strategic future of the Institute. As the Glasser convention of 1996 drew nearer the clouds overhead took on a more ominous look. Understanding the events leading up to the 1996 convention and the controversial decision that

Glasser explained and emphasized at the convention, as well as the Institute's policies following the convention are key to understanding the core of Glasser's mission. The issues were so important that he was prepared, even if all the membership of the Institute disagreed with him, to go it alone. If anything should get the attention of those interested in the life of William Glasser, the events of 1996 should be very, very high on their list.

The pamphlet was really more of a small booklet—16 pages in length—and packed with information. Opening the pamphlet one is struck by the size of the small print that fills the page. The front page of the pamphlet has a picture of Glasser with a big smile. He is wearing a collared shirt like we used to see in the '70s, which makes sense since the pamphlet was published in 1977. In very large print just above his picture the pamphlet reads, Glasser's Approach to Discipline. In smaller print near the bottom of the front page it states, A Report Published by Dr. William Glasser's Educator Training Center. Much of the pamphlet describes Glasser's Ten-Step Approach to School Discipline; however it also shares many testimonials and data in support of Glasser's methods. "Realistic and working," proclaims the pamphlet in reference to the Ten-Steps. "Suspensions decreased 50% to 80% in junior and senior high schools," it claims. "Vandalism decreased 40% to 90% in all of the secondary schools" where the Ten-Steps were in place. A testimonial from Jersey Village High School in Houston, Texas, states "Second-time discipline offenders decreased by 88% and fighting by over 90%. Drop-out rates fell from 18% to 6.3% since the discipline was introduced." For anyone interested in improving school discipline the pamphlet describes in detail how Glasser's program works, what schools can expect when they implement the program, and how to get in touch with the Educator Training Center for more information.

Glasser had gained a reputation for having common sense, helpful strategies when it came to classroom discipline, and the pamphlet was designed to remind educators about the Glasser option. Mary Kay Murphy, a freelance writer from Atlanta, had alerted readers in 1973 to Glasser's classroom discipline prowess. "Dr. William Glasser," she opened, "is a psychiatrist-turned-educator whose ideas about education have been sending shock waves through the schoolhouse." She described how Glasser was veering his approach in the direction of discipline and, in fact, had "taken the initiative to point out ways in which *Schools Without Failure* and discipline are inextricably bound together." Ms. Murphy could not have known when she wrote about this "inextricable bond" that Glasser would come to see the bond, or this connection between discipline programs and student success, in an entirely new light, and that he would ultimately stake everything on breaking this bond. The break wouldn't happen immediately. When Ms. Murphy published her article in *Scholastic Teacher* in 1973, William Powers was just having his book, *Behavior: The Control of Perception* published as well. And when his school discipline pamphlet first appeared in 1977, Glasser was only then reading *Behavior: The Control of Perception* for the first time. He would come to embrace the principles of control theory, which eventually led him to see human motivation and performance in a different way, but this journey took place over a period of years. In the meantime, he wrote articles like the one he contributed to *Learning* magazine in December of 1974, in which he outlined the "ten steps to follow"[3] when working with a difficult student. Others besides Glasser also wrote articles on discipline. One title that caught my attention appeared *in American Educator* in

1978—it was called Mr. Glasser's Gentle Rod.[4]

It may be schools wanted discipline plans, and it may be that for a while Glasser and the Educator Training Center played into their desire for discipline plans, but he soon came to see significant flaws in such an approach. Discipline plans seemed to be a part of the problem, rather than part of the solution, and he didn't want to be known for carrying a rod, gentle or otherwise. For him, this major change was the result of three forces coming together—a positive "perfect storm"—and creating something unique to each of them. The three forces were: 1) the maturing ideas of reality therapy, 2) the new ideas of control theory, and 3) the very new ideas in the management approach of W. Edwards Deming. Reality therapy had always emphasized the need for involvement or a warm connection between people and personal responsibility; control theory underscored these elements and added elements like the quality world, creativity, and total behavior, and in the process identifying the fallacy and the destructiveness of stimulus-response motivational techniques. Deming clarified how damaging coercion and manipulation were in the workplace and how they actually sabotaged productivity. Glasser strongly agreed with Deming and soon thereafter wrote, "Unless we can get rid of coercion, we will not make even a dent in the problems of education."[5]

Glasser recognized elements in Deming's 14 Points for Management that were very similar to the elements of control theory, and he felt that point #8—Drive out fear—was the most important of all. Only as managers were able to create safe and supportive workplaces would workers choose to do their best work; and only as teachers were able to create safe and supportive classrooms would students choose to put forth their best effort in school. In the spirit of reality therapy, schools needed to place a high premium on supportive connections; according to control theory schools needed to recognize that an individual is motivated to meet his or her needs in the best possible way at any given moment; and according to Deming schools needed to relinquish the habit of coercing and forcing students to do school work and behave themselves. So important were these elements, especially the last element, Glasser would write *The Quality School* wherein he described the importance of managing students without coercion. He would later credit Deming with leading him to write *The Quality School.* The point is that as a result of these insights he began to disassociate himself from school discipline programs. "I was trying to get people to think in terms of preventing discipline problems," he later explained, "and if I focused on discipline problems, I, in a sense, would be admitting that they're going to happen, that they're inevitable."

The disassociation process expanded to include even his own discipline plan—the Ten-Step Approach to Discipline. This surprised many since there doesn't seem to be anything remotely coercive in any of the ten steps. When questioned on the need to reject even his own approach Glasser replied, "There's nothing wrong with the Ten-Step plan. It just turns discipline into a cookbook thing." While many felt the Ten-Step Approach was still effective, even in the long term, others felt rejecting his plan was the thing to do. "I think it was smart that he rejected even his own discipline model," Linda Harshman, the executive director of the Institute, offered. "It strengthened his case." Al Katz, long-time Institute member, remembers it from a slightly different angle. "Glasser said that not only do I disavow other discipline programs, I disavow my own. That said a lot about his honesty. He said I made a mistake. I thought it would work, but it's creating the opposite of what I want." What Glasser wanted were schools that cared about kids and wanted to take the fight out of the learning process. The focus needed to be on schools becoming need-satisfying places where students wanted to go.

At the same time Glasser was putting reality therapy and control theory and Deming together and beginning to conclude that school discipline programs were part of the problem, one of his senior faculty, Diane Gossen, was developing a school discipline model called Restitution. Diane was one of the early Glasser disciples and a long-time instructor for the Institute. She received her first training in reality therapy in 1970 and applied her learning in her classes as a College of Education faculty member and then later in the fields of corrections and addictions. Her real epiphany came later, though. "In 1981," she wrote, "I began a kind of learning which I had never experienced before. Glasser introduced me to the work of control theorist William Powers. Studying the model of a self-regulating system as set out in *Stations of the Mind* resulted in a major paradigm shift for me. I began to teach the principles of internal motivation."[6] Invited to teach control theory to the school administrators within the Johnson City School District, Gossen was drawn back into the field of education in 1987. Soon thereafter, she experienced her second significant epiphany, that being Glasser introducing the Deming model in combination with reality therapy and control theory. At the time, the schools of Johnson City, New York, were the epitome of effective, progressive school reform, and for her Glasser's new package—Reality Therapy + Control Theory + Deming = The Quality School—explained the successes that were occurring there. She explained, "Applying Deming's principles to school management and using the ideas of the Quality School enabled me to analyze why previous school change had been transitory and why Johnson City schools were so successful. It became clear to me the discipline model used by most schools focused on the misdemeanor rather than on helping to child learn a better way to behave. As I thought about it, it also became clear that a better way not only made a reparation for a wrong, but it strengthened the child."[7] The Restitution discipline model, based on this way of thinking, was meant to help restructure schools away from traditional methods of discipline. Students could learn to make amends, and in the process learn to become a socially responsible member of the group. For the teacher, Restitution provided a process for students to be redirected. It was designed as a tool to gain control without sacrificing the self-esteem of the individual.

Schools took to the ideas of Restitution and in certain geographic pockets, especially, word of its success rates spread quickly. Australia, it turns out, was one of those pockets. It is interesting that as Glasser was putting reality therapy and control theory and Deming together to come up with *The Quality School* approach, which also began his disassociation with school discipline programs, Gossen was putting the three together and coming up with Restitution, a school discipline program based on the idea of "making it right." As one of her colleagues later shared, "She meant well." Of this, there seems to be no question. And, in fact, for several years after *The Quality School* was published, Restitution workshops were included as part of the Institute curriculum and featured at regional Glasser conferences.[8]

On the surface, Restitution was an accepted part of The Quality School approach. Below the surface, Glasser and others within the Institute were beginning to have questions about its effectiveness with students and especially about the impact it would have on Glasser's overall mission. There isn't room in this chapter to fairly cover the details of the Restitution discipline program, and there is no way we can know the extent to which teachers who had been trained in Restitution were accurately implementing its strategies or reflecting the spirit of the program in the way Gossen intended. For whatever reason, Institute members began to have concerns. One Institute faculty member, putting it bluntly, stated: "I called it bastardizing Glasser's ideas. They would twist people's arms, like what do you want, or is it right? With your arm being twisted you'll say the right answer. I saw Restitution being demonstrated and I thought it was badgering and threatening in tone. If you don't answer the question according to how I saw it, rather than how you perceived it, you just kept answering the question until you answered it right." Jim Montagnes recalled, "When Diane first wrote *Restitution* it was not meant to in any sense be external control. I trained the staff at Huntington-Woods. The first year, Kay Mentley used Restitution. One of my fellow trainers was real big on Restitution. I gave her something once and she replied that now she had to give me something, to restitute, and quite frankly, I was sick of it. Restitution is something that to me has to come from within. It can't be imposed."

Montagnes may have represented a growing concern of a number of people within the Institute over Restitution, however it should be noted that many within the Institute embraced Restitution, especially teachers and principals. Part of the concern had to do with how quickly Restitution was spreading. Educators who welcomed the ideas of control theory into their lives saw it as a natural step to welcome Restitution into their lives as well. After 1990 Glasser wasn't pushing or even offering a discipline plan in support of the control theory approach and teachers saw Restitution as a tangible help toward implementing control theory in their classrooms. One administrator explained, "I guess there's some controversy over Restitution, but all I can say is it helped to turn my school around, and it changed my life, for the better, as a principal."

The behind-the-scenes Restitution drama didn't keep Glasser from writing and in 1994 he published *The Control Theory Manager*,[9] a small book for leaders. Ken Blanchard wrote a cover testimonial for the book that was very supportive, yet prophesied the demise of the title of the book at the same time. Blanchard became very well known in the field of business when he, along with Paul Hersey, developed the concept of Situational Leadership. He would later co-author *The One-Minute Manager*,[10] a very successful book, and be catapulted to the level of international business guru. For Glasser's book he wrote: "I have been a fan of William Glasser's for a long time. I am thrilled that he is beginning to apply his theories to the management of people. Don't get confused by the word control. Dr. Glasser is talking about really empowering your people to do the kind of quality work they really want to do. It's a whole different kind of control. It's control from the worker's standpoint."[11] It's interesting that Blanchard, while being so positive, would also alert readers to a problem with the word "control." It was a problem Glasser had been dealing with for some time.

Even though William Powers had set the stage for Glasser to take the control theory ideas and apply them to behavioral settings, the two of them began to disagree over the best way to teach people about control theory and even over the details of what control theory was and how it really operated. Glasser admitted he and Powers had major disagreements—Powers didn't believe in the basic needs or other things Glasser was teaching and Glasser had given up on the levels of perception—and the partnership that had begun with Glasser's trip to Chicago in 1977, a working relationship that had unofficially ended years before, was now officially on its last legs. Glasser shared with

Bob Wubbolding that he had "always disliked the name control theory,"[12] which could be true. Renaming his book, Take Effective Control of Your Life, to Control Theory would seem to say otherwise, but there could have been a tension within him over the title even then. David Johnson would later agree, "It was unfortunate that he chose the term control theory to start out with,"[13] confirming a growing dilemma within Glasser over the title with which he was so associated, a dilemma that was about to intensify.

In the fall of 1995, at their annual convention in Ireland, the Irish approached Glasser and told him about the "tremendous difficulties" they had with the control theory title. He recalled "the word 'control' in both Ireland and Australia was a bad word, due to the Irish being subjugated and starved and beaten down by the English, and then the English dumping all the Irish convicts and other people in Australia." As far as control goes they threw the Catholic Church in there with the English, too. Men were more frustrated with the control of the church than the women, but control, whether moderate or excessive, was the cause of the frustration. Glasser, already dissatisfied with the title, more than got the point. "The Irish people told me they couldn't live with the word 'control' theory; it was terrible."

The Irish decried the ineffectiveness of the term control theory, but to their credit they also suggested an alternative. Brian Lennon, an early proponent of reality therapy and control theory in Ireland, remembers the moment even more specifically. "A man by the name of John Murphy, who felt the term control theory was just very hard to explain to people, suggested that choice theory would be an improved name." Glasser confirmed that it was Murphy who proposed the new title. "He told me the book was really tough, especially the name of it, because the name means a lot." Others at the convention agreed choice theory was a more accurate and representative title and encouraged Glasser to consider a change. He promised them he would think about it, yet he knew how much a name change would involve.

As Glasser returned to Los Angeles from Dublin he had a lot to think about. He had been feeling for years that control theory wasn't the best title, but now the Irish had really brought the point home to him. A name change may sound simple enough, but it wasn't simple at all. So much effort had gone into the sharing and spreading of control theory. So many classes taught, so many schools in-serviced, so many pamphlets produced, so many journal articles written, and so many books published, all proclaiming the elements of control theory. The year before, in 1994, the Institute name had even been changed to include control theory. Instead of the Institute for Reality Therapy, the organization now became the Institute for Control Theory, Reality Therapy & Quality Management. As his plane landed in Los Angeles, even though it was a very long flight, Glasser still wasn't sure what to do. It had been 10 years since he had adopted the term control theory for his *Take Effective Control* book and now he was dealing with the result. He had gotten himself into this problem, he thought, and he would have to get himself out.

Rarely one to slow down during his career, this may have been a good time to do just that—to ease up and think about the issues facing him. This is not to suggest he didn't adequately think about the decisions that were emerging, but as far as his schedule, his appointments and projects continued unabated. The Quality School program really took off in 1994, with instructors being brought up to speed on helping schools become Glasser Quality Schools; the *Control Theory Manager* was published; and it was in the fall of 1994 that he dove into the Schwab school project in Cincinnati. His relationship with Carleen had become very special, something that doesn't happen without a commitment of time and energy. He published another book in 1995,

Staying Together,[14] and then began his own staying-together relationship when he and Carleen were married that summer. His trip to Ireland came soon after that. His speaking appointments stretched out ahead of him on the calendar, as always, yet one big appointment loomed larger than any of them. That big appointment was a two-month speaking tour in Australia and New Zealand, as well as presentations in Singapore, Korea, and Japan. Most of his time would be in Australia, though, where he was scheduled to give 29 presentations. More than just the sheer number of talks Glasser was going to give, the Australia trip would turn out to be more significant than anyone could have imagined, including Glasser himself.

The term "control theory" may have been on the mind of members in Ireland, but in the months leading up to his Australia tour something else was on the mind of Institute members back in the U.S. The Restitution school discipline program was becoming more popular and with its popularity came more scrutiny. Not all liked what they saw and Glasser began to receive feedback to that effect. The Institute advisory board was among those sharing such concerns. Most of the members were not aware Glasser had been working on the issue behind the scenes for several years and some were beginning to question his leadership. Bob Hoglund, a longtime Institute trainer, remembers how serious and even traumatic the Restitution issue was for the Institute, but he also emphasized, "the whole situation is the best example of Glasser practicing what he preaches. I was on the board at the time," he continued, "and I was privy to some things that others were not. This was going on behind the scenes for four to five years, and every year it was having more and more impact." Glasser didn't want Restitution taught as a discipline program and the Restitution people would say they weren't teaching it as a discipline program, even though their brochure advertised it that way. As Bob remembers it,

"Bill would meet with Diane and others and they would work something out, but after a time Glasser would see they weren't doing what they agreed to, so he would meet with them again." On a flight from Phoenix to Portland, which was routed through Los Angeles, Hoglund ended up on the same plane as Glasser and Carleen. They were on their way to a Quality School Conference during the fall of 1994 in Portland. During the trip Carleen asked Bob to sit by them so they could visit. "I'm going to end Restitution," Glasser began, "and I would like your support. I'm just going to say that Restitution is done. I've wrestled with it and I've wrestled with it and I'm just going to do it." During the conference he must have changed his mind because he didn't do it.

"He didn't follow through," Hoglund explained, still slightly frustrated about it years later. "When he got to Portland, Diane asked to speak to him and he ended up giving her time up front." Glasser allowing Gossen to address the group would seem to reveal the importance of her status within the organization, as well as Glasser's desire to transparently process the growing *impasse*. Along with Gossen's presentation to the general assembly, Glasser decided to host a meeting in his suite and air the issue with those interested. For the 40 or so people in the room the negative tension was palpable. Some questioned how Glasser was about to shut Restitution down and yet they knew nothing about it. Hoglund spoke up and said to the group: "If you were a principal in a Quality School and had a problem with a couple of kids, you wouldn't call a faculty meeting about them. You would talk to the kids. This is what Bill has been doing behind the scenes for four to five years." More questions challenged the way Glasser was trying to handle the situation and again Hoglund came to his defense. "Part of the problem is that Bill is practicing exactly what he says. He absolutely has been a lead-manager behind the scenes. He has maintained the dignity of others and given opportunities to work things out."

Glasser decided he was going to keep an open mind a little while longer. "I won't shut it down yet," he said. There continued to be a unity between those on each side of the Restitution issue, but it was fragile and unsteady. Hoglund felt something ominous was present. "It felt to me that something had begun, that this was a beginning of a group that was in direct opposition to the philosophy of the business—the business being the core values of control theory. Lots of us felt the same as Glasser and saw this development as a problem. Those who agreed with Glasser couldn't believe he waited six years to deal with it."

Bob Wubbolding remembers how Glasser went back and forth on Restitution. Others have indicated that Glasser received pressure from both sides of the issue, but Wubbolding couldn't confirm that. "I'm not sure if he received pressure from those who didn't like Restitution," he explained. "I didn't like it, but I never pressured him." Glasser may have been sure about his position regarding Restitution, but he was torn on what to do about it within his organization and how to go about doing it, whatever "it" was. An example of this inner conflict occurred just prior to his Australia tour. "In February," Wubbolding pointed out, "Glasser actually endorsed Restitution in an Institute newsletter. And then in April he went to Australia, where he was seeing it everywhere."

Posters advertising Glasser as The Rebel Psychiatrist were placed throughout Australia in anticipation of his speaking tour. He would be there over a month and give almost 30 presentations in the process.

Decision in Australia

The Glasser organization in Australia was as solid as any in the world and many reality therapy and control theory inroads had been made into the fields of mental health, counseling, and education. There was a control theory presence in a significant number of schools in Australia. Piggybacking on that success, by the time Glasser arrived in the country for his 1996 tour there was also a significant Restitution presence in many of those schools. One Institute member observed that the Australians seemed to have come to the point where "they saw Restitution as a part of the Reality Therapy process. In other words, they identified that you have to do Restitution if you are going to honor the principles of reality therapy." As a result, as Glasser visited schools there he saw Restitution being used a lot.

Knowing how tenuous Restitution was in Glasser's thinking, Diane Gossen had reason to be concerned during his Australian visit. Glasser later recalled, "Diane sent me a fax or something saying that for God's sake, when you get to Australia you must not mention that you don't have faith in Restitution. We're selling a huge program over there. I wrote her back and said, no, I'm not going to speak out against Restitution, but if anybody asks me a question I'll say that I no longer support it, and I'll explain why, that it's external control." Those supporting Restitution hoped Glasser's visit to Australia, where Restitution was being used in so many schools, would help him see things differently and become more accepting of this discipline program. Their worst fears were confirmed, though, when his observations in classrooms led to the exact opposite effect. The part of the "perfect storm" through which Glasser was now navigating—the part about Restitution and how to respond to its growing popularity—was coming into focused clarity for him. None of the options facing him seemed pleasant, but what to do seemed clear.

The speaking tour actually began in New Zealand. Only a few months before Glasser had been in Ireland, now he was down under where the climate was different as far as the weather goes, but surprisingly similar when it came to the control theory title. The Irish had made an impression on him, and their suggestion of "choice theory" even more so, so it may be that Glasser was especially sensitive to people's reaction to the term control theory. He admits that he noticed a discomfort with control theory in his New Zealand listeners, even before he got to Australia. If the process going on in his mind over the value of control theory as a title for his key beliefs could be compared to a scale, with control theory on one side and choice theory on the other side, control theory was on the verge of being swept away. Glasser had selected control theory as a title out of, what for him was, necessity, yet it was an uneasy selection. The sales of his book, *Control Theory*, had benefited, but he had paid a price among those who embraced the purity of control theory more than he did. And ever since he christened control theory as his title he constantly needed to explain and disclaim elements that people seemed to assume in a title with the word "control" in it. The Irish, graciously yet firmly, urged him to make a change, something he had reflected on for years. The point is that what happened next was not an impulsive decision. What he did shortly after beginning his Australia schedule, as much as it may have appeared to be a decision of the moment, was in fact the culmination of months and years of experience and thought.

Glasser remembers, "It was about the third talk of the 29 that I was scheduled to give. It was somewhere just below Cairns,[15] but before I got to Brisbane. During the talk I noticed that as soon as I said the words control theory that I was kind of losing them. And then I said, no, no, no, no. I've been making a mistake for quite a while and I may as well rectify it right now. I'm giving up calling the thing 'control theory,' because it really doesn't describe the theory and gets them to thinking that it's about controlling others. I said I may still mention the words 'control theory,' but it will be because I have used them so much, and I'll apologize when I do. From now on we're gonna call it choice theory."

Glasser understood the implications of what he just said—the retooling of an international organization, the articles and books that would need to be written or rewritten, and the explanations that would need to be presented at talks he was giving—but few others in the room did. There were no gasps or sighs or applause. The implications would sink in soon, but at the moment, the proclamation was too much of a surprise. He acknowledged that the Irish had suggested the term choice theory and that he agreed with them. "I just thought," he explained, "that choice theory was an extremely accurate term, because if we're choosing what we do, then there's no difficulty whatsoever saying that we're responsible for what we do." The idea of responsibility had been misused a great deal, in his opinion, especially after *Reality Therapy* was published. People were saying you have to be responsible in a stimulus-response or externally controlling[16] way and he described how he pulled back from using the word as much as he once did. The term choice theory, though, brought being responsible back into a more user-friendly context. Even as he said the words, he knew he was going to have to write a book replacing control theory with choice theory.

Within days he had made two decisions that would significantly and permanently affect his mission and his organization and the many individuals who comprised the organization. The second part of the "perfect storm"—the part about fixing the less effective title of control theory and replacing it with choice theory—had entered the fray. The problem he had considered for so long had now been addressed. Somehow during that talk he decided to go for it. Whatever had kept him from making the decision earlier was gone and he acted decisively. And rather than wondering what he had just done and second-guessing what he had just said, his proclamation had the opposite effect. Telling others brought relief and freedom and even more resolve. "I just bit the bullet and did it," he exclaimed, "and I'm glad I did!"

Linda Harshman, executive director of the Institute, remembers Glasser calling her from Australia. "The thing came to a head in Australia," she began. "The Institute board had been bringing concerns to him regarding Restitution and many questions were coming in from around the country. It impressed Bill that schools in Australia were so into the discipline aspect. So he calls me and said he was going to take a stand on this thing, and that he was going to write a memo and send it to her. As faculty we were a little shocked." They saw Glasser as a whatever person and here he was taking this stand." Glasser would, in fact, write three memos while in Australia, each one longer than the one preceding it, and each one becoming more specific and serious in tone. No one would be able to read the memos and afterward continued to see Glasser as a whatever person. In the process he clearly outlined his mission and his vision for the future.

The first memo is dated May 8, 1996, and describes his desire to focus on changing the system and is included here in its entirety.

At last year's Quality School conference, I tried very hard to reconcile my differences with Restitution by saying it would be all right if it led the child to restore school to his or her Quality World. However, it wasn't until I began to work in Australia that I realized that this was not happening. Regardless of its creator's intent, Restitution, which is being marketed as a discipline program, is perceived by teachers as a way to manage misbehaving students while the school is attempting to become a Quality School. I

Decision in Australia 311

believe teachers are getting the wrong message: focus on the student's misbehavior, not on the system. No matter how you do it, when you focus specifically on what a child is doing wrong, instead of putting all your effort into improving your relationship with that child, it is unlikely that the child will ever put you into his or her Quality World.

Just because teachers, who do not know choice theory, want such a program is exactly the reason not to offer it. Initially, the vast majority of teachers do not want to change what they do because almost no one ever wants to give up the S-R system that has been a part of their lives since birth. If we want Quality Schools, we must send the message that we believe so strongly in choice theory, and what I have written in *The Quality School* and *The Quality School Teacher,* that we will offer nothing that dilutes this message. From the beginning, all of our teaching must explain that any program that doesn't totally focus on changing the system will prevent the school from becoming a Quality School.

In a Quality School, discipline problems disappear because the students, the teachers, and the parents put their school in their Quality Worlds. When this happens, that school has achieved the hardest part of the task it set out to accomplish. For these reasons, and many others that I will explain at our convention in Albuquerque, discipline programs, or any program that focuses on student misbehavior, cannot be a part of the teachings of the William Glasser Institute. Even though I am still in Australia, I thought it was important for you to know that Restitution will not be a part of the Quality School Conference in October in Minneapolis.

I hope that you will support me in what I believe. I have worked very hard to support the Quality School Consortium since its inception and all of the schools wanting to become Quality Schools. I am looking forward to seeing you in Minneapolis.

Several key points emerge in the memo. The first is the focus must be on improving the system, rather than on changing a student. He didn't want administrators and teachers viewing students as the problem and felt so strongly about it that he emphasized "any program that focuses on student misbehavior cannot be a part of the teachings of the William Glasser Institute." That statement is significant for two reasons—the first reason being its far-reaching implications and the second being that at the moment he wrote this statement there was no such organization called The William Glasser Institute. At that moment the Institute was still known as the Institute for Control Theory, Reality Therapy and Quality Management. Finally, readers were alerted to the importance of upcoming meetings in Albuquerque and Minneapolis.

The second memo was even more far-reaching and described details that would affect more than just which ideas were teachable. The second memo outlined organizational boundaries that would have profound effects on people, their lives, and even their income. Glasser was far away from his home base when he was making these decisions so it is unlikely that his normal support system was in place. And it could be said that even within his home base the international Institute board was advisory only. In the end, he decided the direction he wanted to go. A great deal of communication was going back and forth from California, where the Institute was located, and Australia, but it isn't clear how much counsel he was seeking through this communication. He wasn't depending on or hiding behind a board or any other group of advisors. He made a set of decisions and went with them.

Something else that may have influenced the nature of these decisions and the speed with which they took place appeared briefly in one of our interviews. We were talking about Deming and the influence of his 14 Points on Glasser's thinking. Glasser talked about how significant the point about driving out fear was to him, but then he also talked about how people thought that TQM, an acronym standing for Total Quality Management, was developed by Deming, but that it wasn't true. "People attribute it to Deming," Glasser explained, "but he hated the term total quality management, because the idea of installing it became more about external control. Other people developed TQM and then they patronized Deming, who by this time was old and feeble, and pushed him on it because TQM is something you can sell. See, it gets back to money." The possibility that people other than an idea's creator could take that idea and craft it to make money for themselves could have been significant in Glasser's thinking as he wrestled with what to do with Restitution. And the possibility he might be perceived as too old and feeble to deal with strong-willed people within his organization could also have been a significant influence as he crafted the second memo, written eight days later on May 16, which follows in its entirety.

A Message to the Faculty
From William Glasser, M.D.

During my recent tour of Australia, visiting schools, meeting with educators, and giving talks mostly to educators but also to anyone else interested in my ideas, I had the opportunity to clarify my current thinking concerning the future of the Institute and what we teach. As a result, I have made the following decisions:

1. I will change the name of the Institute from its current long and cumbersome name to The William Glasser Institute. This is in keeping with the Alfred Adler Institute and Milton H. Erickson Institute. For years, I have been urged by many people to do this but I have resisted the change. But now, as I see my ideas being used by people all over the world, my name is more and more taking precedence over the specifics of what I teach. Since this is the case, it makes good sense that this change should be reflected in the name of the Institute. I also think that with this change it is our responsibility to make it crystal clear that from now on all Institute faculty will teach only my ideas or ideas, that, as of this date, I completely and unequivocally endorse. Also, by making this change, I am much more assured that my ideas will continue to be taught after my death.

2. I have decided to change the name of control theory to choice theory because it is a more accurate description of what I actually teach. I am doing this because I have expanded what I was initially taught by William Pow-

ers by adding the basic needs, the quality world, total behavior, and other points all well-illustrated on the latest, 1996 edition of the blue chart. I have long divorced myself from the levels of perception which are central to Power's teaching. While I believe that it is possible that they are accurate, I do not believe they can be used in our work or in our lives. Finally, since I have taught that we choose all we do before I met Powers and well before he wrote his book, *Behavior: The Control of Perception,* I think it is more accurate for me and more fair to him to stop using the name control theory. Already in Australia, I have started to use choice theory instead of control theory and I encourage all faculty to begin to do the same.

3. Since I am devoting almost all of my present energy to trying to help people create Quality Schools, I have been saddened by the fact that some of our faculty are teaching discipline programs. I believe that discipline programs are S-R based and focus on changing students rather than changing the system from S-R to choice theory. I believe that it is impossible for any school that focuses on discipline to become a Quality School. I believe this so strongly that, well before I stated this clearly in my 1990 book, *The Quality School,* I had stopped teaching discipline practices. Even practices strongly supported by reality therapy including my own, very popular, "The Ten Steps of Discipline."

4. As soon as the name of the Institute is officially changed to The William Glasser Institute, I will ask all present faculty members, who accept the above philosophy to join me in the new Institute. In doing so, they have made the decision to only teach my written or spoken ideas or ideas I presently endorse. To be perfectly clear, if they choose to teach, sponsor, or support assertive discipline, judicious discipline, restitution, or any discipline program, present or future, they cannot be accepted or continue as faculty members of The William Glasser Institute.

What this means is that I am asking all faculty members to make a choice. I value each and every one of you as teachers and as friends. I hope you will decide to stay with the new Institute but, if you do not, I will never criticize your decision to leave or what you choose to do after you have left.

You will be contacted by the Institute as to your decision as soon as the name is changed.

If there were any doubts about how Glasser was going to respond or where he was headed this memo erased them. He was changing the name of the Institute, changing the label of control theory to choice theory, rejecting school discipline programs, and accepting into the new Institute only those who accepted his philosophy and agreed to teach the ideas he endorsed. If the memo lacked anything, it certainly wasn't clarity.

Institute member reaction varied, although even those who had wanted him to do something, anything, were impressed by the scope of his decisions. Many of the members were concerned about the tone of the memo. Linda Harshman, Institute director, remembered fielding lots of communication during that time, emails and phone calls wondering "how is this not boss-management? Isn't this boss-management?" When asked if he had to field accusations of wanting more control or more power, Glasser responded, "No, not very much. They understood it. They understood the reasons for it, most of the people." Exactly how many members supported him regarding the memo or really understood the wording and tone of the memo we'll never know. There is reason to believe Glasser may have been wrong in thinking that most of the members understood. Some saw irony in a memo that announced a new label called choice theory actually limiting or restricting people's choices.

The decisions Glasser made in 1996 and described in the second memo may not have been totally understood at the time, but they certainly provided a platform from which to consider management approaches, especially the management of students, and thorny issues like rules, expectations, and boundaries. Some people learning about choice theory for the first time (usually boss managers) become frustrated in their perception that choice theory approaches don't have any "teeth" and people can basically do whatever they want, whenever they want. Yet here the creator of choice theory declared very specific boundaries with far-reaching effects. Educators refer to a moment in a classroom when circumstances converge to create a special readiness or hunger for learning as a teachable moment. This moment in Glasser's career was and is a teachable moment for those wanting to understand the core elements of choice theory and the options available when boundaries need to be set. In declaring these boundaries Glasser was running a significant risk of being misunderstood, yet something in the issues was important enough that he felt it was worth it.

A third memo, the longest of the three, was sent from Australia on May 22. It was addressed to all Institute faculty, the Quality School Consortium Board, and all of the members within the Quality School Consortium. The Quality School Consortium had, in a very short time, become a significant part of what had been The Institute for Control Theory, Reality Therapy and Quality Management and the Australia memos would have been of special interest to those involved with schools. The eight-page memo described Glasser's journey as he worked with schools—his recognition that positive relationships are a key to student success, and especially his recognition that it was the S-R system that caused so much of the low performance and ultimately rebellion. He pointed out that *Schools Without Failure* "was an early attempt to change the system, but I still did not recognize that the system itself was the cause of the problems." The Quality School and The Quality School Teacher emphasized that the old S-R system must be "completely banished" from the schools, but many teachers did not understand what Glasser was really proposing and were actually using reality therapy as a way to preserve the S-R system. With regard to this Glasser admitted, "I deeply regret ever using my own reality therapy ideas to create the ten steps of discipline. It was an honest mistake. I did it before I realized that it was the system, not the students that had to be changed."

Glasser was aware that teachers struggled to even conceive of a system that isn't based on S-R, yet it was on this point that The Quality School ideas would rise or fall. The day he wrote the memo he was asked by a group of teachers, "Why not use what we perceive to be a reality therapy, choice theory program such as restitution while we are in the process of changing the system?" As a follow-up they pressed him, "If we don't do this, what can we do with the discipline problems we have to deal with until we change the system?" These were teachers in the final week of their Glasser Intensive Week training, their certification week, but they were struggling to really get what Glasser was proposing. "If we teach or imply," he began, "that focusing on problem students is part of what we believe, we will defeat our own goals. The more we do this in the Quality School Program, the less likely teachers are to even take a look at the S-R system that is causing the problems they are so concerned about. This is what I saw happening here in Australia, which got me so concerned about discipline programs. We must be strong enough to resist demands for help with discipline and for discipline programs and offer them lead-management practices."

Glasser alluded to something he may have seen in Australia when he wrote: "What you should never do, because it is not reality therapy, is to insist that anyone, student or adult, be badgered to make a self-evaluation that supports what is in the teacher's quality world, and then be totally coercive by saying to the child, this is what we believe, isn't it? In essence, I cannot support any program that asks a child to try to adjust his or her behavior so that it is acceptable to a coercive person or system." How many times he observed such an interaction we don't know, but even if it was only once, the interaction made a big enough impression on him that it nudged him into memo-writing action. He had tried to accommodate the Restitution approach to discipline, but this scenario may have been the straw, the last tiny straw in a series of events covering months and years, that was one too many for the camel.

Glasser reminded Consortium members about specific lead-management strategies in the memo, however rather than focus on those elements, which can be found in *The Quality School* and *The Quality School Teacher,* what follows is the last page of the third memo just as it was written—

Many of our people fought the introduction of choice theory,[17] but they finally accepted it. For them to do this, I had to explain and re-explain choice theory. I am willing to do this again with my firm belief that we have to distance ourselves from the idea that we can fix people instead of changing the system, or even along with changing the system. If we can do this, we will be unique in a world that has been and, unfortunately still is, more willing to focus on what others are doing than to take a hard look at what we may be doing. Let's be known as an organization that has the strength to look this ancient problem squarely in the face.

I will use the Albuquerque Convention and the Quality School Consortium Conference to explain in detail what I am talking about here. We have a golden opportunity to discuss this crucial issue at our annual general meeting in Albuquerque and at the Professional Development Day. I will have made my presentation and have made myself available during the convention to explain these new ideas. Here is an opportunity for you to deal with me and each other about this important concept. I believe I have led this organization well for many years. I don't think there is one thing I have taught that has not proven useful. I also believe that I have been open to your ideas, and this is the first time I have rejected what any of you have taught. To me, this is so important because It Is a chance for our Institute

Decision in Australia

to take world leadership in improving the way organizations function.

What I am going to do is give all faculty a chance to think about this important decision until January 1997, when it is time to remit your membership dues. As you pay your dues to The William Glasser Institute, you will be asked to affirm what you joined this organization for in the first place: to teach my ideas that I support. As a member of our faculty, you are associated with our ideas. People cannot help but think that what you teach is supported by the Institute. What I have described in this message is what we can support.

Therefore, if you teach what we cannot support, in or out of our Institute-sponsored programs, you are sending a strong message that you do not believe in one of the most crucial things we stand for. This is a dilemma that cannot be solved unless you choose to separate yourself from the Institute. If you do this, your message will be clear, and our message will be clear. The people you teach will be able to know where each of us stands. They have a right to know this. I would expect that anyone who is a member of our faculty will wholeheartedly support what is written in this message. If you cannot support what is written here, I would not expect you to join the new Institute.

As I said previously, I encourage all of you to come to our convention in Albuquerque and to our Quality School Conference in Minnesota where we can talk and ask questions about the contents of my three messages. It is impossible for me to explain fully what I mean and to address all of your questions in the context of this eight-page memo.

Albuquerque brought new meaning to the word "lucky." The regional organizations of the Institute took turns putting on the annual Glasser conventions, each year hoping the venue would attract members and contribute to the event being classified as a success. High attendance could even contribute to the region turning a profit for the convention, which greatly helped meager local budgets based solely on membership dues. Under normal circumstances the organizers of the Albuquerque convention would have been concerned about whether or not national or international Institute members would want to go to Albuquerque, New Mexico, for a conference. They would wonder about the venue and the prices; they would wonder about airfares and convenience of travel; and they would wonder about what there was to do in Albuquerque. Such wondering would have occurred under normal circumstances, though. The Albuquerque convention was setting up to be anything but normal. The drama and importance of Glasser's decisions in Australia, and his call for members to meet him in Albuquerque to discuss the issues, fell in the convention organizers' lucky laps like a fistful of aces. No need to worry about whether or not people would want to attend. Glasser had taken care of that.

The Institute had gone through drama before, but not on the scale of what faced them in Albuquerque. An example of an earlier drama occurred after Glasser first introduced control theory and wanted his trainers to teach and coach the new ideas. "We had a little organizational convulsion around 1987,"[18] Glasser began. "I felt that some of our trainers were using stimulus-response psychology. I was trying to get rid of it and said that I want all faculty members to re-qualify. They had to send in role-play videotapes. Some didn't re-qualify and they got mad and left." Jim Montagnes, a longtime member of the Institute and a senior faculty instructor who had given close to 700 Glasser Basic Week courses, remembers the requalifying well. After talking about one of the individuals who left the Institute over it, Montagnes explained, "To be truthful, I was told that I had to do some work, too. I wasn't as close to Bill as some of the others, but I just picked up my socks and did it." For some, the requalifying seemed a reasonable request; for others it was a personal affront. "Yah," Montagnes continued, "for whatever reason, some chose to be angered, while some of us said, well, gee, I guess we got to improve." Glasser felt especially bad about one of the instructors who he felt needed to re-qualify, but who chose to be angry and leave the Institute rather than submit another videotape. Glasser offered to work with him, and Naomi even went to the instructor's home in an attempt to restore the communication connection, but it was to no avail. At the time this process felt painful, but it involved comparatively few in number. The Restitution issue and the accompanying decisions Glasser made in Australia would ultimately involve the entire Institute membership.

More than just keynotes and break-out workshops, the 1996 convention in Albuquerque would set the course of the Institute into the foreseeable future. The stakes were high and Glasser realized how important it was for members to understand not only the details of his decisions, but also why he felt it was important to do what he was doing. Glasser had a sense that he needed to connect with hearts as well as minds. Even in Albuquerque, behind-the-scenes attempts at negotiation took place, but Glasser was firm in the direction he was headed. He took very seriously the pivotal address he gave at the convention. One colleague remembered that for this talk Glasser stood behind a podium and wore a suit, which he had not done before, and he spoke from notes, which he never did.

Glasser was 71 years old when he stepped up to the podium in Albuquerque and began one of the most important talks of his career. The Institute had come to a fork in the road and he was about to explain the road they were choosing and why they were choosing it. His audience was on high alert, an air of expectancy filling the room. While most people are retired by the age of 70, there was no indication of agedness or slowing down in Glasser as he stepped on the platform. He seemed as charged as the audience, strong and energetic, as he began. The first part of the talk reviewed some of his own life story and the early beginnings of the Institute. He noted how over the years the Institute trainers began to teach some of their own ideas along with his, but that he did not make a big deal out of this since their ideas were not necessarily in conflict with his. As choice theory became better and better understood and as trainers learned to apply the ideas to the full gamut of human experience—business, school, marriage, and personal settings—it also became more and more difficult to fit the information into a short intensive week. In other words, for this practical reason the Institute board had a growing belief that Glasser's ideas should be featured in Glasser trainings. There just wasn't time to cover anything but Glasser's choice theory elements in a short seminar. This part of the presentation served as a reminder to people that he had always been a reasonable, accepting, and flexible leader up to that point and set the stage for the remainder of the talk, the organization-splitting part of the talk.

"In Australia I really became faced with certain things. And these are the things I'm facing today. And these are the things I'm taking a strong stand on. This is something I've never done. Glasser's been known as wishy-washy, and I was really tempted to stay wishy-washy. It took a great, great thing to unwishy-washy me, but I am going to do it." In this case "great" was not used in a positive sense, but rather to alert people to something important. That something was school discipline programs that promised to change children, rather than being focused on changing the system that fostered misbehavior in the first place. Glasser felt the Restitution school discipline program fell within that category, and even though its advocates were not trying to do anything wrong their focus was on changing children. While many within the Quality School Consortium viewed the Restitution program as helpful, Glasser saw something in it that would prove otherwise. "Will Dr. Glasser take Restitution away from me?" he thought aloud, probably reading the minds of many in the audience. "Absolutely not," he continued. "Keep it as long as you want. Use it. It may even work for you. But it will destroy my mission." The words "my" and "mission" are very powerful when you put them together and his audience sensed the presentation becoming more personal and even intimate. Glasser was on a mission, had always been on a mission, a highly challenging mission to change the world and some of its most cherished, yet destructive, beliefs. The mission had begun during his residency back at the veterans' hospital in Los Angeles and had continued through every presentation, every journal article, and every book he had written since. Along the way he was an observer, as much the learner as the teacher, but as he spoke from that Albuquerque podium it became clear his observations had crystallized into convictions. He had become sure choice theory was about guiding yourself, not about changing others, and organizations that believed in choice theory would be committed to providing students or workers with an environment in which they could become the best version of themselves, rather than being manipulated into becoming a puppet of the organization.

Peel through the layers of choice theory and you would come to a layer that proclaimed Change the System. This was one of its key points, one of its non-negotiables. "You can't change the system," Glasser explained, "as long as you're willing to accede to the demands of the teacher. Give us something specific we can do—words to say, specific changes we can make when this kid is here, there, or someplace else—and as soon as we do that, we say to them the system you're using in the school is okay, you've just got a lot of kids that aren't in good shape. People say, well, Dr. Glasser, I recognize that and I understand that, but we gotta have a discipline program until the system changes. The system isn't something out there that's going to eventually change. The system changes the minute the first teacher starts saying to the first kid something different than learn it or we'll hurt you." This was the point on which so much hinged. Glasser had observed that stimulus-response thinking had become so much a part of our lives it was almost impossible to tweak it slightly. People have marinated so long in a world of external control and manipulation and coercion that it is incomprehensible to even imagine a management system that isn't somehow, to some degree, based on these elements. He tried to emphasize this critical reality. "As long as they think," he stated, "as long as we come in there with a program that says we can change the kid while you're in the process of changing the system, they're not gonna change the system." Teachers wanted to mix the two—a lot of choice theory with a little bit of external control—but Glasser believed strongly one could not be superimposed on the other.

He projected into the future and predicted what he felt would happen if the Institute continued to sponsor a discipline emphasis. "The worst thing if the program doesn't work very well, is that you and I, the people from the Institute, are involved in the discipline program and we'll be blamed, and especially I'll be blamed. My name is on the program. My name is on the Institute. Therefore I have no choice but to say to myself, if you want to teach these kinds of programs, do it, they may be valuable, they may be important, the country may need them desperately. All the parts of the country that don't want to change the system are hungry for a better program, and Restitution may be a better program, but it's not a program I can abide by and what we are trying to do." The moment brought new attention and meaning to the phrase "what we are trying to do." People who thought they understood choice theory, and thought they understood how it needed to be applied in a school setting, now wondered if they really did understand it. They paused and wondered what it was about choice theory that had Glasser standing up front in a suit, slowly and clearly outlining these concerns. What had they missed before? What had he missed before?

One of the painful impacts of Glasser's decisions was its effect on relationships within the faculty team of the Institute. Glasser felt strongly about his perceptions of the issues, but others felt just as strongly about their own perceptions. He had made it clear that choice theory and discipline programs could not coexist, which was basically saying faculty members who embrace Restitution and other discipline programs could not be a part of an institute that embraced choice theory. "I don't know what else to do," he admitted with resignation in his voice. "I may lose some long-esteemed and good faculty members, but is it right for me to accommodate this if it's destructive to my mission?" He wanted every Institute member, faculty or otherwise, to continue with him on the journey, but he felt he could not endorse anything that would ultimately confuse or distract people from the core of the principles of choice theory.

At the end of the talk he said something that really put into perspective what he was trying to say. "So that's the dilemma we have," he began to conclude. "On Sunday we'll talk about that dilemma and see if we can come to some resolution that will be satisfying, but the resolution will not be that I can accept any discipline programs, cuz I can't. If it ends up right back where it was with me, and all the rest of the people go, it'll be me and Linda and we'll keep hammering away for the rest of our lives. I feel very, very serious about this. Because I finally recognized what my mission in life is." In effect, he was saying if I have to go on by myself, if everyone believes differently and wants to head another direction, then I will go it alone. As was said at the beginning of this chapter, if anything should get the attention of those interested in the life of William Glasser, the events of 1996 should be very, very high on their list. "Wishy-washy Glasser" had become as hard as a rock, and in the process had put everyone on alert to what really matters.

Glasser had written about it from Australia and as of January 1, 1997, Institute members noticed a difference when they went to reenroll with their annual membership dues. There was a section that asked faculty members to pledge to teach only the endorsed ideas of William Glasser and a line to sign their name as a promise to abide by this agreement. The agreement expected faculty "to teach the ideas of Dr. William Glasser and those endorsed by him; to work with 'approved' faculty of the Institute (i.e. not ex-Institute faculty) and; to specifically teach, sponsor, and promote the prevention of discipline problems in schools through the use of choice theory and lead-management as illustrated, for example, in *Every Student Can Succeed*."[19] The decision had been described in memos and spoken from the podium in Albuquerque, but now the deadline had arrived and the decision had become very real indeed.

A boundary had been set and people could decide on which side of that boundary they would be. Bob Wubbolding agreed with that description and added, "There was a line and you're either on one side or the other." The line was never intended to separate people, just ideas, but as people we align ourselves with certain ideas, certain ways of being or believing, and in doing so we sometimes choose on which side of a line we will be. In this case the line separated people. It separated long-time colleagues and friends. Diane Gossen left her long-time association with the Institute and a number of people went with her. Some thought that money was a prime motivator in this exit, and described how lucrative the Restitution program was, but others disagreed and acknowledged that the principles of Restitution went deep with Diane, even back to her work with aboriginal communities in northern Canada. "Diane meant well," a colleague affirmed, "but Restitution was being marketed as a discipline tool. She was making a fortune on it, which is her right, and Bill said that's fine, just don't do it in the name of Glasser Quality Schools. Bill came a long way and met with them many times trying to work this out. He certainly didn't mean them any ill. And I don't think they meant him any ill. There were just two views on it."

One insider believed that 12 to 15 people left the Institute over the Restitution issue or the other changes that were made. Another felt the number was between 500 and 1,000 who left. While highly discrepant it may be both of these numbers are correct. It may be, for instance, that 12 to 15 key faculty members chose to disassociate from the Institute, while over 500 members, in general, let their membership lapse because of the changes. The Quality School Consortium was dissolved a year later and, while it might appear these two events—Glasser's 1996 changes and the demise of the Quality School Consortium a year later—are connected, a member on the Institute board at the time assured me this was not the case. The Consortium being dissolved could have also contributed to members leaving the Institute. For whatever reason, the Institute membership was adversely affected after the Albuquerque conference and after the January 1, 1997, reenrollment deadline. Glasser later talked about how he "split the organization on Restitution," and referred to "the organization breaking in half over it." The terms "splitting" and "breaking in half" indicate a significant wound to the Institute roster, although he may have been exaggerating to emphasize the separation of the opposing ideas that led to the split. Through whatever lens you want to look at it—through the lens of philosophy and beliefs or through the lens of lowered membership numbers—the events of 1996 were a big deal.

To use a medical analogy, the 1996 surgery was decisive and was meant to cure what ailed the patient, but instead the wound seemed to fester. Members continued to wonder about the changes and would talk to each other privately about their implications. The festering became very public when the spring 2005 edition of the *Journal of Reality Therapy* was distributed at the International Glasser Conference, which was held in July of that year in Dublin, Ireland. Larry Litwack, the journal's founder and editor for 25 years, wrote an editorial that questioned the Institute's need to control what faculty think and teach; questioned the need to have a loyalty oath; and questioned the need to lose long-time faculty members. Quoting from Edward R. Murrow, Litwack wrote, "We must not confuse dissent with disloyalty," and then described the inconsistency of attempting to control the purity of the ideas taught by Institute faculty. "To some," Litwack continued, "this seemed an inherent contradiction to and violation of the basic concepts of internal control psychology as exemplified by choice theory."[20]

The journal editorial caused quite a stir at the Dublin conference with those in attendance once again talking about the Institutional changes proclaimed in Albuquerque. When I asked one old-timer if he was at the 1996 Albuquerque conference and if so, did he remember what Glasser had said, he answered he remembered it clearly. "Glasser explained that Restitution was coercive," he recalled, "and then his solution was coercive." Other Institute members said flatly they signed the oath year after year, but that it did not keep them from teaching what they needed to teach. These people were not troublemakers and are incredibly supportive of Glasser, but his response in regard to Diane Gossen and Restitution did not sit well with them even nine years later. At the same time, there were people at the Dublin conference who felt Litwack's editorial was inaccurate and inappropriate.

When asked what his thoughts would be if faculty members, to some extent, resented the loyalty oath, Glasser answered, "Well, that's their privilege," and explained again he saw nothing wrong with asking them to teach the things in which he believed. He pointed out that other great teachers, like Stephen Covey, have huge organizations and he tells you exactly what you have to say. When reminded he had been flexible on the basic needs, that a person could take one away or add one as long as they made it clear that this was their thinking and not Glasser's thinking, yet was inflexible when it came to Restitution, he quickly affirmed his position. "Yes, because Restitution is an idea and choice theory is an idea and to me these ideas cannot coexist within my mind and within my Institute. I said to people, 'If you want to teach this, you know, go in good health, but you cannot do it within the Institute. I will make no effort to discredit you. I will make no effort to stop you from doing anything like that. And I will make no effort to stop you from teaching my ideas, but you're teaching them within your own framework, not within mine.'"

One longtime Institute member felt it was very unfortunate so many people left the organization because of the changes. "The organization is really Christian in nature and it is painful to lose a brother. Of all the individuals who have been a part of this organization over the years that I can think of, I can't think of one that I would say it's better they're gone. Everyone came here to add to others, not subtract. I love Bill and I love all the people who have left. I'm not going to sit in judgment of any of them. I just wish we were all here today."

Tom Amato, acknowledging how high the stakes were and how important the topic was, explains, though, how impressive it is to him that Glasser was willing to argue with himself on his journey in search of truth. "Others felt they had arrived," he pointed out, "but Glasser kept going."[21] In this case he kept going even though it adversely affected his relationship with colleagues and Institute members. As painful as the events and decisions might have been, they provided Glasser with a reason to clarify his beliefs and ultimately a platform from which to emphasize them. He said as much at the end of his pivotal talk in Albuquerque when he stated, "Seventy-one years old in Australia standing upside down I recognized this. I shoulda gone there sooner."

NOTES

1. The song was first recorded by Wynonna and Naomi Judd in December of 1990.
2. Junger, S. (1997). *The perfect storm*. New York: W. W. Norton & Company.
3. Glasser, W. (1974). A new look at discipline. *Learning, 3(4)*, 6-11.
4. Lipman, V. (1978, August-September). Mr. Glasser's gentle rod. *American Education*.
5. Glasser, W. (1990). *The quality school: Managing students without coercion*. New York: Harper Collins. p. 69
6. Gossen, D. (1996). *Restitution: Restructuring school discipline*. Chapel Hill, North Carolina: New View Publications, p.x.
7. Gossen, D. (1996). *Restitution: Restructuring school discipline*. p. xi, xii.
8. In 1994, I personally attended a Restitution workshop taught by Diane Gossen as part of a Glasser conference sponsored by the Evergreen School District in Vancouver, Washington.
9. Glasser, W. (1994). *The control theory manager: Combining the control theory of William Glasser with the wisdom of W. Edwards Deming to explain both what quality is and what lead-managers do to achieve it*. New York: Harper Collins.
10. Blanchard, K. and Johnson, S. (1982). *The one-minute manager*. New York: William Morrow and Company.
11. Blanchard, K. (1994). Cover testimonial for *The Control Theory Manager*, by William Glasser, and published by Harper Collins.
12. Wubbolding, R. (2000). *Reality therapy for the 21st century*. Philadelphia, PA: Brunner-Routledge, p.58.
13. David Johnson interview, June 29, 2004
14. Glasser, W. (1995). *Staying together: A control theory guide to a lasting marriage*. New York: Harper Collins.
15. Cairns is located on the coast in the northeast corner of Australia in the state of Queensland.

16. Glasser felt that it was during the Australia tour that he began using the term external control in the place of stimulus-response.
17. This actually was referring to the introduction of control theory, but he was staying true to the promise he made in northern Australia that he was going to start using the term choice theory.
18. Bob Wubbolding remembers this taking place in 1983.
19. Taken from the 2003 Programs, Policies & Procedure Manual of The William Glasser Institute.
20. Litwack, L. (2005, Spring). Editor's comments. *The Journal for Reality Therapy, 24(2)*, 4.
21. Tom Amato is the director of the Napa Valley Youth Advocacy Center in northern California.

13
WARNING

"I believe that the title may actually be understated."
—*Glasser's response to an interviewer who pointed out that*
Warning: Psychiatry Can Be Hazardous to Your Mental Health
was a provocative title.

When Glasser began to write the manuscript that would become the *Warning*[1] book it had been almost 50 years since he began his career as a psychiatrist. During those 50 years, as the field was pulled and pushed to the views of psychobiology, psychiatry would continue to create its identity. In June of 1954, the month before Glasser began his psychiatric residency, *Time* magazine ran an article on the new wonder drug of the year. Sounding more like an advertisement than an article it stated that "chlorpromazine hydrochloride[2] is now the most exciting new drug seeking recognition in the world's pharmacopoeias," and that it "is a versatile and fantastically interesting drug to medical researchers."[3] It was a "star performer" (the article's exact words). Those reading the article, though, would learn the "star performer" had the ability to "produce the effects of hibernation" and that "patients who were formerly violent or withdrawn lie molded to the bed." A spokesman for Smith, Kline & French, the drug company marketing the drug as Thorazine in the U.S., described how "it is as though the patients said I know there's something disturbing me, but

I couldn't care less."

It may be difficult, years later, to appreciate how chlorpromazine could have generated such glowing pronouncements and affirmations. Having people lying molded to the bed doesn't strike us as being the breakthrough drug of the year. Interestingly, the article did admit, "There is no thought that chlorpromazine is any cure for mental illness."[4] Yet the article ended on a high note, pointing out to readers that at that moment there were 400 research projects under way—"testing chlorpromazine on man and beast"—and that later that month, 12,000 doctors would be heading to the AMA convention in San Francisco, where they would have a chance to see exhibits on what had been learned about the drug. In June of 1954 the bandwagon was just being built, being readied for everyone to jump on it.

By the time Glasser began writing *Warning* in 2002, the brain-drug bandwagon had become a behemoth. Early signs of the pharmaceutical industry's success, described in previous chapters, were seen during the 1960s and '70s, but no one could have predicted the success that awaited these companies during the decades of the 1980s and '90s. Prescription drug sales exploded in the early '80s, reaching sales of 200 billion dollars a year in the U.S. alone, which ranked pharmaceutical companies as the most profitable in the country. To begin to appreciate what this meant, consider that in 2002 the combined profits of the top 10 drug companies were greater than the profits of all the other 490 Fortune 500 companies put together.[5] Pfizer had profits, not overall sales, but profits of 7 billion dollars in 2001, a figure that exceeded the profits of the home-building, apparel, railroad, and publishing industries combined. In 2003, Pfizer's profits soared to $12 billion.[6] As Charles Barber declared in *Comfortably Numb: How Psychiatry is Medicating a Nation*,[7] "the size and reach of the psychiatric drug industry is staggering." Examples he shared of this size and reach include—

- 33 million Americans were prescribed a least one psychiatric drug in 2004, up from 21 million in 1997.[8]
- The spending on antidepressants rose from $5.1 billion in 1997 to $13.5 billion in 2006; and on antipsychotics from $1.3 billion in 1997 to $11.5 billion in 2006.[9]
- The third best-selling antidepressant, Lexapro, has been on the market only since 2002, yet 15 million Americans have already taken it.[10]
- Zoloft's American sales—$3.1 billion in 2005—exceeded those of Tide detergent that same year.
- The worldwide sales of one drug for schizophrenia, Zyprexa—$4.7 billion in 2006—were greater than the revenue generated by the Levi Strauss Company.[11]

The numbers that reveal the size, scope, and influence of "big pharma,"[12] as Jacky Law describes it, are almost too big to comprehend. Several factors have contributed to this success. One factor is the emphasis that drug companies put on marketing. The pharmaceuticals would like us to believe that high drug costs are due to the high costs in creating and developing new drugs. The numbers reveal, though, only 10%-12% of their budget goes to research and development, while almost 40% goes to marketing.[13] This marketing includes advertising directly to the consumer through television commercials and popular magazines like *People* and *Time*, as well as giving gifts and incentives to physicians to prescribe specific drugs. Put in real terms, pharmaceutical companies spend $21 billion a year on promoting their products, of which 88% is directed to physicians, with the remainder spent on direct-to-consumer advertising. Given that there are 600,000 doctors in the U.S. this means the equivalent of $30,000 was spent on every one of them.[14] Another factor has to do with favorable government regulations for which the drug companies have lobbied. Angell[15] describes how the drug companies emphasize and repeat words like "research," "innovation," and "American." "Research. Innovation. American. It makes a great story," she admits, "but while the rhetoric is stirring, it has very little to do with reality. First, research and development is a relatively small part of the budgets of the big drug companies—dwarfed by the vast expenditures for marketing and administration. Second, the pharmaceutical industry is not especially innovative. Only a handful of truly important drugs have been brought to the market in recent years. The great majority of 'new' drugs are not new at all but merely variations[16] of older drugs already on the market. Third, the industry is hardly a model of American free enterprise, since it is utterly dependent on government-granted monopolies in the form of patents and FDA-approved exclusive marketing rights. If it is not particularly innovative in discovering new drugs, it is highly innovative—and aggressive—in dreaming up ways to extend its monopoly rights. Drug companies have the largest lobby in Washington and they give copiously to political campaigns. Legislators are now so beholden to the pharmaceutical industry that it will be exceedingly difficult to break its lock on them."[17]

These regulations, combined with aggressive marketing, have contributed to pharmaceutical companies achieving a profit margin not even closely approached by any other industry or company on earth. "In 2001, the 10 U.S. drug companies in the Fortune 500 ranked above all other US industries in average net return, whether as a percentage of sales (18.5%), of assets (16.3%), or of shareholder equity (33.2%). These are astonishing margins. For comparison, the median net return for all other industries in the Fortune 500 was only 3.3% of sales."[18] These levels of profit are also due, of course, to the high cost Americans pay for drugs. Drugs are more expensive in the U.S. than in any other country in the world. The pharmaceuticals bemoan that it takes $800 million dollars to discover a new drug, a position thoroughly refuted in a book by the same name—*The $800 Million Pill: The Truth Behind the Cost of New Drugs*.[19] The truth is that drug companies, motivated by a desire to make a great deal of money, do just that.

Aggressive marketing and favorable government regulations, while important, could not on their own have created, though, the kind of profits the pharmaceutical companies have achieved. An insatiable appetite by the public for pills that will apparently fix what ails them is the essential ingredient. The appetite for pills didn't occur overnight. In fact, there was a time when people, including physicians, were wary of medication and prescribed or took as little of it as possible. That attitude changed, though, as two important pieces of this complex puzzle simultaneously fell into place. The first piece had to do with the "physicalizing" of mental symptoms into brain disease. The second centers on what Whitaker describes as the modern-day alchemy[20] of brain drugs being perceived as curative. As people became convinced that brain disorders were based on faulty biology, and there were pills to address this biology, the acceptance of and push for medication increased significantly.

There are two groups that stood to gain from brain symptoms being the result of a physical or biological abnormality—the drug companies that make the pills and the psychiatrists who prescribe them. As already mentioned, the drug companies have made and are making a great deal of money based on the public's belief that brain symptoms are due to biological causes. What psychiatry stood to gain involved money, to a degree, but the motive went deeper than that. It is true psychiatrists, in general, usually do not make as much money as most of their doctor colleagues, and that simply prescribing brain drugs increases the number of patients a psychiatrist can see each day. Talk therapy takes time: prescribing and monitoring medication much less so. Money was a factor in the field of psychiatry participating in the creation of the biological model of mental illness, however psychiatry stood to gain even more from the biology of brain disease. Psychiatry stood to gain an identity, something for which it had been in search for a long time.

The care of the mentally ill has a dark history of misunderstanding and mistreatment. Early attempts to deal with those with crazy behavior included locking them in foul-smelling cells and physically disciplining them into submission with whips, fetters, and other methods that could only be described as torture. Crazy people were little more than brutes—animals that needed to be dominated and broken. Physicians of the day were leaders in these approaches. Patients, if they could be called that, were bled, given purges, emetics, nausea-inducing agents, even for overextended periods of time; they also were placed on near starvation diets; had mustard powders applied to their scalps which produced blisters, into which a caustic was then placed that produced pain beyond imagination. These kinds of strategies were intended to get the crazy person thinking about something other than his craziness. These and other treatments too terrible to mention, rather than being helpful, caused more pain and more craziness.

At the beginning of the 19th century, a French physician, Philippe Pinel, began to change this brutal approach. He recognized "if the insane were not treated cruelly, they behaved in a fairly orderly fashion."[21] Pinel developed what he called, *traitement morale,* a humane approach in which he talked with his patients and listened to what they had to say. His methods were effective and patients began behaving well enough to be discharged. As a result, he came to the conclu sion "if a nurturing environment could heal, then insanity was not likely caused due to an organic lesion of the brain. Instead, he believed that many of his patients had retreated into delusions or become overwhelmed with depression because of the shocks of life—disappointed love, business failures, or the blows of poverty."[22]

Thanks to the Quakers of Pennsylvania, a humane approach to mental problems also developed in the U.S. After one of their own died in an asylum due to mistreatment, rather than noisy complaints, they decided to open their own retreat center for the mentally ill. Guided by their religious values, rather than medical wisdom, they "would treat the ill with gentleness and respect" and be more concerned with the needs of the patients over the needs of the caregivers.[23] Whitaker describes:

The Quakers, humble in nature, did not believe that their care would unfailingly help people recover. Many would never get well, but they could still appreciate living in a gentler world and could even find happiness in such an environment. As for the path to true recovery, the Quakers professed 'to do little more than assist nature.' They wouldn't even try to talk the patients out of their mad thoughts. Rather, they would simply try to turn their minds to other topics, often engaging them in conversation about subjects their patients were well versed in. In essence, the Quakers sought to hold to their patients a mirror that reflected an image not of a wild beast but of a worthy person capable of self-governance."[24]

Quietly, without fanfare, the Quakers' moral treatment approach led to impressive results. During the retreat's first 15 years, 70% of the patients recovered; even of those who had been chronically ill before entering the retreat, 25% recovered. Others took note of moral treatment methods and the approach's influence grew during the early 1800s.

During this time a tone was being set by society on how to respond to the mentally ill. A major part of this response was to build asylums where treatment could occur. Along with asylum building, though, the period is noteworthy for the battle that took place over who would guide or even control society's response to insanity. On one side were those who sought to be true to simple, humane, moral treatment methods, while on the other side were physicians who wanted to emphasize scientific methods. It is interesting that those who believed in the moral treatment approach did not want physicians involved with asylums at all. In fact, some asylums didn't even want physicians on their governing board. Moral treatment had risen as a reaction to the scientific or medical model. As a result, physicians saw moral treatment methods as a threat and took steps to take back territory they felt they had lost. Instead of embracing patient-centered ideas and practices, physicians sought to return to the "scientific" practices of bloodletting, the use of drugs like opium and morphine to sedate, and the use of physical restraints like mitts, straightjackets, and small cages. Most important, they fought to make sure only a physician could be superintendent over an asylum. As key states such as New York and Massachusetts agreed to this arrangement the tide of moral treatment was turned and the medical model for treatment of the mentally ill was confirmed and more fully formed.

The term psychiatry, first coined in 1808, comes from the Greek—*psych*, which means mind, and *iatry* for medical treatment—and stands for the medical treatment of the mind. Medicine, in general, is concerned with pathology or disease and treats symptoms that are apparent due to injury or that can be identified from a physical test such as a blood test. Psychiatry has wanted all along to join their medical counterparts in treating ailments that are as valid as setting a broken bone or removing a non-functioning gall bladder. This validity could be achieved only if mental symptoms were "physicalized" into medical diseases. Breggin puts it simply, "The idea that these extremes of irrationality are due to a disease is inseparable from the survival of psychiatry as a profession. If irrationality isn't biological, then psychiatry loses much of its rationale for existence as a medical specialty."[25] This has been the connection—that broken biology is the cause of mental illness—psychiatry has fought to create and maintain.

With the stakes being so high for the field of psychiatry, with its identity depending on psychiatrists' diagnoses being as "medical" as other specialties, it is easy to see how psychiatry could get caught up in the pharmaceuticals' web of influence. At their core the issues have always been the same, even if the biological medical model is presently in the driver's seat. Is mental health an inside/out process or is it really outside/in? Can people learn to create and maintain good mental health from the inside out or, when mental health goes awry, can it only be fixed from the outside in? Because psychiatry believes irrational mental symptoms are the result of broken biology, it has embraced the view that mental health repair is an outside/in process, a position the drug companies are all too happy to support.

To achieve the total package—one in which physicians, and psychiatrists in particular, saw mental symptoms as diseases with biological pathologies and also that pharmaceutical companies produced drugs that affected brain chemistry and mood—the brain drugs would have to be perceived as the only viable option, the only real cure. For the public, though, to see brain drugs as the best option with even curative powers an alchemy needed to take place. Chemicals like chlorpromazine—which started out in dyes and insecticides, moved to anti-vomiting agents, and then calmed manic patients to the extent that it was referred to as a chemical lobotomy—had to somehow be changed into the Wonder Drug of 1954. Dross had to be turned into gold. Pharmaceuticals cannot be blamed for this alchemy more than the psychiatrists, nor can it be the other way around either. They formed an alliance in which both got what they wanted—profits for one, identity and respect for the other.

WG

From the moment in Australia that he decided to change the label of his theory, Glasser knew he was going to be involved in another writing project. "When I talked about changing it in Australia I knew I was going to have to write a book replacing *Control Theory* with *Choice Theory*." With the controversy of the Albuquerque conference behind him, Glasser seemed to take on a new level of energy that was impressive even for him. He admitted the negotiations leading up to the conference and the conference itself were painful for him, and he emphasized he didn't want anyone to leave the Institute because of the changes, but he also admitted he was glad when some of the members left. "I was tickled pink when they left the Institute, because they were exhibiting so much external control. They were causing a lot of problems, even at the conventions leading up to 1996, and I was relieved when they were gone. It was liberating." Another factor in this burst of creative energy was his relationship with Carleen Floyd. They had recently married in 1995 and Carleen, an experienced choice theorist in her own right, knew how to support Glasser in his writing, speaking, and traveling, while at the same time keeping in mind his high need for freedom.

The book *Choice Theory*,[26] published in 1998, was intended by Glasser to be a comprehensive summary of his ideas. As with almost all of his previous writing, *Choice Theory* was written in simple language so that, as he had written in his first book, "any interested person could easily gain a basic understanding of psychology"[27] and on how our brains work. He readily acknowledged he had "continued to use the name 'control theory' for too long" and that the new focus on choice was a more accurate name with which to work. From the beginning he had wanted a theory that would explain why his approaches were effective. Now, whether for his reality therapy counseling strategies or for his Quality School improvement ideas, he believed choice theory provided the theoretical framework to anchor these approaches. "Reality therapy is a practice that I discovered," Glasser explained. "*Choice Theory* is the theoretical support for the practice." Or as he wrote in 2008, "The train track is choice theory and the train is reality therapy."[28]

Confirming the importance of her role in their new relationship, Glasser dedicated the book to Carleen. "This book is as much hers as mine," he emphasized. "I wrote it, and she gave input to every page, literally to every word. I love her very much and wish I had the words to describe our marriage." He then quoted a passage from *Far From the Madding Crowd*, an 1874 novel written by Thomas Hardy, to try and capture what he was trying to say.

> This good fellowship—camaraderie—usually occurring through the similarity of pursuits is unfortunately seldom super-added to love between the sexes, because men and women associate, not in their labours, but in their pleasures merely. Where, however, happy circumstances permit its development, the compounded feeling proves itself to be the only love which is as strong as death—that love which many waters cannot quench, nor the floods drown, besides which the passion usually called by the name is as evanescent as steam.

It would have been difficult to give her a higher tribute. There was nothing fleeting or fading in their relationship. Instead, Glasser had come to see how effective they were at working together.

He would come to refer to *Choice Theory*, the book, as the mother ship, with everything in his prior work pointing forward to it and everything in the work that followed pointing back to it. The mother ship metaphor emphasized the importance of choice theory as the central premise on which his other ideas were built. It wasn't that choice theory was radically new in terms of Glasser's approach, however everything now would be seen though its lens. An example of this occurred when the hardcover book, *Reality Therapy in Action*,[29] was republished in paperback as *Counseling with Choice Theory: The New Reality Therapy*.[30] At its core the new reality therapy wasn't really new at all. The same principles that had been in place since the beginning were still in place, yet for some the new terminology was troubling. Those who felt skilled in reality therapy techniques had come to feel loyal to it as a therapy. Because of that some were not excited about the arrival of this new mother ship. Linda Harshman, executive director of The Glasser Institute at the time, reminded Institute members. "To be associated with Bill Glasser means you are going to continue to grow and that change is a part of the culture. The system never becomes permanent." Most, though, welcomed the new terminology and agreed with Glasser that the term "control theory" required unnecessary explanation.

That Glasser was able to get *Choice Theory* written and published less than two years after announcing the birth of the new name in Albuquerque is remarkable, especially when you consider what else was going on during this period. Near the end of 1997 Glasser gave a talk to the Corning, New York, school district on his Quality School ideas. It was a special treat for Glasser to return to Corning. Thirty-six years earlier, in 1961, he had been invited to Corning to be a part of the Second Corning Conference, which had as its goal to assemble 100 of the greatest minds from different parts of the world and representing different vocations and walks of life. "The central question of the Corning Conference," as described in one of its brochures, "will be the extent to which the traditional ideal of significance and dignity of the individual is vital and viable under the conditions of the emerging world: and Industrial Civilization."[31] In the conference program Glasser was affirmed for his expertise in working with juveniles within the California Youth Authority system and for his then recent book, *Mental Health or Mental Illness?* To be invited to such an esteemed event, even before his resume had really begun to gain notoriety, was a significant honor. Now, as he was trying to put the finishing touches on a manuscript that would finally summarize his ideas, ideas that had traveled over a million miles in presentations and trainings, and had been fine-tuned in hundreds of articles and 13 books, he returned to Corning. Although primarily directed at those associated with Corning's school district—administrators, teachers, and parents—the presentation was so successful it piqued the interest of the larger community. What started as a desire for school improvement led to a commitment by the entire town to begin the Choice Theory Community Project. By 2003 the project had even gotten the attention of *The New York Times*.[32] As 1998 progressed, Glasser was fully engaged in this new and exciting endeavor.

Unfortunately, even in the midst of a new book being written and an entire town wanting to embrace his ideas, 1998 also brought pain as Joe, Glasser's eldest child, passed away. Unbeknownst to anyone until it was too late, Joe was being lethally affected by a rare condition known as Wilson's Disease, an inherited disorder that does away with the body's ability to deal with copper. As copper deposits build up in the body, certain organs, including the liver, brain, kidneys, and eyes are especially affected. Eventually these organs stop working correctly.

Joe Glasser was 47 years old when he died. He had struggled during his life to make it and to be a success, and at the end of his life he was struggling to survive.

"Even before Joe's undiagnosed Wilson's Disease," Bob Glasser, a cousin, remembered, "he just wasn't able to keep a job. Marie and I always liked Joe. He was a really nice guy. We would see him when we could. He would always have an idea; well, I'm gonna do this or I'm gonna do that. Nothing ever panned out. Why? That's beyond me."[33] Fitzgeorge Peters, a colleague and close friend of the Glassers, explained, "Joe seemed to want to follow in his father's footsteps, but he couldn't pull it off."[34]

Glasser loved Joe, yet Joe frustrated him, too. As time went on he didn't talk about Joe much. One colleague described, "Bill never mentions him, never mentions Joe," but other colleagues who were closer to the family recount how much of a reader Joe had been and how much he wanted to be close to his family. Glasser remembers Joe wanting to go with him when he gave talks and he fondly remembers when, while visiting his sister, the two of them played golf together and Glasser hit a hole in one. "We were playing golf on a little course where my sister lives, a little three par, and I'm not much of a golfer, but I hit the ball on about a hundred and, maybe about a hundred and ten yard hole, maybe even less, but anyway, you hit up over a hill, you couldn't really see the green, but you knew where it was, and when I got there I couldn't find the ball. And I looked and looked and looked and all of a sudden, I was playing with my son Joe, he says, 'Look in the cup, Dad, and there it was.'" Glasser emphasized Joe was a very intelligent person, yet also admitted Joe "fitted the description in the book *Choice Theory* of the 'workless.' Joe never really ever succeeded in work. He tried to work and he got jobs and I got him jobs, but for some reason he would just get totally panicked about, oh, I can't do it and things like that. So Joe was a talker but not a doer. And in our family, especially in my wife's family, there were a lot of talkers who weren't doers. So it's kind of a genetic thing, and I really felt that genetically in terms of the five basic needs Joe had really no strong need for survival. Therefore never felt the inclination to work. He had a strong need for power, and when you have a strong need for power and a low need for survival, then when you go to work you want to start at the top. And of course you can't start at the top, even with the advantages he had, and even when he got his PhD."

I interrupted him at this point in the interview, maybe surprised that Joe completed his doctorate. "He got his PhD," Glasser continued, "but he wouldn't have got it if I hadn't made a special trip to Florida and worked with him for about a week and convinced him that you got to do the work and everything else. Joe was a great talker. People liked him and they liked his intelligence. So he got away with a PhD probably not doing nearly the work that most other people do."

"What did he get his PhD in?" I asked.

"Counseling psychology. And then, he, he just didn't want to get a job. He tried to start a private practice and, of course it didn't work, and, and he really never, never worked at any job that I could ever remember. He got Wilson's Disease, which is the inability to excrete copper and that killed him. And we didn't know about it. It was diagnosed too late. But that doesn't mean if he hadn't gotten it Joe would have done miraculous things with his life, because I don't think he would. Even my brother, who didn't do much work until about 40-some years of age, eventually started working and made some money. That was pretty good, but before that my parents supported him and his whole family. So 'workless' genes run in both my wife's family and my family, and I think there's 'workless' genes in almost every family." Glasser was prepared and willing to support Joe for as long and in whatever way was necessary, but he also hoped that in the same way his older brother, Hank, had eventually kicked into a "work" gear, Joe would find that "gear," too. It is possible Wilson's Disease was the cause of Joe's life struggles. Typically, the disease appears in people before they turn 40 years of age, but symptoms can show up in children by age 4. Wilson's symptoms can include confusion, dementia, difficulty walking or stiffness when moving arms, emotional and behavioral changes, personality changes, phobias, and weakness.[35] This list might explain what Joe was dealing with.

WG

With *Choice Theory* now firmly established within the covers of its own book, Glasser entered a zone of publishing productivity unmatched by any other time in his career. In the year 2000 alone Glasser published four books—*What Is This Thing Called Love?*,[36] a small book that he and Carleen wrote for young, single women; *Every Student Can Succeed*,[37] the last book of five books that he wrote on education and teaching and learning; *Getting Together and Staying Together*,[38] an update of the book *Staying Together* that Bill and Carleen wrote as a team; and *Reality Therapy in Action*,[39] a 243-page hardcover printed by Harper Collins. These books were quickly followed by three more—a book on fibromyalgia[40] from a choice theory perspective in 2001; a Harper Collins hardcover entitled *Unhappy Teenagers: A Way for Parents and Teachers to Reach Them*[41] in 2002; and another Harper Collins hardcover in 2003 with the eye-catching title of *Warning: Psychiatry Can Be Hazardous to Your Mental Health*.[42] And this list doesn't include the many journal articles he authored and the interviews he fulfilled. Glasser was 78 years old when the *Warning* book was published, yet his pace remained intense. Still playing tennis a couple times a week with his regular set of playing partners, he continued to talk about inroads he still needed to forge in the field of psychology. The general population seemed content to accept the bill of goods that psychiatry, the pharmaceutical industry, and the media were pushing. With a fervor similar to a religiously motivated evangelist, Glasser wanted to spread the good news that people, rather than being prisoners of a psychological disease, could begin to take responsibility for their lives and break the chains that were holding them.

As had happened many years before, when he received Powers' book from a friend in New York City, Glasser received a neatly packaged book in the mail. The return address on the package indicated it was from Ireland and the book, *Beyond Prozac*[43] by Terry Lynch, was inside. It was not unusual for Glasser to receive books or articles from friends. He had always been a voracious reader and was forever on the lookout for a good story or a thoughtful article. Some materials he skimmed; others he read carefully. Within just a few lines of beginning to read *Beyond Prozac,* Glasser knew this was going to be a book that he read very carefully. Drawing on his experience as a physician, as well as his graduate degree in psychotherapy, Lynch acknowledges the widespread acceptance of emotional distresses being classified as mental illness and the widespread belief that these mental illnesses can only be treated with drugs, but he then shares case study after case study that show how effective a sympathetic ear and a helpful counseling session can be. Lynch explained how a person's distress, rather than being a sign of craziness, actually has deep meaning, and that instead of medicating or numbing this distress away, the distress must be understood. Lynch writes in a voice that is patient and reasonable and Glasser was impressed with the way *Beyond Prozac* addressed such important, and even charged issues. As he read the book, Glasser was inspired.

It was early 2002 when the package containing *Beyond Prozac* arrived. Glasser's most recent manuscript, *Unhappy Teenagers,* would soon be hitting bookstores and apparently he was ready for his next project. *Beyond Prozac* echoed what Glasser had been saying for decades, yet it was unique, too. Lynch had a distinctive voice. For one thing, *Beyond Prozac* was packed with examples, the stories and case studies of people working through their distress and reaching for something better. These stories are compelling, not because Lynch somehow dramatizes them, but because he does just the opposite. The stories are similar to the stories of people we know; they are similar to our own experiences. Another thing that caught Glasser's eye was the way Lynch took on the field of psychiatry, the drug industry, and the governmental policies and agencies that promoted ineffective mental health treatments. Lynch didn't mince words, yet his points came across as rational, rather than aggressive.

When Brian Lennon put *Beyond Prozac* in the mail he couldn't have known how significant the book would be to Glasser. As it turned out, *Beyond Prozac* was the final nudge, the finger that touched the domino that set in motion Glasser's writing another book. Glasser said as much in the book's dedication. "When you sent me Terry Lynch's book, *Beyond Prozac: Healing Mental Suffering Without Drugs,* I was on my way."[44] Lennon had been one of the earliest adopters of reality therapy and the concepts of choice theory in Ireland and Glasser had come to appreciate him deeply. "Since we met many years ago," Glasser wrote at the beginning of the dedication, "I have felt your mind is a mirror image of mine." Irishmen are rarely speechless, but Lennon later described, "The *Warning* dedication came as a massive surprise. I was in Bled, Slovenia, and a friend, John Brickell, had a copy of the book, which I had only seen in manuscript up to that point. As I flicked through the pages I came upon the dedication for the first time and, also for the first time, I was speechless!"

The book, for Glasser, would come to be a collection of his most assertive thoughts on the problems of mental illness and the real treatments needed if people were to become mentally healthy. Some felt the project was not only assertive, but also aggressive, starting with the cover of the book. In bold letters meant to resemble the life and death warning on a pack of cigarettes, the title proclaimed WARNING: PSYCHIATRY CAN BE HAZARDOUS TO YOUR MENTAL HEALTH. When the manuscript was close to going to press a colleague approached Glasser and expressed what a mistake the title was. "He was scared to death," Glasser recalled. "He said, 'My god, the whole psychiatric establishment is going to turn against us.' I said 'I hope so.'" Part zealous, part confident, part assertive, and part aggressive, Glasser was reentering the fray with a different language and tone.

Terry Lynch wrote the foreword for the *Warning* book, which effectively set the table for Glasser to make his points. Together they reminded readers that decades of intensive psychiatric research have failed to establish a biological cause for any psychiatric condition and treating mental distress through a medical approach assumes this connection is nothing more than presumption. Researchers now concede antidepressants like Paxil, Prozac, and Efexor are barely more effective than placebos. "Psychiatry," Lynch wrote, "has walked itself into a cul-de-sac from which it is unwilling to return."[45] In stronger terms, Lynch states, "It is time to examine the psychiatric monopoly on mental health. It is essential that no stone be left unturned in our efforts toward effective mental healthcare. Not only is psychiatry leaving many stones unturned, it is doing its best to ensure that stones remain unturned."

Glasser was driven to inform the world that mental health can be taught to people. The world was on a course that embraced just the opposite—that we really can't take care of ourselves—and he wanted people to know the truth. "There is a vast difference," he began in *Warning*, "between seeing yourself as mentally ill, believing you can't help yourself, and seeing yourself as unhappy, but tending to believe you can help yourself."[46] He was convinced that people could learn how to be mentally healthy. He also became convinced that understanding the importance of happiness in our lives was key to our mental health. People are confused, he felt, about what true happiness is and about the thinking and behavior that leads to real happiness.

"A key component of mental health," Glasser wrote, "is knowing the difference between happiness and pleasure. As much as these two experiences may seem to be the same—both feel very good—they are very different. Happiness is feeling good because you are choosing to behave in ways that keep you close, or get you closer, to the important people in your life. Pleasure, often associated with addicting drugs, gambling, or casual sex, may, for short periods, feel better than happiness. But we should not be fooled; pleasure is not happiness. It is another experience altogether."[47]

We want to be truly happy, which involves a number of factors. It involves our connected and committed relationships with others; it involves a sense of satisfaction from being who we want to be; it involves self-respect that comes from recognizing our power of choice and continually learning from those choices; and it involves feeling good. Problems develop when we are willing to settle for feeling good, without working toward the other factors that lead to really being happy. In search of this "feeling good" state, people become "self-medicators." As we discover what helps us to feel good we become our own personal psychological pharmacologists, ready and willing to prescribe as much of an experience as we need to feel better. Soon, a person becomes addicted to the behavior that leads to feeling better, even if only for a fleeting moment. Self-medicating behaviors can be destructive habits, like alcohol and eating disorders, or they can involve seemingly innocuous behaviors like shopping or even working. Whatever the behavior may be it begins to take on a life of its own. The behavior or experience becomes all-important and other parts of our life begin to take a back seat, including our relationships with people, even our relationships with our closest friends and family. It has been said that which we don't control, controls us, and when it comes to pleasure that is not an overstatement. We become slaves to the behavior that brings us pleasure, even though it doesn't bring us happiness.

"It is virtually impossible to be unhappy for five or six weeks and remain symptom free."[48] Glasser stated. From the beginning, he emphasized the significance of good relationships when it comes to mental health. In fact, he believed broken relationships are at the core of all mental health problems. Staying unhappy for an extended period can lead to a cycle of events that often includes the following steps:

o When our relationships become broken and stay broken, especially with someone close to us like a spouse or a child, we become unhappy. If the relationship doesn't improve, our unhappiness becomes deeper and more nagging.

o We seek to fix the problem, usually by trying to control or manipulate the other person into acting how we want them to act, but it only makes it worse. After a time, our unhappiness is significant enough that psychological symptoms begin to occur—stress, anxiety, fear, and anger. We begin to feel trapped in a bad situation, and fearful of our own anger we begin to shut down, to depress our frustration in a way that won't let it escape. If our unhappiness persists, our creativity also begins to involve physical symptoms like headaches, stomachaches, and intestinal problems, backaches, and even aching joints. The power of our creativity can be very impressive.

o Of course, when we are unhappy we want to do something about it. We don't feel good and we want to feel better.

o We often already know about behaviors that help us feel better or we are on the lookout for such behavior. Either way, we behave in ways that help us feel better, even when the behavior offers only short-term pleasure. Because the pleasure doesn't really address the cause of our unhappiness, and because it is not unusual for the pleasure behavior to actually make the cause of our unhappiness worse, the destructive symptoms persist.

o Eventually our symptoms scream loud enough that, often reluctantly, we become convinced we need expert help. We approach a doctor, who probably will prescribe many tests in the hope of discovering a pathology to treat, but the tests are not conclusive. He recommends an anti-depressant to help control our moods and maybe also recommends we see a psychiatrist. If the doctor has not prescribed a brain drug, the psychiatrist certainly will. As Breggin confirms, "When the patient reaches out, the psychiatrist puts a pill in his hand."[49]

o The drugs mute or numb our feelings. The pain or frustration is not so sharp. Yet while these drugs can numb the feeling, the symptom has not gone away and continues to affect our mental and physical health. Within our psychological and physical body systems, pain exists for a reason. Pain lets us know that something is wrong and needs to be addressed. It may mean that an area in our body needs to be cared for or protected. Taking a pill that numbs the pain may be counterproductive if it leads to thinking the problem is better, when it is not, or if it leads to continuing to live our lives in a way that actually hurts us.

This cycle of events was one of the key reasons Glasser wrote the *Warning* book. "I wrote the *Warning* book," he explained, "because society is looking for a chemical cure to an unhappy problem." This was a huge point to him. During one of our interviews, just as the *Warning* book was first published, he emphasized: "This is the most gigantic medical fraud that's ever been perpetrated in the United States—the fraud of mental illness. I mean it's gigantic!" The drug industry masquerades as mental health's best friend, but Glasser reminded us it was just that, a masquerade. However, as long as people believed in mental "illness" as defined by the pharmaceutical/psychiatric machine, they would become, in Glasser's words, "one of the millions of geese that lay the golden eggs."[50]

Another author wrote of this fraud in terms just as strong as Glasser's. "We are being recruited into mental illness faster than the speed of light. The trouble with mental illness is that it is not measles; it is whatever a psychiatrist or psychologist says it is." And what they say it is, is too often self-serving. "First psychiatry sells us a disease," she observes, "then they sell us a cure." In other words, as she states firmly, "We are being sold our own insanity."[51]

Glasser agreed with such convictions regarding the brain drug industry, but more than that he wanted people to understand how these drugs affected their lives. "The drugs are prescribed," he wrote, "with the idea that feeling better is all you need. But it isn't all you need. It's even worse than all you need, because you mistake the pleasure of the drug for happiness. You may feel better but you are just as lonely as you would be if you were in a bar drinking alone. That loneliness will soon overcome the pleasure the drug provides." And then he shares what may be one of the key points of the book, and maybe of his career. "There is no happiness drug, legal or illegal, that brings people closer together."[52]

This is the choice with which members of the human family are constantly faced. Do we pursue real happiness and the work that it involves or do we settle for short-term pleasure and a feeling of pseudo-control? Most people have not identified their struggle in such simple terms and may not even be aware they are making these choices, but know it or not, this is the reality they are trying to negotiate. "You can only find happiness," Glasser emphasized, "in choosing to change the way you relate to the important people in your life." This is where the work lies. How we relate to our present circumstances, which usually has a lot to do with the people we are closest to, is where answers can be found. Relating to this, Glasser gently warned (after all, it is a *Warning* book): "Once you feel good on a drug, prescribed or self-prescribed, the incentive to do anything other than take the drug and enjoy the pleasure is diminished or removed."[53]

And so the cycle goes. Many, many people experience the cycle every day. Many feel something very serious must be wrong with them. Their drug, whether a self-prescribed behavior or a drug prescribed by a doctor, briefly numbs the pain or frustration, but does not help them address the problem. They become convinced they are suffering from a mental illness and that drugs offer their only relief. Glasser offered hope to those living through this cycle. Rather than being trapped, he reminded readers: "Keep in mind that unhappiness, not mental illness, is your problem. You can find happiness if you understand the importance of choice in your life."[54]

One of the reasons the pharmaceutical industry has reaped incredible amounts of profit is that society prefers the disease option. This view was starkly portrayed in the opening line of Patty Duke's book, *A Brilliant Madness,* where she begins, "A DISEASE? THANK GOD!"[55] She was relieved to find she had an illness and her depression and her behavior had not been her fault. Many people struggling with mental and physical symptoms feel the same way. They, too, are relieved that the medical profession, which they assume is backed by science, has identified their symptoms as a disease that is beyond their control to affect or alter. Someone offering a hopeful alternative is fine, to a degree, but not when they start mentioning responsible choices.

One of the key pieces in the "mental symptoms as science" view is the bible of psychiatry, the *Diagnostic and Statistical Manual of Mental Disorders,* also referred to as the DSM-V. The first DSM was published in 1952, with major updates taking place in 1968, 1980, and 1994. As far as the field of psychiatry is concerned, it would be difficult to overstate the importance of this very thick book. The DSM, quite simply, is the final word on whether a symptom represents a mental disorder or not. The fact that the manual is made up of more than 900 pages suggests many, many behaviors and symptoms have crossed over into the disorder category. The DSM represents the American Psychiatric Association's claim that they have jurisdiction over what mental illness is and is not. Such a claim is no small thing. For one thing, and this is where psychiatry and the drug companies get their power, it has come to determine whether or not a treatment is covered by health insurance. At a deeper, personal level, in the process of staking this claim, the DSM has guided how we as a society should think about our troubles.[56]

Much has been said about the DSM and its views on mental illness. While I do not want to take a lot of space talking about the DSM, I think a couple of passages from the book *Making Us Crazy* are helpful here. One passage describes that while it is well-known the pharmaceutical companies fund the American Psychiatric Association's conventions and major journals, it is less well known that drug companies contribute to the development of the DSM. "These companies," the authors begin, "have a direct financial interest in expanding the number of people who can be defined as having a mental disorder and who then might be treated with their chemical products. For this reason, drug companies are disturbed by the findings of many surveys that have found a majority of people whom DSM would label as having a mental disorder neither define their own problems as mental illness nor seek psychiatric help for them. For drug companies, these unlabeled masses are a vast untapped market, the virgin Alaskan oil fields of mental disorder."[57] And indeed the "disorders" and "diseases" in the DSM have increased with each update of the manual, so much so that Glasser chuckles as he points out their goal is to get every one of us eventually categorized as being mentally ill. This quote, though, is a serious allegation involving exploitation and manipulation, themes the authors cover throughout the book. "After 17 years of studying the constant revising of DSM," they continue, "we have difficulty reconciling what the APA claims about the manual with what actually happens in its creation. The story told here is not the conventional one of science triumphing over the mysteries of nature. Rather, we trace how the psychiatric profession struggles with various political constituencies to create categories of mental disorder and garner support for their official acceptance."[58] If this is true, the manual is nothing more than a description of symptoms which self-serving "experts" christen as mental illness, not as a result of credible scientific research, but as the result of opinions formed under social and political pressure.

Glasser points out that instead of the DSM being viewed as the bible of mental illness it should be called the Big Red Book of Unhappiness.[59] As a book describing behavioral symptoms, the DSM was fairly accurate. "I don't deny the reality of their symptoms," Glasser said of those experiencing mental distress. "I deny that these symptoms are an untreatable component of an incurable brain malfunction. I do not see their symptoms as mental illness, but as an indication they are not nearly as mentally healthy as they could learn to be."[60] This was the theme to which he kept returning—people can learn to become and stay mentally healthy.

Similarly to what he described at the end of *The Identity Society* (1972), where he wrote about community involvement centers, Glasser again described a more local solution to an international problem. For him it came down to the creation of local choice theory focus groups, in which a local facilitator would help participants discuss how their choices were contributing to their mental health or mental distress. The *Warning* book itself was meant to serve as a resource for individuals to use on their own, but Glasser was hopeful small groups would spring up around the country and implement what he had described. "This book is my attempt to provide this opportunity for the majority of people diagnosed with disorders listed in the DSM-IV, and to provide it free or at very small cost."[61]

When I asked him if he had an outline in his head when he gives lectures, some of them going for several hours and all of them without notes, Glasser explained there were four areas he keeps in mind—the basic needs, the quality world, creativity, and total behavior. To begin to understand human behavior these were the four major areas that, for Glasser, must be understood. For instance, understanding the power of our creativity can help people who are struggling with the idea they might be choosing their painful or distressing symptoms. "Unhappiness is the force that motivates the creativity inherent in our brain to come up with, not only the symptoms described in the DSM-IV, but also aches, pains, fatigue, and even some or most of what is seen when our immune system attacks a normal tissue in our body as in autoimmune disease. Creativity, helpful or harmful, good or bad, can be expressed in all four components of our total behavior."[62] Some respond that such a view might be well and good to explain things like stress headaches or worried stomachs, but it is too much of a stretch for such an explanation to address major mental illness symptoms like schizophrenia. Glasser held to his position even with serious mental symptoms, although he admitted his theory was difficult for many to accept. "It is hard for anyone, even for a psychiatrist, to conceive of the creative potential of our brains," he began. "If you can hear voices, your brain can create voices. If you can see, it can create visual hallucinations. If you can feel pain, it can create pain, often in greater duration and severity than you would ever experience from an illness or injury. If you can feel fear, it can create disabling phobias. If you can think rationally, it can go beyond rationality and create supernormal mania."[63]

In other words, psychological, and even physical, symptoms, instead of being the result of illness or disease, is the brain's way of signaling us that something is wrong, similar to pain receptors telling us to move our hand when we touch something hot. Glasser said as much when he stated, "I believe all symptoms, painful, frightening, crazy, disabling, possibly even symptoms of a disease like arthritis, are your brain's way of warning you that the behaviors you are presently choosing are not satisfying your basic needs."[64] It's not that we choose headaches or that we choose craziness, but that we choose behaviors are so unsatisfying that headaches are one of the results.

Glasser realized not all of his ideas were original, but he did feel at least one of his ideas was very important and very original. That idea was the concept of total behavior. Others may have felt just as strongly as Glasser—that there was no such thing as mental illness; others felt a positive relationship with the patient was important, and that present behavior, rather than the past, should be the focus; and others had decried the growing dependence on chemicals as the answer to mental distress. But in the idea of total behavior, Glasser was unique. The idea of total behavior was based on the assumptions (Glasser called them "axioms") that all we do from birth to death is behave; that all behavior is a total behavior; and that all behavior is chosen or purposeful. By total behavior Glasser explained every behavior is made up of four parts—one part thinking, one part acting, one part feeling, and one part physiology. No matter what we are doing, those four parts are always involved. Whether we are quietly reading one moment or cycling up a steep mountain road another moment, the four parts of a total behavior will be present. While reading, the physiology part of our total behavior will have a normal heart rate and our skin will be comfortably dry, while with cycling up a steep hill the physiology part of our total behavior will have an elevated heart rate, very moist skin, and heavy breathing. While reading, our feelings will be unique to that moment, to the content we are reading, and to the context for our reading in the first place. Reading a novel while on vacation carries with it different feeling from reading notes a half hour before a high-stakes examination. For Glasser, one of the keys to total behavior is the idea that people have direct control of the thinking part and the acting part of behavior; while only indirect control over the feeling part and the physiology part. I might not be able to directly tell my heart, okay, go up to 160 beats per minute, but I can directly choose the behavior to run up a steep hill, which will definitely influence my heart to reach and surpass the 160 beats per minute. Ultimately, Glasser accepted the metaphor and graphic of a car as a representation for total behavior, with the front wheels, the wheels we actually intentionally steer, representing our thinking and our acting, and the back wheels representing our feeling and our physiology. Total behavior is a very empowering belief. It's true that such a model carries with it a great deal of personal responsibility, but the implications of having so much control over our thinking and our acting are quite remarkable! We are free, free to choose how we will think and act, free to set our course.

The *Warning* book, with its focus on personal freedom and responsibility, is a moral book. Glasser did not shrink from morality or from right and wrong. For him, moral behavior was not based on religious ideology or on a spiritual concept of God, but rather on the idea of a person meeting his or her own needs, while at the same time not keeping others from meeting their needs. There is a Golden Rule familiarity of such an approach, a concept Glasser is fine with. He liked the Golden Rule. The *Warning* book, though, is also a pragmatic book that comments on the reality of our present healthcare situation. "The unwillingness of the medical profession to come to grips with the creativity of an unhappy brain," Glasser points out, "costs billions of dollars every year. If we wait for the medical profession to take the lead here, we will wait forever. My goal in this book is to bring the idea of total behavior and creativity directly to the public."[65] The "billions of dollars" estimate was actually too low, as an average of $6,000 per year is spent on healthcare for every American ($1.7 trillion annually), with almost all of it going to cure rather than prevention.[66] In one of our interviews Glasser explained how the country needed to apply medical care to only medical diseases. "Attempting to provide medical care for every symptom that comes up is really not possible."

Within the pages of the *Warning* book, Glasser supported the idea proclaimed in the title that psychiatry could be hazardous to your mental health, but there was a reasonableness in his writing. He was more interested in the good fight of mental health than the bad fight of psychiatry, the DSM, and brain drugs. During our interviews a couple of years after *Warning* was published, when he was already on to his next project, the idea that mental health was a public health issue rather than a medical problem, I asked him about his "moving on" from the emphasis in the book. The *Warning* title seemed to sound the battle cry for a full-on, prolonged assault on the psychopharmacology system, yet apparently he had discovered significance in another approach. Thinking out loud to me, almost in a tone that suggested let's move on, he explained, "I'm damning psychiatry as much as I'm gonna damn it. I'm saying they diagnose diseases that don't exist, they give drugs that can harm you, and they tell you that you can't help yourself. That's about as good as I can do."

NOTES

1. Glasser, W. (2003). *Warning: Psychiatry can be dangerous to your mental health.* New York: Harper Collins.
2. Alias 2601-A, trademarked Thorazine in the U.S.
3. Time magazine. (1954, June 14). The wonder drug of 1954?
4. *ibid.*
5. Angell, M. (2004, December 7). Excess in the pharmaceutical industry. *Canadian Medical Association Journal, 171(12).*
6. Surowiecki, J. (2004, February 16). The pipeline problem. *The New Yorker.*
7. Barber, C. (2008). *Comfortably numb; How psychiatry is medicating a nation.* New York: Pantheon Books.
8. Brown, A. (2006, July 9). Questions raised about drug Yates was taking. *Houston Chronicle.*
9. NDC Health. (2005, March). Top 200 drugs for 2004 by U.S. sales.
10. CBS News Health Watch. (2003, July 16). Mother's little helper turns 40.
11. Drug Topics. (2007, March 5). Top 200 generic drugs by units in 2006.
12. Law, J. (2006). *Big pharma: Exposing the global healthcare agenda.* New York: Carol & Graph Publishers.
13. Angell, M. (2004). *The truth about the drug companies: How they deceive us and what to do about it.* New York: Random House.
14. Kassirer, J. (2005). *On the take: How medicine's complicity with big business can endanger your health.* New York: Oxford University Press.
15. Marcia Angell is a physician who for two decades worked at the New England Journal of Medicine and who saw firsthand the growing corruption in the pharmaceutical industry.
16. These variations or copycats of older drugs already available became known within the industry as Me-Too drugs.
17. Angell, M. (2004). *The truth about the drug companies: How they deceive us and what to do about it.* New York: Random House. p. xvi
18. Angell, M. (2004) and Law, J. (2006)
19. Goozner, Merrill. (2004). *The $800 pill: The truth behind the cost of new drugs.* Los Angeles: University of California Press.

20 Whitaker, R. (2002). *Mad in America: Bad science, bad medicine, and the enduring mistreatment of the mentally ill.* Cambridge, MA: Perseus Publishing.
21 Whitaker, R. (2002). *Mad in America: Bad science, bad medicine, and the enduring mistreatment of the mentally ill.* Cambridge, MA: Perseus Publishing.
22 *ibid.*
23 *ibid.*
24 *ibid*, p. 24
25 Breggin, P. (1991). *Toxic psychiatry.* New York: St. Martin's Press.
26 Glasser, W. (1998). *Choice theory: A new psychology of personal freedom.* New York: Harper Collins.
27 Glasser, W. (1960). *Mental health or mental illness?: Psychiatry for practical action.* New York: Harper & Row Publsihers.
28 Glasser, W. (2008, Summer). *William Glasser Institute Newsletter.*
29 Glasser, W. (2000). *Reality therapy in action.* New York: Harper Collins.
30 Glasser, W. (2000). *Counseling with choice theory: The new reality therapy.* New York: Harper Collins.
31 The Second Corning Conference, Corning Glass Center, Corning, New York, May 18-20, 1961. The first Corning Conference had been held in 1951.
32 Foderaro, L. (2003, July 12). Corning by the book: Utopian or Orwellian? *The New York Times.*
33 Robert Glasser interview, November 5, 2004.
34 Fitzgeorge Peters interview, July 18, 2004.
35 As found at www.ncbi.nim.nih.gov/pubmedhealth/PMH0001789/
36 Glasser, W. and Glasser, C. (2000). *What is this thing called love?* Chatsworth, CA: William Glasser, Inc.
37 Glasser, W. (2000). *Every student can succeed.* Chatsworth, CA: William Glasser, Inc.
38 Glasser, W. and Glasser, C. (2000). *Getting together and staying together: Solving the mystery of marriage.* New York: Harper Collins.
39 Glasser, W. (2000). *Reality therapy in action.* New York: Harper Collins.
40 Glasser, W. (2001). *Fibromyalgia: Hope from a completely new perspective.* Chatsworth, CA: William Glasser, Inc.
41 Glasser, W. (2002). *Unhappy teenagers: A way for parents and teachers to reach them.* New York: Harper Collins.
42 Glasser, W. (2003). *Warning: Psychiatry can be hazardous to your mental health.* New York: Harper Collins.
43 Lynch, T. (2001). *Beyond Prozac: Healing mental distress.* Douglas Village, Cork: Mercier Press.

44 Glasser, W. (2003). *Warning: Psychiatry can be hazardous to your mental health*. New York: Harper Collins.
45 Glasser, W. (2003). *Warning: Psychiatry can be hazardous to your mental health*. New York: Harper Collins. From Lynch's Foreword.
46 Glasser, W. (2003). *Warning: Psychiatry can be hazardous to your mental health*. p. 9, 10
47 Glasser, W. (2003). *Warning: Psychiatry can be hazardous to your mental health*. p. 57
48 Glasser, W. (2003). *Warning: Psychiatry can be hazardous to your mental health*. p. 39.
49 Breggin, P. (1991). *Toxic psychiatry*. New York: St. Martin's Press.
50 Glasser, W. (2003). *Warning: Psychiatry can be hazardous to your mental health*. p. 20.
51 Curtiss, A. (2001). *Depression is a choice: Winning the battle without drugs*. New York: Hyperion.
52 Glasser, W. (2003). *Warning: Psychiatry can be hazardous to your mental health*. p. 59.
53 *ibid*, p. 60.
54 *ibid*, p. 61.
55 Duke, P. and Hochman, G. (1992). *A brilliant madness: Living with manic-depressive illness*. New York: Bantam Publishing.
56 Kutchins, H. and Kirk, S. (1997). *Making us crazy: DSM: The psychiatric bible and the creation of mental disorders*. New York: The Free Press.
57 Kutchins, H. and Kirk, S. (1997). *Making us crazy*. p. 13.
58 Kutchins, H. and Kirk, S. (1997). *Making us crazy*. p. 18.
59 Glasser, W. (2003). *Warning: Psychiatry can be hazardous to your mental health*. New York: Harper Collins.
60 *ibid*, p.xxi.
61 *ibid*, p.xxvi.
62 Glasser, W. (2003). *Warning: Psychiatry can be hazardous to your mental health*. p.113.
63 *ibid*, p.116.
64 *ibid*, p.110, 111.
65 Glasser, W. (2003). *Warning: Psychiatry can be hazardous to your mental health*. p. 121.
66 Snyderman, R. (2005, March 6). *San Francisco Chronicle*.

14
STILL LOOKING AHEAD

"They asked Frank Geary, the great architect, a question that really resonated with me. They said to him, 'Frank'—he's a very unprepossessing guy, a very modest guy—they said, 'how do you know when a building is finished?' And he thought for a little bit and said, 'In my mind they are never finished. I keep working on them as long as I think about them.' And my answer to that question from a choice theory perspective is that, in my mind, choice theory is never finished."
—William Glasser

As the 737 descended into Los Angeles airspace, final preparations for landing were well underway. Passengers had been reminded seat backs should be in the full upright position and that their tray tables should be up and fastened in the seat backs in front of them. Trash was being collected by the cabin attendants and people had been reminded to turn off their electronic devices. The flight had originated in Kansas City and William Glasser, one of the passengers, was returning from the 2004 American Counseling Association convention. He had received the ACA's Legend in Counseling award and had been invited to give the President's Address, but it had turned out a bit different than he expected. Instead of the President's Address being scheduled so that most of those attending the convention could hear the talk, it was scheduled as just one of the many break-out options. "A lot of people came to our booth," Glasser remembered, "and I thought I was going to have a huge audience. I was never so disappointed in my whole life when I got to my talk on Saturday afternoon, which I thought would be an ideal time. I was supposedly giving the Presidential Address, and I suspected there would be a few other talks going at the same time, but there were like 49 other presenters talking at the same time." In the end, more than 150 people came to his talk and he felt better after his presentation went well. He thought about the talk as the plane continued its descent. In spite of the pressure-regulated cabin his ears popped as the plane dropped closer and closer to sea level. Commercial passengers have a sense they are descending as they get closer to their destination airport, but most don't realize they are dropping at over 800 feet per minute. The plane made occasional gentle turns as it coordinated with other planes in lining up perfectly with the runway, still miles away. To onlookers at ground level, large jets about to land seem to be barely moving, but this is an illusion. Going at over 200 miles per hour as they approach the airport, flaps fully extended to increase the lift over the wings, they will "slow" to 175 miles per hour as their wheels gently touch down on the runway pavement. While others scrambled to exit the plane as it came to a stop at the gate, Glasser had been on enough flights that he knew there was no need to hurry at this point. He, along with everyone else on the plane, would exit when his or her row's turn came to exit, and that was that. He glanced out his small window again and thought about what he needed to do. There may not have been as many people at his talk as he had anticipated, but the talk had clearly outlined where he would head for the remaining years of his career.

I interviewed many of Glasser's friends and colleagues as I prepared to write his biography and all of them, except for one, enthusiastically supported the process. The one who declined was, ironically, Donald O'Donnell. Ironically, since O'Donnell, more than anyone else involved with Glasser, had always been so eager to share his story and the history of the Institute. One possible reason for O'Donnell's not visiting with me may have had to do with Glasser's interest in the present and the future, instead of where he had been in the past. I had to deal with this myself during my interviews with Glasser—the bulk of the interviews taking place between 2003 and 2008—as he was much more interested in talking about what was going on right then in his life. O'Donnell and Glasser had been very close friends for many years and it was hard to see this closeness diminish. Their association had made each other better. O'Donnell had become an even better school principal because of Glasser's coaching and Glasser's insights into the educational realm were much improved because of O'Donnell's input and influence. Glasser wrote extensively about O'Donnell's school in his widely read book, *Schools Without Failure*, in 1969. Their friendship was tested in the mid-'90s when O'Donnell wanted to put increasing amounts of energy and resources into a documentation of the past. Glasser conventions began having a history room or area where people could look at pictures or artifacts from Glasser's or the Institute's past. Glasser's heart was not in it though, and it contributed to a kind of distance between them. When I asked Glasser if he and O'Donnell had had a falling out, he replied, "No, not really. It's just that he was much more interested in the history of the organization. He thought I should have supported the history of the Institute, and it's just that I'm not really that interested in the history thing." When I followed up by pointing out he really didn't like looking back very much, he responded simply, "No, I don't."

A year later, in 2005, he admitted, "I'm so involved in what I am doing now that it's hard to focus back." He did have a lot going on.

He was consistently doing radio interviews around the country; he had just finished writing a series of plays for fourth-graders; one of the premier Glasser Quality Schools, Kay Mentley's school in Grand Traverse, Michigan, had received a $1.6 million grant to train teachers and track the results of choice theory implementation; he was dialoguing with Sam Gladding, president of the American Counseling Association, about a new emphasis for the ACA; he was in contact with Nicholas Cummings, who was president of the Cummings Foundation for Behavioral Health, about a chapter Glasser had written for a book Cummings and a colleague had edited entitled *Destructive Trends in Mental Health*[1]; he was getting very involved with Loyola Marymount University, both in the teaching and the researching of his ideas; and he was developing his next big focus, that mental health needed to be treated as a public health problem rather than a medical problem. These activities and projects did make it harder to focus on the past; they also might have made it harder to focus on the future, the future, that is, of the Institute.

Some referred to this topic, the future leadership of the Institute, as the 800-pound gorilla sitting in the corner of the room. It was a gorilla of Glasser's unintentional making. He turned 80 years old in 2005 and he was slowing down. His creativity seemed as present as ever, but he was less able to travel. There were key people who had been involved with the Institute for many years who potentially could have begun to take Glasser's place, but for whatever reason Glasser did not initiate this process. At times, Glasser even seemed resigned to the Institute riding off into the sunset. "Linda (Linda Harshman, Executive Director at the time) tells me we're not doing as much business and we can hardly keep going. I said, 'Look, we'll go as long as we can go and then, that's it, that's all.'" He thought aloud about how the Institute used to be a bigger deal, but now not as many people were involved. There were two boards for the Institute—one was an advisory board made up of regional members from around the U.S. and the world, and the other was the official board or legal board made up of only three members--Glasser, Carleen, and Linda Harshman. Glasser expressed some frustration at the advisory board for not working as hard as maybe they could have worked, but he acknowledged again they were an advisory board only. When I asked him directly what would happen to the Institute when he was no longer involved, he couldn't really say. While Linda Harshmann and Carleen were insightful in the ways of choice theory, Glasser didn't see either of them, both approaching or basically already enjoying retirement, leading the Institute into the future, a likely complicated future with people trying to figure out what to do without his involvement. In 2004, at 79 years of age, he stated matter-of-factly, "I should be around another 10 years or so..." Then his voice trailed off into quietness. It was his way of saying 'we don't have to worry about this right now.' After a moment of silence, he continued quietly with what was even more on his heart than the leadership question. "I'm just not sure if others are as enthusiastic about choice theory as I am."

During our interviews we also talked about his legacy. How did he want people to remember him? And which of his ideas did he especially think it was important for people to understand and embrace? When asked about his greatest contribution he replied, "Well, if we're talking about one thing I've contributed, which I think is my greatest contribution, it's the concept of total behavior. I think if you really understand that concept and use it in your life, that if you can live your life and move it on the front wheels, you're going to be much more effective than if you live your life on the rear wheels." During another interview he explained he "wanted people to think of him as a thinker who has helped a great many people to lead happier lives than they're leading now. I want to be known as the one person who helps people to deal effectively with the one human component that other mammals don't have, which is the need for power. Regardless of where you see it—whether it's in Iraq and the war going on there, whether you see it in marriages, or whether you see it in a company and how employees treat one another—it is the need for power and it has led to all kinds of serious human problems. I would like to be known for helping people understand how to deal with their need for power."

WG

During the 2005 Evolution of Psychotherapy conference in Anaheim, California, I asked Glasser if, with so many of the presenters emphasizing choice, responsibility, internal control, and the dangers of psychotropic drugs, he felt like less of a maverick. "Yes," he replied. "I do feel like less of a maverick." From one perspective, that others had joined him or were saying the same things he was saying, being less of a maverick was a good thing. From another perspective, though, that you were no longer viewed as leading the way, or worse, you weren't given credit for the leading you had done, being less of a maverick was a painful thing. One of Glasser's colleagues described it this way: "He's continually changing and, frankly speaking, I think he likes to be a step ahead of everybody. He just enjoys that. He's always operated as a solo pilot and been a maverick in the profession."

"Ever since he wrote his first book," Bob Wubbolding pointed out, "he's been regarded as a kind of guru." Over the years a great many people read or listened to Glasser's ideas and those ideas made a significant impact on their lives. People came to treat Glasser with a special respect and even awe. Wubbolding, a loyal colleague for many years, reminded people, though, that while Glasser was a maverick and incredibly insightful when it came to human behavior, things needed to be kept in perspective. "Some people say that you live choice theory," he began. "Others, myself included, say this is a psychological theory. Let's not make it more than that. Let's not make it the only way to live. In a spiritual sense, there is a whole other level that this doesn't touch on. And maybe it shouldn't touch on. Spirituality can build on this system, but it is a limited system. That makes the founder the developer of a psychological theory, but let's not make him more than what he is."

Glasser himself emphasized he wasn't perfect. "I've tried to live a good life," he offered, "but I'm not a perfect person. I've made mistakes." Similar to what Bob Wubbolding was trying to say, Glasser was clarifying that choice theory doesn't make people perfect. Choice theory offers excellent explanations as to why we do what we do, either good or bad, effective or ineffective, responsible or irresponsible. Choice theory explains motivation and, to an extent, behavior. It doesn't predict behavior, control it, or perfect it.

Still, even as he admitted he felt like less of a maverick, and even as he admitted he was not perfect, Glasser matter-of-factly pointed out: "I've had quite an effect on many people. I've made so many presentations for so many years, and from those presentations I've gained a modicum of prominence, you know." It was a humble way of describing his place in the world, especially in the fields of psychology and education. As he entered the twilight of his career, it struck those close to Glasser how consistently his behavior was marked by grace and optimism. When I suggested as Albert Ellis got older he got crankier, but that didn't seem to be the case with him, Glasser replied, "No, you see, I believe my ideas are happy ideas."

Even as Glasser felt less of a maverick in that moment, he was in the midst of leading-edge efforts in two important areas. The first area had to do with his groundbreaking message to the more than 50,000 members of the American Counseling Association. The second area had to do with his growing belief that real solutions to the pandemic levels of unhappiness, and the mental distress that accompanies it, would be found in the public health model, rather than in the medical treatment model in which society was so heavily investing. The implications of his ideas, both for the counselors and for society, in general, were huge. It may be hard to understand how he could have felt like less of a maverick even as these ideas and efforts were put in play, but maybe he had been on the leading edge for so long it felt old hat for him.

As Glasser realized more and more the field of mental health really didn't focus on mental health at all, but instead focused on labeling behavioral symptoms as mental illness and disease, he became convinced the focus needed to shift to helping people realize their own potential for becoming stronger, happier, and mentally healthier. The field of psychiatry had been focusing on the mental illness model for decades, and in the process had embraced brain drugs as the answer to behaviors they labeled as incurable, lifelong diseases, and to mental conditions that could be somewhat stabilized, but not cured. Those involved with counseling, though—psychologists, therapists, family counselors, marriage counselors, and social workers—had continued to focus on talk therapy as their main way to treat clients. As the brain drug wave grew to tsunami proportions in the 1990s and swept over society in a flood of advertising and sales, it began to affect even those who had previously been so committed to talk therapy treatment. Counselors with doctorates or with the necessary certification were more and more seeking the ability to prescribe drugs as a part of their treatment methods. When Glasser presented at the 2004 American Counseling Association conference, the desire of the counselors to be able to prescribe drugs had only increased. It seemed a growing number of counselors viewed it as a credibility issue. Clients wanted the drug option and some counselors felt they would simply go to another therapist to get it. It wasn't a majority of counselors who felt this way, but the number seemed to be growing. Glasser was convinced this represented a perfect opportunity for ACA members to differentiate themselves and establish their credibility based on a foundation of mental health, rather than mental illness. "I'm trying to persuade the counselors," he explained, "to move away from mental illness and drugs, to mental health and happiness. That's where I am. I believe there is such a thing as mental health."

Glasser felt a majority of the counselors "pretty much embraced" choice theory, but he wanted them to do it officially. He was energized by his efforts to gain a breakthrough in this area, whether with regional counseling associations or with key individuals: "I think we're on the verge of making some big dents in the whole thing." In the months leading up to our interview on this topic he had been to ACA state meetings in Kentucky, North Carolina, South Carolina, Maine, Michigan, and New Mexico, each time wanting to remind them of the special niche counselors had and that they didn't have to follow in the footsteps of psychiatry and the DSM-IV. He wanted them to realize they could have a successful practice on the basis of choice theory and on the basis of mental health. "I spent maybe a half hour on this," he recalled from his talk in New Mexico, "saying you can start a practice and you can advertise that you focus on mental health, that you don't believe they are mentally ill, that they are not as mentally healthy as they would like to be, but you can focus on that."

During our interviews in 2004 and 2005 I heard the name of Sam Gladding a lot. At the time, Gladding was president of the American Counseling Association and Glasser was hopeful Gladding would be key to the mental health breakthrough. The two of them seemed to be in regular communication. He always brought me up to date on their latest conversations or emails. During one of these updates he said: "The counselors should put out a statement that we practice, you know, our practice is based on mental health. We don't believe you have a mental illness. There's nothing wrong with your brain. It would be nice if people could go to the phone book and find counselors who focus on mental health and who will help you to be mentally healthier, or help your child to become mentally healthier. This is something I am really thinking about. I haven't had a big public relations breakthrough with this stuff. I mean it's not that I have been working on this idea for a long time. The mental health stuff has only been a couple of months now. But I think the mental health idea would get me a public relations breakthrough. So I am gonna ask Sam Gladding to perhaps contact the media for the ACA and say we're having a very interesting presentation on mental health, and that counselors are very interested in this, and that maybe you ought to listen to what Dr. Glasser has to say."

Gladding and Glasser would eventually take the stuff of their private conversations, the emails and phone calls, and share their ideas publically in articles they each wrote for *The Family Journal: Counseling and Therapy for Couples and Families.* Glasser made his case for the ineffective state of psychiatry, the preponderance of brain drugs, and the preponderance of people being diagnosed with mental illness, as well as a brief description of how choice theory could help people in distress. He concluded his article with a call for purpose and action. "I believe," he began, "that counselors need an identity if they are to successfully pursue their goal of being a recognized force in the world. The identity that I offer is mental health through choice theory." Some might misunderstand him on this point. He wasn't trying to "sell" choice theory to the counselors. He truly believed that choice theory accurately explains why people do what they do and he wanted the American Counseling Association to tap into that accuracy. As far as he was concerned, psychiatrists had abandoned the concept of mental health, and in the process had created an identity almost completely associated with mental illness and brain drugs. The time was perfect for the ACA to claim a uniquely powerful position. His clarion invitation continued, "If the American Counseling Association would adopt the mental health mantle, which is up for the taking, I believe they could have an easy-to-understand, unique identity that could serve them well. The danger of psychiatric drugs is now coming out of the closet. The mantra of counselors could be Effective Mental Health Without Drugs, and at a cost far less than the billions of dollars being spent on drug treatment now. If a group as large and as prestigious as the American Counseling Association would formally accept and promote these ideas, I believe the world would listen carefully."[2]

The level of interest and support from Gladding may have led Glasser to see him, especially as the current president of the ACA, as a real opportunity for systemic change. As it turned out, Gladding's support was somewhat more muted. In the same *Family Journal* that Glasser's article, A New Vision for Counseling, was published, Sam Gladding wrote a response to that vision. Gladding's article title declared, The Potential and Pitfall of William Glasser's New Vision for Counseling. It was less than an endorsement, yet the article identified some key decisions for the counseling profession. Gladding acknowledged Glasser as a pioneer in the field of mental health and for the soundness of reality therapy and choice theory. He further commended Glasser for highlighting the problems with pills and the field's overdependence on the medical model for solutions. A part of Gladding seemed to see the sense, even the brilliance, in what Glasser was saying, but a larger part of him was filled with questions about the implications of his ideas. "The question becomes," he began, "can we live without a reliance on drugs as a primary source of happiness, wholeness, and wellness in our profession, as well as in society? Should we, as counselors, and the American Counseling Association take on a unique identity adopting the mantra Effective Mental Health Without Drugs? I am personally sympathetic to an affirmative answer to both questions. Yet I am realistic too in recognizing that we as counselors, and we as the American Counseling Association, are very diverse in our backgrounds, beliefs, and practices. As a group of counselors, we use various theories and some of us, I think, legitimately need medications. As an entity, we are diverse in regard to what we believe as well as what we embrace as valid. Thus, the question is not, 'Will we respond positively to the challenge in William Glasser's article?' but rather, 'Can we?' Do we have the will to break from the herd of mental health providers and be different and distinct in what we offer and why? Is such a course the most prudent one we should take? The question Glasser has raised should be discussed and debated because of its complexity and possible outcomes to us individually and collectively."[3]

Like G. L. Harrington 40 years earlier, Gladding could not put all of his eggs in Glasser's basket. Harrington participated with Glasser in the events that led to the writing of *Reality Therapy*, but he pulled back when *Reality Therapy* took off like a cannon shot. He didn't want to risk his professional standing by fully embracing Glasser's approach. Harrington, in effect, wanted others to decide for themselves whether or not *Reality Therapy* had merit. Similarly, while he admitted Glasser's approach provided a good alternative, Gladding did not position it above other approaches. In effect, Gladding was asking questions that each counselor would have to answer for himself or herself.

From a cynical viewpoint, one might surmise Gladding was expressing interest in and expressing support for Glasser's ideas in the hope that he could get Glasser to participate in the 2004 ACA convention. Authors and speakers as popular as Glasser experience such flattery on a regular basis. But I don't think that was Gladding's motivation. Gladding seemed to be drawn to Glasser's approach, but for some reason he couldn't fully buy into them. Glasser said as much when I asked him about Gladding. "He really supports it," Glasser emphasized at first, "but, you know, I'm a little too much for him." At another time, reflecting on the different people during his career who had written forewords or testimonials for his books, he admitted he had probably made too big a deal out of it. "I probably have overestimated the value of support from other people. I've always thought it's very important, and it is, but, but in the end it doesn't seem . . ." He paused, his voice trailing off, "Anyway, you've just got to stand on what you write, that's all."

The decision Sam Gladding faced as an individual and the American Counseling Association faced collectively is basically the same decision every individual faces when dealing with unhappiness and mental distress. Has our life been hijacked by some psychological virus over which we have no defense other than a pill to moderate our symptoms, or are we able to recognize and treat our own unhappiness? Are we victims of outside illnesses that attack and overwhelm us or have our thinking and behavior in some ways led to our dysfunction? In another periodical Gladding wrote that the implications of Glasser's approach are monumental. The word "monumental" seems appropriate for this discussion.

From my visits with Glasser in 2005, two stories are noteworthy. The first because it is one more example of Glasser's creativity; the second because, well, because it was just so special. As one of our interviews was getting started Glasser was describing an important person with whom he was in touch, a person with access to a lot of money, regarding an idea. I got the recorder set up and wanted him to clarify what he was talking about. He proceeded to explain he had written this guy a letter challenging him, asking him to offer a reward of $100,000 to anyone who can prove that mental illnesses have a pathology. Such proof did not exist as of 2005 and Glasser was confident it never would exist. In the end, after lawyers weighed in on the possibilities, the offer was never developed, but it shows how Glasser was always on the lookout for a breakthrough angle.

The second story could easily be a book of its own. During one of my interview trips to Glasser's house, while looking through old scrapbooks piled in an office closet, I made a remarkable discovery. Carefully pasted and taped into the scrapbook were 40-year-old, yellowed newspaper clippings that described an event that was simultaneously fascinating, frustrating, and awful. The clippings alerted me to a story I briefly alluded to in Chapter Five of this book. During the 1965/1966 school year at Oxnard High School in southern California, a young vice-principal was forced out of her job for managing student discipline infractions with Glasser's reality therapy principles in mind. Her name was Adrienne Nater and the articles documented her views regarding student discipline and described how her theories were supported by better results; that she was forced to resign by an administration that felt she "just wasn't suited for the job"; that local editorials came to her defense; and students and parents fought to keep her and her ideas at the school. It was all for naught, though, and at 32 years of age, out of her job, she headed out to make a positive difference elsewhere. When I showed Glasser and Carleen the scrapbook they were as intrigued by the tale as I was. "She's probably still alive," Glasser thought aloud, a thought that hadn't even crossed my mind. "And she may still live in the area," Carleen chipped in, which I privately felt had almost no chance of being true. Convinced that it was a real possibility, Carleen picked up the phone and called directory assistance. There were several possibilities within the greater Oxnard area and Carleen asked the operator to connect her to the first number on the list. When a woman answered the phone Carleen explained she was married to William Glasser, and described the newspaper clippings that had led to her making the phone call. Was there any chance, Carleen wondered to the person on the other end of the line, that she might be the Adrienne Nater referred to in the articles? To my amazement, and to the joy of the three of us—Glasser, Carleen, and me—around their kitchen table, she indicated that she was indeed that Adrienne Nater. Moments later Carleen handed the phone to Glasser, whereupon a conversation like none I had ever witnessed took place. To think of the pain of her forced resignation in 1966 and the twists and turns her life may have taken after that, and to picture her so many years later receiving a phone call, out of the blue, from the very person whose ideas she felt were important enough to lose her job over, it was just an amazing moment. For me, it was one of the most memorable moments of the biography project. Less than two months later, Glasser had a speaking engagement in Ventura, California, and the two of them were able to meet.

From the very beginning of his career Glasser desired to make a basic understanding of human psychology accessible to every person. And to that end he wrote in a clear and simple voice. He didn't feel psychological problems were all that mysterious and that people could become skilled at not only looking after themselves, but also able to lend a psychological hand to others experiencing distress in its varied forms. At the end of *The Identity Society* (1972), for instance, he described the idea of Community Involvement Centers in which "each community would have its own organization to help its failing people, no matter what symptoms they exhibit."[4] Again later, in the *Warning* (2003) book, he described the concept of choice theory focus groups in which people learning about choice theory could support one another in the process. "It's not like what I'm saying is very hard to do or cost a million dollars or something," Glasser explained during one of our interviews. "It's just that we're so stuck in the tradition of the external control world we live in that we're almost paralyzed against really changing the way we deal with people, and even deal with each other – as in marriage. There's no reason for half the people that get married to get divorced. That's a totally absurd statistic!"

Some may want to make it more complicated, but Glasser identified basic unhappiness as the reason for mental distress and the psychological symptoms that come out of that distress. This unhappiness is almost always because of relationship problems with other people. We have a need to get along with others; to be valued and affirmed; to make contributions and have them recognized; and to listen and to be heard. The more important the relationship is—such as with a spouse or partner, or with a child, or with a boss or colleague at work—the more important it is to us the relationship be need-satisfying. We want to be happy, and when we aren't we struggle to become happy. Without insight or tools to help us, we often retreat into coping or surviving. Such unhappiness is not insignificant, and as mentioned earlier, Glasser stated clearly: "It is virtually impossible to be unhappy for longer than five or six weeks and remain symptom free."[5] Many will pause here and wonder if it can really be this simple. Can the pandemic of psychological and emotional distress be attributed to simple unhappiness? Glasser answered yes to that question and reminded me: "It's not like there's a hundred problems in the world. There's only one."

When, in 1960, his first book was titled *Mental Health or Mental Illness?* Glasser could not have known that over 40 years later the title would capture the driving question he wanted, for the world's sake, to answer. Are our psychological symptoms the result of illness or disease, or are they the result of our unhappiness? The title also called attention to the idea that there is such a thing as mental health. As obvious as this may sound, Glasser felt mental health professionals, and by extension, society in general, were so focused on mental disease and illness they had lost sight of the mental health target. The focus was so much on minimizing or numbing the bad effects of distress symptoms that there was no focus on achieving real mental health. "I'm saying something to the world," Glasser clarified. "Look, what you call mental health right now is really mental illness." The field may refer to itself as the mental health field, but based on their approach, based on their literally forcing people into treatments for which there was no pathology, Glasser stated it was more accurate to refer to the field as the mental illness field.

He wanted people to focus on the good fight of mental health, rather than the bad fight of mental illness. When I pressed him to say more about this he reminded me he had already explained it. "What I'm saying," he began, "is that there is such a thing as mental health and I can define it." It was true. He had written in the *Warning* book that happiness is mental health, and then provided the following definition: "Happiness or mental health is enjoying the life you are choosing to live, getting along well with the people near and dear to you, doing something with your life you believe is worthwhile, and not doing anything to deprive anyone else of the same chance for happiness you have."

With this definition of mental health and happiness in mind, as he thought more and more about it, Glasser became convinced the focus really could be on health, rather than on illness; that people could be taught to be happy, rather than labeling their unhappiness as mental disease and giving them pills to moderate their moods. The light bulb began to go on in Glasser's head. The medical model was helpful when dealing with actual pathology, but it was actually counterproductive when dealing with psychological symptoms for which there was no pathology. A better model for helping people learn how to deal with their own unhappiness, and the psychological symptoms that resulted from their unhappiness, was and is the public health model. "Unhappiness is a public health problem," Glasser explained to me. "What we need is a public health education program to educate people as to how they can reduce their psychological symptoms and become happier."

Throughout 2005 Glasser talked about this new emphasis, especially after something he had written was ready for distribution. "I finally crystallized my ideas on what I call mental health," he said as he walked to his desk, "and I have written a little booklet, which I'm gonna sell for five dollars. So it's cheap enough that anyone would buy it, and short enough so anyone could get the idea by reading it." He had retrieved a booklet from his desk and showed it to me. *Treating Mental Health as a Public Health Problem* was clearly labeled across the front. I interrupted him as he went on about the price of the booklet and the marketing and tried to bring him back to the actual focus of the booklet. "I'm not saying to stop the drugs, stop all that. I'm saying use a different model. Look at smoking," Glasser pointed out. "Smoking in the United States has dropped in the last 20 years from 56% of the people smoking then to, uh, 19% who are smoking now. That's a huge drop! Think about how many lives have been saved because of that drop. Have they been saved by doctors? Absolutely not! Doctors smoke themselves in many cases. They've been saved by a public health education program to educate people to the dangers of smoking. So what we need is a public health education program to educate people to how they can reduce their psychological symptoms and become happier."

Given the overwhelming burden that healthcare costs are placing on our personal, corporate, and national pocketbooks, it would seem people might take note of Glasser's suggestions. Billions and billions of dollars are being spent every year for unnecessary or inconclusive medical tests in an effort to discover a pathology that doesn't exist.[6] "I want the people who spend the money for health in this country to stop wasting their money on mental illnesses and instead spend their money on developing a delivery system for mental health, which we basically have already done." He meant here that a public health system was already in place. "Others," he continued, "like Albert Ellis, and Aaron Beck, and Alfred Adler, may have good ideas and even deliver ideas. Any mental health ideas that help people to realize you don't have to go to a therapist for a long period of time are probably helpful ideas. The one I suggest, choice theory, is the one I've used to deliver mental health, but I don't claim it's the only one. What I do claim is that we should be moving from a medical delivery system to a public health delivery system." Glasser was adamant regarding the need for this shift, yet he recognized just how much the healthcare system, especially the pharmaceuticals, wanted things to stay the same.

Glasser's enthusiasm for his new thinking on the public health model was fueled toward the end of 2004 when he became aware of a proposal that came out of his old *alma mater,* Case Western University School of Medicine. Glasser shared with me a presentation given at a faculty retreat by Ralph Horwitz, Dean of the School of Medicine at Case Western, entitled A for Radical Reform of Medical Education. Horwitz stated, "the disciplines of public health and medicine must be united in a single, complementary program of study." Further, he declared: "To meet this objective, Case Western Reserve University proposes to create a School of Medicine and Health with the goal of enabling the professional integration that must be a core strategy in addressing the current crisis in the inter-professional relationships between medicine and public health. Through our recreation of the medical school, we will educate physicians to understand the interplay between the biology of disease and the social context of illness; between the care of the individual patient and the health of the public; and between clinical medicine and population medicine. The physicians who emerge from this experience will be individuals whose leadership in science, practice, and healthcare policy will reflect the interplay among the most enduring and salient themes in health and healthcare. The Case School of Medicine and Health will challenge the profession of medicine to re-imagine itself as responsible not just for the care of patients with disease, but also for the prevention and control of diseases in individuals and communities, and ultimately for the health of people in the United States and across the globe. Our proposal is intended not simply to reform medical education, but to shift existing paradigms in order to reinvent it."

Glasser must have been astounded when he first read these bold statements. Maybe he pinched himself to see if he was actually dreaming. Here was somebody speaking Glasser's language. Horwitz's proposal did put the words "medicine" and "public health" in the same sentence, but stopped short of including "mental health." Glasser was pleased his own *alma mater* colleague was apparently thinking in similar ways to himself and wrote a letter to Horwitz that explained his vision for the future. "I agree completely with what you are proposing," he began, "but I am concerned that while you focus on public health, you do not specifically include public mental health in that focus." The psychiatric establishment was not leading in this effort and in Glasser's opinion paid only lip-service to the idea of mental health. He described how huge numbers of symptomatic people were being diagnosed as "mentally ill" and that two things needed to happen to address the situation. "First," he continued, "we must be able to explain what is causing their psychological symptoms, and second, we need to put in place a system of public mental health in which millions of people with serious psychological symptoms can be effectively treated." The medical model attempted to do this, but fell woefully short. Glasser pointed out, "People are diagnosed with clinical depression, bipolar disorder, schizophrenia, and especially ADHD, even though there is not a shred of evidence of any pathology in their brains." This lack of brain pathology in people exhibiting serious mental symptoms and distress comes as a surprise to many, but as yet no definite biological connection has been made between crazy behavior and a diseased brain.[7]

Glasser saw it as a problem of common sense and hoped Horwitz and his colleagues at Case Western would be a part of helping people come to their . . . well, come to science at least. "We are presently struggling unsuccessfully with a huge epidemic of misdiagnosed mental illnesses," he wrote, "because the scientific community has, for a variety of reasons, many of them monetary, replaced science with common sense. Common sense can be defined as a belief that seems so obvious it should be accepted without question. Unfortunately, however, many of these 'obvious' beliefs have with time been proven wrong. Examples of common sense in medicine are widespread. George Washington was bled to death by physicians using common sense. More recently millions of tonsils and adenoids were unnecessarily removed based on common sense, even after antibiotics became widely available."

Glasser wanted Horwitz to see "psychiatric common sense" had led to people being diagnosed with brain illnesses for which there was no pathology, and powerful drugs were being administered for these so-called illnesses. People may suffer from the symptoms listed in the DSM-IV, but that does not make them mentally ill. Glasser believed relationships were so important to the human psyche that when relationships were damaged or missing altogether it would ultimately affect our ability to successfully process life. "I am one of the few psychiatrists," he explained to Horwitz, "who are vitally concerned with mental health as completely separate from what is now called 'mental illness.' Like almost all mammals, we are social creatures; we need each other, both to be happy and when we are small to help us survive. To do this we have to learn how to get along well with the important people in our lives. We also need to learn to get along better with ourselves by learning to accept there are limitations to what we can do."

People could literally learn to be happy; could learn to get along well with the important people in their lives; and could become aware of the onset of mental distress symptoms and how to address them. In

Still Looking Ahead

the same way "couch potatoes," people less than physically healthy, could become healthier through better diet and exercise, Glasser believed that unhappy, symptomatic people, people less than mentally healthy, could become healthier through a public mental health program that taught them about how their brain works. "If this approach to unhappiness through public mental health programs were supported by a medical school such as Case," he wrote toward the end of his letter, "it could positively affect the mental health of huge numbers of people at little cost to anyone. It could literally save millions of dollars by reducing unnecessary visits to doctors' offices and emergency rooms and give doctors more time to treat people who need medicine and surgery."

Written in September of 2004, the letter represented what Glasser was coming to see as his final great push, based on the idea that the medical model was being misapplied to psychological symptoms and the public health model was really the only systemic way to begin to make a positive difference. It wasn't that the medical model was bad in and of itself. What it is designed for it does well. It just wasn't designed to take on psychological symptoms for which there is no pathology. Writing the letter to Horwitz, almost seven pages in length, spurred Glasser into stating his public mental health position more descriptively and definitively, and once again he sat down at his computer and laid out the problem and what he saw as the solution.

Originally labeled *Treating Mental Health as a Public Health Problem*, within a year it would be relabeled as *Defining Mental Health as a Public Health Issue*.[8] Almost obsessed with keeping his writing short and simple, the booklet was only 35 pages long, and ultimately, rather than selling for five dollars each, they were given away to anyone interested in the information.

The information was more important than that, more important than a give-away booklet, and Glasser kept looking for opportunities to share his public mental health vision. Some recognized and understood the importance of his ideas—the principles of choice theory and the concept of teaching the principles through a public health model—and threw their support into making the vision a reality for as many people as possible. I witnessed an example of this level of support while attending the 2005 Glasser International Conference in Dublin, Ireland. Glasser's ideas have made significant inroads into the counseling approaches in Ireland, with many in the helping professions taking the choice theory training. By the summer of 2005, the ideas had reached to the higher levels of Irish government. Tim O'Malley, then Minister of State, with Special Responsibility for Mental Health, opened the Glasser International Conference with a supportive introduction of Glasser and a speech in support of his approach. O'Malley, who was a pharmacist before entering his government role, had read *Warning: Psychiatry Can Be Dangerous to Your Mental Health* and agreed with what it said. In the same year that it was published, 2003, O'Malley established an Expert Group on Mental Health Policy, a committee on which Terry Lynch, the author of *Beyond Prozac*, served.

Another example of support for Glasser's ideas came out of Loyola Marymount University, in Los Angeles, California. His connection to the university and the positive things that resulted from that connection actually came out of something pretty routine -- jury duty. In February of 2006, Carleen Glasser was fulfilling her jury duty summons. After roll was taken, a process in which everyone's name is called out publicly, a gentleman approached her and wondered if, by any chance, she was related to William Glasser, the well-known psychiatrist. She replied that she was married to him. The chance encounter was fortuitous for several reasons. The gentleman who approached Carleen Glasser was Brad Smith, a program coordinator in public health studies at Loyola Marymount. Smith, like many others quietly working within the helping professions, had been taught about reality therapy and control theory and read Glasser's books for himself. He knew the ideas worked from firsthand experience. Equally important, Smith was a high energy, can-do person who quickly sought to get Glasser involved in his classes at Loyola. Just as quickly, Glasser became excited about the potential of this new opportunity.

By 2006, when he began to get very involved at Loyola, Glasser was beginning to slow down. He was taking on fewer speaking appointments and, in general, was traveling less. He also was driving less on the busy southern California roads that surrounded his house and Santa Monica, recognizing he felt less and less comfortable navigating the traffic, especially at night. Few people knew of his physical ailments. He quietly and matter-of-factly stayed on top of his diabetes, describing himself as someone who ate to live, rather than lived to eat. Few people would also know of the open-heart bypass surgery he would undergo just a couple of years later. Through it all, though, Loyola was a bright spot in his life. We never talked without the latest upcoming development at Loyola. And when I visited him in southern California for further interviews I would always be invited to go with him to Loyola and observe the class he was teaching. Besides the individual students who were helped in these classes, two important thrusts developed as a result of Glasser's involvement at the university.

The first thrust had to do with Loyola's desire to research Glasser's ideas, to put them to the test, and study the extent to which they are effective. Glasser was in full support of this and the structure slowly came into place to create research questions and studies that would lead to objective results. An example of this research involved deans and resident assistants in the freshmen dorms being taught choice theory, with the idea of studying the frequency of dysfunctional student behaviors. They knew, for instance, how many times during the previous year that ambulances had pulled up in front of one of the dorms to care for students with alcohol poisoning. Would at-risk behaviors decrease if adult and student leaders in the dorms knew about choice theory?

Momentum for choice theory seemed to build at Loyola and a Glasser Research Center was being discussed. I attended a banquet on Loyola's campus in March 2008, held in honor of Glasser, at which he was invited to speak about his public mental health vision. At one point in the proceedings a man went to the podium and called Glasser forward to join him, whereupon he presented Glasser with a large, attractive certificate stating that he was publicly pledging $100,000 to the William Glasser Fund at Loyola Marymount, in appreciation for what Glasser's ideas had done for him personally. I learned later the man had struggled for a long time with alcohol addiction and he credited choice theory for beginning to restore self-control to his life. There was also talk of an endowed chair at Loyola in Glasser's name. I was pleased that an academic institution was apparently going to take on the housing of Glasser artifacts and materials, as well as the study and research of his ideas. This was a component that had been missing from what Glasser had to offer—the component of research to back up his ideas. It was the component to which critics of his ideas pointed.

Interested in how the research element was going, I visited Loyola during the summer of 2010 and experienced the second important thrust that came out of Glasser's presence there. Prior to my arrival, students from one of Brad Smith's courses, a course in which they themselves had learned choice theory, had been regularly going to the prison for women[9] in Chino, California, and teaching choice theory principles to inmates there. During one of the days I spent at Loyola I got on the bus with Smith and students from his course and traveled to Chino to visit the prison and see and hear for myself the results of the choice theory emphasis. What I experienced there made a profound impression on me. Inside the large prison campus, which housed as many as 2,500 inmates, was a comparatively small portable classroom that served as the center for the Choice Theory Connection Program. Several prison staff members, including Les Johnson, the principal of the El Prado Adult School within the prison, had taken the reality therapy/choice theory course work and had become certified choice theory instructors. Through their efforts, along with the support of the students from Loyola, more than 150 inmates had received choice theory training and there was a waiting list of over 120 inmates wanting to enroll in upcoming trainings. I had the privilege of sitting around in a large circle of women inmates and listening to them share about how the choice theory ideas had changed them. Some around the circle would be getting out within a couple of months, while others, some whom had been convicted of murder, would never be getting out. Yet, regardless, the women consistently talked about the power and freedom they now understood was theirs. One woman expressed thankfulness for the ideas, because in a short time she would be released and be at home again with her children. She had not known how to relate to them before, however with her new understanding of choice theory she felt more ready to listen to them and guide them. Another woman, a lifer, described how when she woke up in the morning, even though she was locked up in the prison, she felt free for the first time in her life. It was a very powerful testimony.

A research team from Loyola also became involved at the

women's prison with the intent to discover or document whether or not choice theory ideas worked. Dr. Cheryl Grills, an associate dean from Loyola and the coordinator of the prison research project, stated her response to the research plainly. "At LMU we have developed an assessment of the Choice Theory Connection Program, and as researchers, we have been stunned! As researchers, the preliminary results have quite literally blown us away!"[10] At a presentation she gave at the International Glasser Conference during the summer of 2012, Dr. Grills described how their assessment battery included standardized scales such as the Emotional Regulation Scale, the Well-Being Scale, the Depression/Happiness Scale, as well as specific assessment tools related to Choice Theory topics. They also measured changes in self-knowledge, attitude, perceptions of stress, mindfulness, behavior, body-awareness, and interpersonal relationships.

"What did we find?" she asked the audience. "We found that in every single measure the women changed! In the research world we want to know if the change is statistically significant, that is, does it measure a change of .05% or greater from the standard? We found that in every single measure the women changed to a much greater degree than .05%. Not only did they change, but there was a transformation which is hard to get at in paper and pencil measures. Our students saw it, others saw it. People know when they are in the midst of transformation." Sitting around the circle on the day I visited the prison, I certainly saw it too.

The success of a good approach or idea within an organization is dependent to a great extent on good leadership. This seems to be especially true when it comes to implementing choice theory. The pull back towards external control—manipulating through reward and punishment—is very strong and without positive, gentle intervention that is the direction human beings head. As it would turn out, the Choice Theory Connections Program continued for years, in spite of budget cuts and other common administrative challenges. The plans at Loyola were not so fortunate. Years later the Glasser Research Center had still not been created; an endowed chair had not been created; the $100,000 gift had not been received, and momentum in general had slowed considerably. Even ideas as powerful as choice theory need buy-in from multiple organizational levels to gain a foothold and then make progress over time. An elementary school, for instance, that is making fantastic progress toward becoming a Glasser Quality School can find their gains in reverse when a key person, such as a principal, leaves.

Glasser admitted after learning about control theory in the late 1970s it took him about two years to shift away from automatically thinking and behaving in stimulus-response terms. It is challenging for a person, even Glasser, to shift away from trying to manipulate others to behave how you want them to behave, or to stop being the victim and blame others for your own unhappiness. Needless to say, it is even more challenging for a group of people, like the staff of a company or a school, to make this shift at the same time. External control habits run deep, but change is possible. Caring lead-managers and commitment to choice theory principles will lead to a shift toward real quality. This kind of nurturing leadership will keep the focus of a home, school, or business on becoming and remaining a need-satisfying place where people get along well and operate at the highest levels. Without this kind of leadership important elements fall by the wayside.

Although at times I wondered if Glasser cared about the future of The Glasser Institute and the structure that had for so many years organized the trainings for reality therapy and choice theory, in the end he spoke and wrote more clearly about what he thought it would take for the Institute to successfully navigate the future. During a speaking tour in Japan, Glasser described his concept of public mental health, and on his return from Japan he reiterated: "If the concept of public mental health takes hold it will move mental health from where it is now—a commercial way to push psychiatric drugs that can be very harmful to those who are prescribed them—to a way that unhappy people can be taught to put choice theory to work in their lives and, in doing so, live happier and more productive lives." He became more and more sure about the need for this approach to mental health. His most definitive statement about this and the future of the Institute appeared in a letter he wrote to the Institute board of directors.

"It is very important to me," the letter began, "that the ideas I developed are preserved to most accurately reflect the way they evolved and I believe the most current of this evolution, the new field of Public Mental Health, will play a critical role in the survival of the William Glasser Institute. We need to attract a new audience for our product and I think this idea has universal appeal. Everywhere we go people seem genuinely enthusiastic about the concept. I would like to see the WGI programs for Reality Therapy Certification reflect a concentration in Public Mental Health. The evolution of my ideas in my lifelong work has grown to include first the development of Reality Therapy, then the addition of Choice Theory, and finally a culmination of the two applied to the entire field of helping professions, which I have decided to call Public Mental Health. We teach this now in our Reality

Still Looking Ahead

Therapy Certification programs. However, I believe it is important to emphasize how practice of the procedures and teaching Choice Theory to groups and individuals in a Public Mental Health program is critical to the survival of the William Glasser Institute."

Many within the organization had wanted Glasser to become clearer about his organizational preferences and set a course for the future, and the board letter, to some extent, did that. Maybe it says something about him that his clearest statements were idea-focused, rather than person-focused. He emphasized what should be focused on, rather than who would lead the Institute toward that focus. The word "survival" is used more than once in the letter, which indicates he may have understood the seriousness of the situation. Time would tell if the public mental health focus would carry the Institute into the future, or if the right person would lead the Institute into the post-Glasser era.

Bill and I watched Super Bowl XL together. Carleen had gone on an errand and we had the downstairs living room to ourselves. Pittsburgh was playing against Seattle and we looked on as the Steelers slowly took the game under control, winning 21-10, although Seahawks fans must have been frustrated with the referee decisions that didn't go their way and contributed to the Pittsburgh victory. It was Seattle's first time ever in the Super Bowl, while for Pittsburgh their victory gave them five Super Bowl victories, tying them with San Francisco and Dallas for Super Bowl wins. (Three years later, Pittsburgh would pass San Francisco and Dallas by beating Arizona in Super Bowl XLIII.) Other than the game and, of course, the commercials, the house was quiet. After the game we went out to eat together. He thought of a place near his house that had good vegetarian choices for me and we both ended up getting the food we wanted. Earlier in the day we had conducted one of our regular interviews, my small recorder documenting his thoughts as I studied notes for the next question. But as we ate at the small neighborhood restaurant there was no recorder on the table, just our food.

As I interviewed him during those two days, February 5 and 6, 2006, it became apparent to me Glasser was at a unique point in his life. He would turn 81 years of age in a couple of months and he had slowed down. Yet, in spite of this he was still writing and speaking and traveling. He acknowledged he was slowing down, something he hadn't done before, and pointed out that he wasn't playing tennis anymore. "I just can't hit the ball like I used to," he admitted. (I actually kept track of the times Glasser said, "I'm going to play tennis today," and the last time he said that to me was on September 7, 2004. We didn't talk every day, so he certainly could have played after that, but by early 2006 he was done with one of his all-time favorite activities.) Still, during the same interview he admitted his tennis playing days were over, he also described how well he was doing. When I expressed to him that I was about to take on a more demanding job that I anticipated would suck up more of my time and energy, and I was concerned it would possibly keep me from writing, he quickly replied that it was all right with him. "I'm in the most productive time of my life right now," he replied. "I'm still making history." I was feeling pressure to get the biography done, yet he was saying why rush to complete the biography when he was still producing?

A year later he described how he had shifted from playing tennis to walking on his treadmill. "I can burn almost 200 calories when I walk in the morning. I like to walk at 2.8 miles per hour. I can kick it up to 3.0 miles per hour, but it's just not comfortable. I would rather walk a little longer at a speed that's good for me." He liked listening to music when he exercised, although his choice of music—John Philip Sousa band music—may not have appealed to others. He held onto the treadmill handrails as he walked and did fine, even when it was cranked up to 3.0 miles an hour, but what seemed easy on the treadmill was getting less so around the house or on errands around town. The handrails were fixed to the treadmill and couldn't go wherever he wanted to go. Others were noticing the change and he was noticing it too. "I'm just. . . I'm just a little unsteady on my feet, a little tiny bit, but not much." The words were matter-of-fact, yet there was something in his voice that said he didn't want to admit this. "I went to a neurologist and he ran all the tests and all the tests came back normal. My blood sugar was a little high, but I don't worry about that because I take that myself, and I only take my blood sugar once a day before I go to bed. If I eat a lot of sweets before I go to bed, like last night I got carried away with a good-sized piece of watermelon. So it was a little bit high."

Since most of the interview work was behind us and I was working on the writing part of the project, I didn't communicate with Glasser as much as when we were visiting almost once a week. Having not been around him as often I was not aware of the unsteadiness on his feet and wanted him to catch me up a bit more. "You were mentioning," I began, "the unsteadiness on your feet. You seem sharp. Your mind. . ."

"My mind is fine," he quickly answered. "The neurologist said it's probably a little bit of old age. I walk on the treadmill every day. I did it today and it keeps my blood sugar down."

I asked about other everyday activities like getting around town for errands and driving. "I have a speaking appointment coming up in

San Diego. I'm shaky about driving. I just drive locally now. It's just that I'm okay if I know what I'm doing, but if suddenly things happen, I don't like it. Linda will drive us. She's a good driver."

As these changes slowed him down, he continued to be positive, friendly, and gracious. Before long he would depend on a walker and by the 2012 International Glasser Conference, held in June of that year at Loyola Marymount University, he would be confined to a wheelchair. It was hard for people who knew him, especially those closest to him, to see him in this life transition. He had been an invincible force for good for so many years, with an energy and strength that often seemed unbounded, yet now the bounds were clear. We come onto the stage of life and after a time we leave the stage of life. For Glasser, his stage represented an amazing journey, an important performance that inspired others to improve their own journeys. It certainly worked that way for me personally. His ideas helped me to be a better teacher, a better principal, a better father, and a better husband. I have felt sadness as the process of his winding down leads to its ultimate conclusion, but I have felt thankful too. I have felt thankful for how his beliefs have strengthened me and others. I have felt thankful I have had the privilege to pick his brain on writings and topics that span his career. And, practically speaking, I have felt thankful that we began when we did. Almost all of our interviews took place when he was totally present, totally sharp. It feels like it was just in time.

To the end of his career, Glasser seemed inconsistently aware of the impact he had made on the world. He was more often dimly aware of his notoriety. This point was driven home to me again as Glasser described how he had found someone to write a foreword for the *De-*

fining Mental Health as a Public Health Issue booklet. "He's a psychiatrist," he explained with a note of enthusiasm. "He's been a psychiatrist. He's semi-retired now, but he still teaches at the Stanford Medical School Department of Psychiatry. He read *Reality Therapy* a long time ago, and liked it, but more recently he read one of my articles and got in touch with me. So we've been talking and I asked him, 'Would you, as a psychiatrist, give me some psychiatric support and write the foreword to the booklet?' And he did it. It was a real nice foreword. So, so that gives me some credibility. I'm not just out there alone, a voice crying in the wilderness. He's a clinical professor of psychiatry, Stanford University. That's good."

It struck me that Glasser saw David Burns, the semi-retired, associate professor from Stanford as confirming his credibility. It struck me later how he had described himself, because of this endorsement, as not being alone. How much did he think about being alone during his career? He was constantly surrounded by crowds of people during his presentations and demonstrations, but one can be alone even in a throng. He had a loyal following, to be sure, but again, one can be alone when you're out in front discovering the next mountain to scale. To what extent did he see himself as a single voice crying in the wilderness? He often was a man alone in his thoughts, seemingly most comfortable with a pen and yellow pad in his hands, or later sitting in front of his computer, his fingers typing out the books and magazine articles that would attract so many to his messages of love, self-worth, personal freedom, and happiness. For whatever reason, the man who helped so many to more effectively connect with the important people in their lives sometimes struggled to connect himself. With Glasser now stepping down from the stage, his legacy lies firmly, yet quietly, in place. There is abundant literature and other media documenting his contributions. As his voice grows quieter the voices of others will need to pick up where he left off. His legacy may be firmly in place, but others will need to keep it evolving and relevant. Ideally, his message will be one of many gathering voices proclaiming a vision about mental health that empowers people around the world to seek and create the best versions of themselves.

Something else came out of this interview that is maddening and, in a bookend kind of way, appropriate all at the same time. Because of Glasser mentioning Whitaker's book, *Mad in America*,[11] in several of his articles, Burns went out and got the book and read it for himself. Glasser described how during one of their conversations Burns wondered aloud why no one had told him about this book. "He said it was like hidden," Glasser remembered. "I said, 'Well, you know, it's not hidden, but Whitaker has a great deal of difficulty getting people to support it.'" Glasser paused here before continuing. "And then Burns told me something. He said to me, 'Would you consider coming up to Stanford and doing a grand round?' A grand round is an important teaching component within a medical school. Usually a patient's case will be presented, with someone like myself addressing the case in front of medical school faculty, residents, and even people from the community. I told him, 'Yes, I would like to do that very much.'" Glasser paused briefly again. "And then Burns says, 'Yah, but there could be a problem.' I said, 'What's the problem?' Cuz he's not a real big shot there. But he's on the staff. And he said, 'Well, at Stanford before anyone presents at grand rounds they have to be approved by the drug companies that give us so much money for our program.'"

I was shocked by this and said, "I'm almost speechless."

"You wouldn't think that at Stanford, would you?" Glasser asked. "Actually, when I asked him to write the foreword for the booklet, at first he said he didn't know if he could. When I asked what that was about, he explained it would have to be approved by the drug companies, too."

It is maddening companies pushing powerful brain drugs in search of profits would be given that kind of influence in a medical school supposedly dedicated to the well-being of its patients. However it is a fitting reminder of the issues and decisions that face everyone involved with present mental healthcare practices. And it is a kind of bookend that encloses the end of Glasser's career. Glasser began his psychiatric residency in 1954, at almost the exact same time in which Thorazine came onto the U.S. market. Thorazine marked the beginning of psychiatry's pursuit of brain drugs as the answer to psychological and emotional distress. Fifty-one years later, Glasser and the drug companies looked across the divide between them, each realizing that success is dependent on the value that others place on their approach. Psychiatry and the pharmaceuticals hope people will continue to see mental distress as a problem of biology, beyond a distressed person's ability to fix; Glasser and the concept of choice theory see mental distress as a response to the problems of life, and offer people a message of hope. It is up to us, the people, to choose the option in which we will invest.

The Glasser International Conference held at Loyola Marymount University in Los Angeles during the early summer of 2012 turned out to be a very special event. It wasn't really decided until January of 2012 to go ahead and schedule the conference in June, which is barely enough time for people to make international travel plans. There seemed to be a recognition, though, of the significance of this particular conference and the reservation requests began to pour in. People from around the world "got it." They got why the conference was being held in Glasser's hometown. As in the movie Field of Dreams, it can be said of this conference, if you plan it, they will come. Yes, there were various presentations and break-out sessions from which people benefited, and yes people wanted to reconnect with colleagues and friends, but the real reason people attended was to say thank you to Glasser. They knew that his health was failing, that he was more than slowing down, and they came to let him know how much he meant to them. Coming from near and far, representing every continent except Antarctica, they arrived from New Zealand, Australia, South Africa, South Korea, Japan, Saudi Arabia, Iran, Croatia, Germany, England, Ireland, Columbia, Canada, and from all around the United States.[12] Glasser's ideas had changed their lives and ultimately helped them to help others change their lives too.

Throughout his life Glasser was matter-of-fact to a fault. He just didn't seem to process certain events, be they especially wonderful or difficult, in a way that most would expect. Yet this trait seemed to have changed by the time the conference occurred. I say this because on more than one occasion I saw him filled with emotion in response to things people were saying to him. He was touched and at times he struggled for the words to express his thoughts and feelings. In a wheelchair, not always able to hear everything he wanted to hear, hunched over just a little bit, he was pushed to the different conference events. Many still sought to have their picture taken with Glasser, often two people, one on each side of him, or a group of people surrounding him from behind, bending over to get into the frame with him. As he said more than once, choice theory is a happy way to live your life, and he graciously played along with the photograph seekers. He didn't always recognize people who approached him, even some who you would have expected him to, but he seemed to appreciate people's efforts to be near him nonetheless. More important, he got it. He got the love, appreciation, and respect that those in attendance were trying to express to him. He got the thank-yous that people were saying by their presence there.

Newsweek ran an article entitled, America's Top Killer: Us[13], that points out "America's top killer isn't cancer or heart disease, or even smoking and overeating—it's our inability to make smart choices that leads us to engage in those and other self-destructive behaviors. Each year," says Duke University's Ralph Keeney, "more than a million people needlessly die because of their own personal decisions." The author of the article, Tony Dokoupil, believes Keeney's work raises a philosophical quandary, and wonders: "If we continue to kill ourselves with poor decisions, are we consciously opting for short, zestful lives over long, abstemious ones? Or is it that we simply need a stronger hand prodding us to make better choices? Keeney and a number of public health advocates say the answer may be more governmental guidance in everything from what kind of food we buy to whether we contribute to our retirement savings. And if Keeney is right, and much of our health and life expectancy is a reflection of our own decisions, are these things we can change, or choices shaped by genes and other forces outside our control?"

In the design of the study Keeney wrestled with just how much choice individuals have, specifically questioning suicides as death by personal decision. Is it fair, Keeney wondered, to label suicide as a choice if someone is suffering from a mental illness of genetic or physiological origin? In the end, though, he came to believe people could have saved their own lives if they had taken a different path. "If it's under a person's control," he states, "I say it's up to them."

The article admits we don't know why so many of us make such lousy decisions, even ones that kill us. Its themes are all too familiar. Why do we behave in ways that hurt others and ourselves? Can we control our behavior or are we the victim of genetic or physiological forces beyond our control? In what ways should outside agencies, like the government or our employer, attempt to support or even manipulate our making better choices? Would we benefit from interventions? One suggestion is that our children need to learn how to make good choices. "However the experts explain our tendencies to self-destruct," concludes Dokoupil, "they all agree that we could use some help negotiating these choices better—and that government can provide it. For Keeney, it's by adding 'decision making' to the standard curriculum in public schools so that more children grow up empowered to recognize and mine all their options, rather than accept those presented by others. 'Imagine if they taught World War II as decision making,' he says. 'That'd be fabulous!'"

It may seem too simple to say it this way, but Glasser's story is really about decision-making. It's about recognizing the depth and breadth of our ability to make choices. It is about learning to choose better options. Although concerned enough to say, "The world is now hanging kind of by a thread," Glasser remains firm in his optimism and belief in the future. "I see the world as a fixable place if they would learn some new things to do. So that's why our thing is to try and teach the world choice theory. To me it is a noble occupation, and I have enjoyed every minute of it."

NOTES

1. Wright, R. and Cummings, N. (2005). *Destructive trends in mental health: The well-intentioned path to harm*. New York: Routledge Publishing.
2. Glasser, W. (2004). A new vision for counseling. *The Family Journal: Counseling and Therapy for Couples and Families, 11(X)*, 1-3.
3. Gladding, S. (2004). The potential and pitfall of William Glasser's new vision for counseling. *The Family Journal: Counseling and Therapy for Couples and Families, 12(4)*.
4. Glasser, W. (1972). *The identity society*. New York: Harper Collins Publishers.
5. Glasser, W. (2003). *Warning: Psychiatry can be hazardous to your mental health*. New York: Harper Collins.
6. A report from the Institute of Medicine appeared in Your Life section of USA TODAY in September, 2012, stating that "The U.S. healthcare system wastes $750 billion a year on unneeded care, useless paperwork, fraud and other failures, and could make changes that would both save money and improve health. The bluntly worded report says that if banks ran like the healthcare system, ATM transactions would take days and if airlines ran like the health system, pilots could design their own pre-flight safety checks or not do them at all."
7. Dr. Timothy Scott in *America Fooled: The Truth About Antidepressants, Antipsychotics and How We've Been Deceived* did a great deal of research and states unequivocally: "The truth is that there is no objective test for determining depression, schizophrenia or any purely mental disorder— no blood test, urine test, or brain scan" (p.45). He also debunks the "chemical imbalance myth" on which so much of our biological emphasis is based. Other important books that explain the myths of mental illness and brain pathology include *Beyond Prozac*, by Terry Lynch, *The Truth About the Drug Companies*, by Marcia Angell, and *Ritalin Nation*, by Richard DeGrandpre. *Ritalin Nation* confirms the large-scale biological myths associated with Attention Deficit/Hyperactivity Disorder.

8   Glasser, W. (2005). *Defining mental health as a public health issue: A new leadership role for the helping and teaching professions.* Chatsworth, CA: William Glasser, Inc.
9   Known more formally as the California Institution for Women.
10 Choice Theory Connection Program newsletter, August, 2011.
11 Whitaker, R. (2002). *Mad in America: Bad science, bad medicine, and the enduring mistreatment of the mentally ill.* Cambride, MA: Perseus Publishers.
12 Not a complete list of countries represented at the conference.
13 Dokoupil, T. (January 5, 2009). America's top killer: Us. Retrieved from www.newsweek.com.

Epilogue

William Glasser passed away on August 23, 2013. He was 88 years old.

I had wanted to hand him a copy of this book while he was still with us, but it was published just a couple of months after he died. He had read portions of the manuscript and was pleased with the tone and the content. And during the summer of 2012, at the International Glasser Conference in June, he was at two presentations I gave on his biography and was able to see and hear for himself the interest that those in attendance had in his life and his career. I was scheduled to give just one presentation, and had shared 75 percent of the material in my notes, but those who were at the session wanted to hear it all and requested a second session as well. Glasser witnessed that affirmation, for which I am thankful.

Glasser was not a stranger to affirmation, as he was a successful author and respected and sought-after speaker during his very active lifetime. As described in the biography he also received a number of awards for his professional contributions. Right before he died, though, he received an award that he cherished especially, and he received it in a place that was particularly significant to him.

The award, an official recognition from the California State Senate, was worded as follows:

CALIFORNIA SENATE

By the Honorable Carol Liu, 25th Senatorial District; and the Honorable Loni Hancock, 9th Senatorial District; Relative to Commending:

William Glasser M.D.

WHEREAS, Dr. William Glasser, a distinguished Los Angeles resident and highly esteemed member of the medical profession, has brought great credit and distinction to himself through his professional and public achievements, and in recognition thereof, it is appropriate to highlight his many accomplishments and extend to him the special honors and highest commendations of the people of California; and

WHEREAS, a world-renowned psychiatrist who employs a nontraditional approach, Dr. William Glasser has been recognized since 1989 as a member of the distinguished faculty of pioneers in the psychological professions by the Evolution of Psychotherapy Conference of the Milton Erickson Foundation; and

WHEREAS, in his early years as a psychiatrist, Dr. Glasser obtained experience at the Veterans Administration Hospital in Los Angeles, and in 1967, he founded The Institute for <u>Reality Therapy</u>, which was renamed The Institute for Control Theory, Reality Therapy and Quality Management in 1994, and The William Glasser Institute in 1996; today, the institute, which is headquartered in Tempe, Arizona, has branches throughout the world; and

WHEREAS, the recipient of numerous honors and awards, Dr. Glasser was presented the American Counseling Association's 2004 Legend in Counseling Award for his development of reality therapy and, in 2005, was awarded the prestigious Master Therapist designation by the American Psychotherapy Association, and over the course of his stellar career, he has shared his expertise as the author and co-author of numerous chapters and books, including *Take Charge of Your Life*, *Choice Theory*, and <u>*Eight Lessons for a Happier Marriage*</u>; and

Epilogue

WHEREAS, intelligent and articulate, aware and involved, Dr. William Glasser is a fine example of a public-spirited citizen willing to assume the responsibilities of leadership, and through his remarkable personal and professional achievements, he has become a legendary figure who is admired by people throughout the State of California and beyond; now, therefore, be it

RESOLVED BY SENATORS CAROL LIU AND LONI HANCOCK, that they recognize and thank Dr. William Glasser for a lifetime of achievements and meritorious service to humanity, and convey sincere best wishes that his indomitable efforts will continue in the years ahead.

Member Resolution No.643- May 11, 2013

Glasser had received his previous awards in front of large audiences of fellow professionals. This award, though, the California State Senate resolution, was conferred during a graduation ceremony, held July 26, 2013, inside the California Institution for Women, the women's prison just outside of Corona, California. The setting was smaller than the national conferences in which Glasser had received his other awards, yet somehow it felt more right, more significant. Those in the prison gymnasium on that day were there to see 112 women graduate with a choice theory certificate of internal empowerment coaching, as designated by Loyola Marymount University. Les Johnson, the Director of the Choice Theory Connection Program, gave the award to Carleen Glasser, who attended the graduation on her husband's behalf. Glasser was struggling with pneumonia symptoms and the respiratory issues that ultimately took his life.

It is so fitting that the last award Glasser received was given to him at a women's prison. He began his career at the Ventura School for Girls, a correctional facility of the California Youth Authority. Now, less than a month before he died, he was recognized for his work throughout the state of California and beyond, and especially for his work right there in the prison.

As of September 2013, 618 women inmates had completed choice theory training. Over the last four years, 175 of the 618 have been paroled. Of the 175 parolees, only five of them have been re-incarcerated. That is a recidivism rate of 2.9 percent, compared to the average statewide recidivism rate of 70 percent. I am convinced that nothing would have made Glasser happier than the women parolees successfully returning to society. Knowing him, he would have wanted to talk with the five who returned to prison and help them to set up a new success plan. One of the keys to reality therapy is, Never Give Up.

Acknowledgements

Thank You . . .

Bill Glasser for creating and refining ideas that so many people have found helpful in their own lives. Your interest in the interview process and your encouragement throughout the project made our work together a pleasure. That we became friends, as we talked through so many issues, means a great deal to me.

Carleen Glasser for your graciousness and optimism. As much as anyone you have wanted the biography to be a quality product, a story that accurately captures the life and ideas of the man you loved so much.

Maggie Roy, for helping me to become a better choice theory husband and father. In a lot of ways the biography was a team effort between us. Being able to count on your complete honesty as you read first drafts of chapters was so significant to the book's success. May the partnership continue forever!

My incredible family—Rachel, Jordan, Sean, Katy, Liam, and Charlie. Your belief in the importance of the biography and your supporting me, even as I kept odd hours in an effort to get the writing done, and even as I brought books and journals and my computer wherever we went, including on vacations, was huge for me. Liam and Charlie, may you continue to grow up surrounded by choice theory.

Tom Amato for being as good a friend as a person can have. When I wondered if I would get it done, or if I could get it done, you never wavered. Never.

Tim Mitchell for getting me unstuck more than once. Your checking in with me and your willingness to so carefully read the chapters kept me on the track of productivity.

William Glasser International, Inc. for your support for this project from the start. Many of you sat for interviews and shared all kinds of artifacts with me. The biography would not have been possible without people such as: Sue Brown, Linda Harshman, Bob Wubbolding, Al Katz, Fitzgeorge Peters, Brad Greene, Bob Hoglund, Suzy Hallock-Bannigan, Jean Seville-Suffield, Lynn Sumida, Maggie Bolton, Brian Lennon, Rhon Carleton, Tom Parish, Brandi Roth, Maureen McIntosh, Jeff Tirengel, Bradley Smith, Bob Sullo, Jim Montagnes, and Jim Coddington, to name a few.

John Collins and the Archie Tonge Education Fund for your early support of the project. When circumstances made the task harder, your support was incredibly meaningful to me.

Tom Lee and the team of people in the Education Department at Pacific Union College with whom I am so fortunate to work. As colleagues, I appreciated your rooting for me to get the book finished.

Ron Bunch, Gary Galusha, Doug Cooper, Bob Hoffman, Laffit Cortes, Ed and Teri Boyatt, and Dick and Anita Molstead. Your friendship has helped me tackle this project, as well as other projects, too.

Barry Karlan for your belief in the value of Glasser's ideas and for taking the initiative to get in touch with the Milton Erickson Foundation to see if they would be interested in publishing Glasser's biography.

Jeffrey K. Zeig, Founder and Director of the Milton H. Erickson Foundation, Suzi Tucker, editor of the manuscript, and Chuck Lakin, designer for the book. Jeff's decision to publish Glasser's story represents the essential moment in this book's life. Everything else, at least as far as this biography is concerned, hinged on that decision. And Suzi's editing made the story better, clearer, easier to follow. Although her editing indicated that occasional changes were needed in the manuscript, I could tell she wanted the book to retain my voice and the words I had chosen in an attempt to capture Glasser's legacy. Chuck had to take the marked up manuscript and turn it into the book you now have in your hands. The font and overall design added to the book's appeal.

Thank you loved ones, colleagues, friends, and choice theory advocates. If I have left someone off this list, it was unintentional.

INDEX

ACA (American Counseling Association), 374-380
Addictions, 175-180, 198-199
ADHD, 167-168, 259
Amato, Tom, 330
American Educator Magazine, 295-296
Angell, Marcia, 336
Apollo High School, 248-256
Applegate, Gary, 221
Army career, 40, 44-45
Awards,
    CA Member Resolution No. 643, 409-412
    Legend in Counseling, 4, 367
    Master Therapist, 5, 376
    Professional Development, 4-5
Barber, Charles, 334-335
Basic Needs, 86,107, 160, 225-226, 245
Bassin, Alex, 125-127, 184, 239-241, 262
Beehive (play), 155
Behavior: The Control of Perception (Powers) 186-191, 194, 196-201, 222
Blanchard, Ken, 301
Boffey, Barnes, 262
Boss managers, 255, 315-316
Boys of Summer, 175-176
Brain drugs, 165-166, 199-200, 333-363, 374-380
    History, 58-59, 333-342
    Pharmaceutical stake in, 333-337, 355-358, 403

    Psychiatrist stake in, 337-341, 351-359, 363, 403
Buchholz, Sam, 125-126, 184-185
Burns, David, 401-403

Caughey, John, 39, 50, 257
Choice Theory Community Project, 345
Choice Theory Connection Program, 393-395
Class Meetings, 142-146
Community Involvement Centers, 170, 359, 382
Competition, 177
Control, external/internal, 23, 166, 225, 250, 259-261, 307-312, 324
Control systems, 186-188
Control Systems Group, 233-234
Control theory
    Education and, 240-246
    Evolution into choice theory, 223-236, 301-314, 318-326
    Glasser and Powers, 192-201, 219-222, 232-234
    Origins 186-191, 194, 196-201, 222, 232
    Reality therapy and, 217-222
Control Theory in the Classroom (Glasser), 240-246
Control Theory Manager, The (Glasser), 301

Cooperative Learning, 242-246
Corning Conference, 343-345
Counseling with Choice Theory: The New Reality Therapy (Glasser), 344
Creativity, 225, 359-362
Curtiss, Kathy, 280

Daytop Village, 184
Deming, W. Edwards, 247-250, 264-265, 296-299, 312-313
Depression, 89-90, 163-164, 177
Discipline, 80-83, 140-141, 241-246, 259-261, 294-297, 314-317, 322-325.
    Restitution model and, 298-300, 304-307, 310-313, 322-329
    Ten-Step Approach to Discipline, 294-297
Disney Conference, 242-243
Dokoupil, Tony, 405-406
Dolan, Bea, 64, 83-84, 100, 257-258, 261-262
Dollard, John 85-86
Drug therapy. *See* Brain Drugs
DSM, 357-360, 388
DuBois, Paul, 100-101

East LA School System, 128-130, 142
Education and Degrees, Glasser
    Case School of Applied Science, 39-40, 70
    Case Western Reserve University, 46-47
    Case Western Reserve University Medical School, 49-56, 60-69
    Educational theory, overview, 135-142, 254-256
    Grades, 137-139, 145-146, 157-159
    Origins, 54-55, 78-83, 87-88, 106, 127-136, 142-144
  Educator Training Center, 127, 132, 146, 154-156, 256, 294-295
Ego, 86-90, 164
Ellis, Albert, 231-232
Emotions, 141

Failure, 54-55, 81-83, 135-159, 168-169

Gladding, Sam, 376-380
Glasser, Alice, 61-62, 172
Glasser, Ben, 17-19, 24-30, 33-36, 51-53, 100, 178, 203
Glasser, Betty 18-19, 21-22, 24-30, 33-36, 51-53, 178, 203
Glasser, Carleen (Floyd), xiii-xiv, 211, 277-289, 303-305, 342-343, 348, 371, 381, 390-391
Glasser, Hank, 19, 25-27, 33, 240, 348
Glasser, Joe, 56-57, 172-174, 239-240, 277, 345-348
Glasser, Martin, 98, 172-174, 262, 277
Glasser, Naomi (Silver), 41, 44-45, 51, 53-57, 61-62, 98, 131-132, 179, 258, 262-263, 267-279, 321,
Glasser Quality Schools, 257-259
Glasser, Robert, 91, 179, 275, 276, 346
Glasser, Ruth, 19, 26, 53, 178
Glasser's Personal History
    Childhood, 1-36
    Education and Degrees:
        Case School of Applied Science, 39-40, 70
        Case Western Reserve University 46-47
        Case Western Reserve University Medical School 49-56, 60-69
Glasser Research Center, 292, 395
Good, Perry, 221, 262
Goodman, Sanford, 34
Gossen, Diane, 262, 298-300, 304-307, 326-327

Gough, Pauline, 234
Green, Brad, 248-249, 256, 290
Grills, Cheryl, 394
Grimes, Jim, 250
Guilt, 111

Happiness/Unhappiness, 12-13,108, 112-114, 352-356, 359-360, 374-375, 382-384
Hardy, Thomas, 23, 343
Harrington, George, 64-69, 97-108, 112, 115-118, 133, 195, 378-379
Harshman, Linda, 262, 269-270, 280, 297, 310, 325, 344, 370-371
Harshman, Ron, 221
Hawes, Dick, 221, 262
Hawkins, Gordon, 169
Henderson, Joe, 178
Hoglund, Bob, 11, 304-306
Homosexuality, 90, 113-115
Huntington Woods Elementary School, 257-258
Hyperactivity, 167-168, 199

Identity, 149-150, 153, 157-172
    Success/Failure Identity, 138-139, 158-160, 165-166, 170, 222
Identity Society, The (Glasser) 156-172, 224
Ideological Shifts, 90, 112-115, 141-142, 295-298, 316-319
Insanity defense, 170
Institute for Control Theory, Reality Therapy & Quality Management, 301-303, 311-312. See also William Glasser Institute

Institute for Reality Therapy, 7, 131. See also William Glasser Institute
Johnson, David, 1, 10-11, 242-245, 302
Johnson, Les, 393, 411

Johnson, Roger, 10, 242-243
Journal of Reality Therapy, 203, 231
Kaiser, Helmuth, 102
Katz, Al, 126-127, 156, 185, 217, 269, 297
Keeney, Ralph, 405-406

Laborint, Henri, 58-59
Lead Manager, 255, 260, 395
Learning Teams, 242, 245
Lennon, Brian, 123, 170, 229, 302, 350-351
Lennon, Laura, 271
Levels of perception, 186, 194-198, 220-221, 301, 314
Litwack, Larry, 231-232, 328-329
Loneliness, 160-166
Loyola Marymount University, 390-395, 403-404
    Glasser Research Center, 392, 395
    William Glasser Fund, 392, 395
Lynch, Terry, 349-352, 390

Mad in America (Whitaker), 101-102, 402
Making Us Crazy (Kutchins & Kirk), 358
Maslow, Abraham, 193
Mental Health, 11-14, 351-354, 383-384
    ACA and, 374-380
    As Public Health, 174-175, 257,370, 374-379, 384-390, 396-397
Mental Health or Mental Illness? (Glasser), 6, 85-92, 150, 383-384
Mental Illness, 11-14, 86-89, 103, 106-107, 109-110
    DSM and, 357-360, 388
    History of care, 338-342
    Pharmaceuticals and, 1-2, 58-59, 333-342, 355-359
    Psychiatry and, 11, 337-342, 351-359,

363, 403

Moral medical treatment, 100-102, 339-340
Morality, 109-110, 113, 362
Montagnes, Jim, 300, 320-321
Morris, Norval, 169
Murphy, John, 302
Murphy, Mary Kay, 295

Nater, Adrienne, 119-120, 380-381
National Committee on Violence, 169
Naylor, Doug, 127-132, 262
Needs. *See* Basic Needs

O'Donnell, Donald, 95-99, 119, 127-128, 131-134, 159-160, 262, 368-369
Orders of Perception, 186-187, 197-198

Perry, Mary, 64, 75, 83-85, 100, 221, 262
Pershing Elementary, 95-99, 240
Peters, Fitzgeorge, 125-127, 156, 185, 270, 346
Pharmaceutical Industry
    History, 58-59, 333-342, 355-359
    Profits, 333-337
    Psychiatry and, 337-341, 351-359, 363
    Stanford University and, 402-403
Positive Addiction, (Glasser), 175-179.
    Runner's World questionnaire, 178
Powers, Mary, 192, 230-233
Powers, William, 184-204, 220-221, 230-233, 241, 301
    Glasser/Powers collaboration, 192-202, 219-222, 232-234
    Glasser/Powers schism, 230-233
Psychiatry, traditional, 87, 109-110, 118-119 363
    DSM and, 357-360, 388
    Pharmaceuticals and, 58-59, 337-341, 351-359, 363, 374-380
    Mental illness and, 11, 337-342, 351-359, 363, 403
Public Health and Mental Health, 174-175, 257, 370, 374-379, 384-390, 396-397
Punishment, 78-83, 87-88, 112, 168-169, 258-259
Purdy, Robert, 128

Quakers, 339-340
Quality School, The (Glasser), 254-255, 297
Quality Schools, 250-259, 310-319
Quality School Consortium, 254-256, 327
Quality World, 197, 253-254
Quality World Workbook, My (C. Glasser), 279

Reality Therapy in Action (Glasser), 344
Reality Therapy, origins, 73-84, 96-110
Reilly, Sue, 154-155, 180
Relationships, 102-104, 110, 160-161, 246, 254, 316, 353, 382-383, 388
Responsibility, 107-108, 162-170, 196-200
Restitution Model, 298-300, 304-306
    Glasser's rejection of, 310-314, 317-318, 321-329
Santee, Harold, 130, 134,

Schools, Glasser's work in
    Apollo High School, 248-256
    East LA School System, 128-130, 142
    Loyola Marymont University, 390-395
    Pershing Elementary, 95-99, 240
    Schwab Middle School, 285-286
    Ventura School for Girls, 63-64, 73-92, 106, 110-112, 134-135, 257

Schools Without Failure (Glasser)
    Origins, 54-55, 134-137, 142-144
    Concepts. *See* Educational theory, overview

Schwab Middle School, 285-286
Selye, Hans, 201-202
Sharpe, Billy, 131-132
Smith, Brad, 391-393
Spirituality/religion, 226-227
Stations of the Mind (Glasser), 194-202, 219-223
Smith, Brad, 391-393
Staying Together (Glasser), 271,274,287
Stone Foundation, 131-132

Take Effective Control of Your Life (Glasser), 223-236
TEC Seminars, 230-231
Television, 167-168
Total Behavior, 361-362

Ventura School for Girls, 63-64, 73-92, 106, 110-112, 134-135, 257

Warning: Psychiatry Can Be Hazardous to Your Mental Health (Glasser)
    Lynch and, 349-352
    Mental health and relationships, 353-354, 356
    Mental symptoms as science, 337-338, 357-360
    Psychiatric/pharmaceutical connection, 337- 338, 354-355
Whitaker, Robert, 101-2, 337-339
William Glasser Institute,
    Founding, 7, 131-137
    Names/name changes, 7, 311-315, 233, 303
    Theoretical Evolution, 154-156, 312- 328, 370-371, 396-397
Wubbolding, Bob, xiv, 155, 221-223, 270, 274, 279, 302, 306, 326, 372-373
Wubbolding, Sandie, 270, 274,282

About the Author

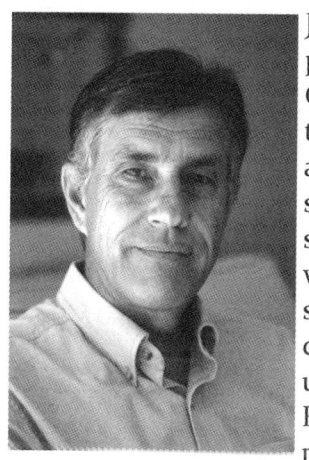

Jim Roy is a professor in the teacher education program at Pacific Union College in northern California. Throughout his 35 year career as a teacher, principal, associate superintendent, and teacher educator, he has sought progressive solutions to the traditional barriers that keep students and schools from thriving. He has worked with Glasser's ideas within the school setting for the past twenty years, which included receiving training and becoming a faculty member of the William Glasser Institute. Roy's dissertation, in which Glasser participated, focused on the history of the development of Glasser's ideas. Roy's first book, *Soul Shapers*, described how the principles of choice theory can help a school go from good to great. The author can be contacted at jimroyglasserbio@gmail.com